Essentials of Pharmacoeconomics

SECOND EDITION

Karen L. Rascati, PhD

Eckerd/Turley Centennial Professor of Health Outcomes
and Pharmacy Practice
University of Texas College of Pharmacy
Austin, Texas

Wolters Kluwer | Lippincott Williams & Wilkins
Health

Philadelphia · Baltimore · New York · London
Buenos Aires · Hong Kong · Sydney · Tokyo

Acquisitions Editor: Sirkka Howes
Product Development Editor: Jennifer Verbiar
Marketing Manager: Joy Fisher-Williams
Production Editor: Alicia Jackson
Design Coordinator: Holly McLaughlin
Compositor: S4Carlisle Publishing Services

Library of Congress Cataloging-in-Publication Data

Rascati, Karen L., author.
  Essentials of pharmacoeconomics / Karen L. Rascati.—2nd edition.
      p. ; cm.
  Includes bibliographical references and index.
  ISBN 978-1-4511-7593-6 (paperback)
  I. Title.
  [DNLM: 1. Economics, Pharmaceutical.   2. Costs and Cost Analysis—methods.   3. Models, Economic.
  4. Pharmaceutical Preparations—economics.   5. Pharmaceutical Services—economics. QV 736]
  RM263
  338.4'76151—dc23

                                                                            2013022615

DISCLAIMER

Care has been taken to confirm the accuracy of the information present and to describe generally accepted practices. However, the authors, editors, and publisher are not responsible for errors or omissions or for any consequences from application of the information in this book and make no warranty, expressed or implied, with respect to the currency, completeness, or accuracy of the contents of the publication. Application of this information in a particular situation remains the professional responsibility of the practitioner; the clinical treatments described and recommended may not be considered absolute and universal recommendations.

The authors, editors, and publisher have exerted every effort to ensure that drug selection and dosage set forth in this text are in accordance with the current recommendations and practice at the time of publication. However, in view of ongoing research, changes in government regulations, and the constant flow of information relating to drug therapy and drug reactions, the reader is urged to check the package insert for each drug for any change in indications and dosage and for added warnings and precautions. This is particularly important when the recommended agent is a new or infrequently employed drug.

Some drugs and medical devices presented in this publication have Food and Drug Administration (FDA) clearance for limited use in restricted research settings. It is the responsibility of the health care provider to ascertain the FDA status of each drug or device planned for use in their clinical practice.

To purchase additional copies of this book, call our customer service department at **(800) 638-3030** or fax orders to **(301) 223-2320**. International customers should call **(301) 223-2300**.

Visit Lippincott Williams & Wilkins at: www.lww.com. Lippincott Williams & Wilkins customer service representatives are available from 8:30 am to 6:00 pm, EST.

*I dedicated the first edition of this book
to my mother, Glenna Rupp Lewis,
who at that time was an active volunteer at
VITAS Hospice in the Central Florida area.
She passed away in 2012, and, in her memory,
I am dedicating all author royalties
of this second edition to this worthwhile cause.*

Reviewers

Norman V. Carroll, RPh, PhD
Professor of Pharmacy Administration
School of Pharmacy
Virginia Commonwealth University
Richmond, Virginia

Raymond W. Hammond, PharmD, BCPS, FCCP
Associate Dean for Practice Programs
University of Houston College
    of Pharmacy
Houston, Texas

David A. Holdford, RPh, MS, PhD
School of Pharmacy
Virginia Commonwealth University
Richmond, Virginia

Donald G. Klepser, PhD, MBA
Assistant Professor
College of Pharmacy
University of Nebraska Medical Center
Omaha, Nebraska

Mark P. Okamoto, BS, PharmD
Professor and Chair
College of Pharmacy
University of Hawaii at Hilo
Hilo, Hawaii

Ryan M. Quist, PhD
College of Pharmacy
Western University of Health Sciences
Pomona, California

David Alexander Sclar, BPharm, PhD
Boeing Distinguished Professor
    of Health Policy and
    Administration
Professor of Marketing;
    Pharmacotherapy, and
    Statistics
Director, Pharmacoeconomics
    and Pharmacoepidemiology
    Research Unit
Washington State University
Pullman, Washington

Fadia T. Shaya, PhD, MPH
Associate Professor, Associate
    Director
Center on Drugs and Public
    Policy
Pharmaceutical Health Services
    Research
University of Maryland School
    of Pharmacy
Baltimore, Maryland

Mark V. Siracuse, PharmD, PhD
Creighton University School
    of Pharmacy and Health
    Professions
Omaha, Nebraska

Audra L. Stinchcomb, PhD
Associate Professor
College of Pharmacy
University of Kentucky
Lexington, Kentucky

Preface

✦ NEED FOR THIS TEXTBOOK

The term "pharmacoeconomics" first appeared in the literature in the mid-1980s. Pharmacoeconomics incorporates methods from more established disciplines to help estimate the value of pharmacy products and services by comparing costs and outcomes. Pharmacoeconomics is included in the curricula of more than 90% of US colleges of pharmacy, although often as part of a course rather than as a whole course.

The Accreditation Council for Pharmacy Education (ACPE) has developed standards and guidelines for professional programs in pharmacy leading to a PharmD degree (Version 1 adopted in January 2006 and effective as of July 2007; Version 2 adopted in January 2011 and effective as of February 2011); these include an outline of the subject matter that should be included in pharmacy school curricula. The following three topics are listed in the ACPE document (see https://www.acpe-accredit.org/standards/default.asp) under the Economics/Pharmacoeconomics heading: (a) economic principles in relation to pharmacoeconomic analysis, (b) concepts of pharmacoeconomics in relation to patient care, and (c) applications of economic theories and health-related quality of life concepts to improve allocation of limited health care resources. This book covers the application of economic-based evaluation methods to pharmaceutical products and services and includes examples of how pharmacoeconomic evaluations relate to decisions that affect patient care and how health-related quality of life (HRQoL) is assessed and valued. Understanding these principles helps providers and decision makers improve clinical and humanistic outcomes based on available resources. Also, highlighting the importance of this topic, in 2010, the North American Pharmacist Licensure Examination (NAPLEX) added pharmacoeconomics to their competency statements (see http://www.nabp.net/programs/examination/naplex/naplex-blueprint).

✦ INTENDED AUDIENCE

Essentials of Pharmacoeconomics is designed for the true beginner—a student or practitioner who may not have even heard of the term "pharmacoeconomics." The purpose of the book is to introduce the fundamental topics, define the terminology used in pharmacoeconomic research, and give many examples in evaluating published research so that readers can evaluate literature relevant to their future or current practice. When readers have completed the book, they should be able to understand, interpret, and determine the usefulness of pharmacoeconomic research articles. This textbook can be used for PharmD students at any level of their professional education.

The distinction of this textbook, compared with other textbooks on the subject, is that it is written at an introductory level and provides many practical examples.

Another advantage of the book is that it was written by one author. This helps ensure a clear flow in providing the information and an elimination of the unintended redundancy sometimes seen in textbooks with multiple authors.

Please note that this is not intended to be an economics textbook, nor is it intended for graduate students who would need to know more about the theory of economics and the statistics or mathematical computations involved in the analyses. Moreover, the purpose is not to train a future pharmacoeconomics researcher, but to give a current or future practitioner the knowledge and skills needed to understand and use pharmacoeconomics research (conducted by someone else) in his or her decision making.

✦ ORGANIZATIONAL PHILOSOPHY

This book follows the outline of a course taught to PharmD students by the author for more than 15 years (and updated annually). Part I (Chapters 1 through 8) covers the basics of pharmacoeconomics. The author recognizes that not all colleges of pharmacy have a whole course devoted to pharmacoeconomics. If this book is used in a course that includes other topics and time allotted to pharmacoeconomics is limited, Part I of the book could stand alone as an introduction that covers the essential topics outlined by ACPE. Part II (Chapters 9 through 14) includes additional topics that are more complex (e.g., modeling) or may be of further interest to the reader (e.g., international use of pharmacoeconomics).

Part I: Basic Topics

Chapter 1 serves as an introduction, stressing the importance of the use of pharmacoeconomics to compare costs and outcomes of pharmacy interventions. The chapter discusses four basic types of pharmacoeconomic research: cost-minimization analysis (CMA), cost-effectiveness analysis (CEA), cost-utility analysis (CUA), and cost-benefit analysis (CBA). All four analyses include the measurement of costs, but differ in the methods used to measure outcomes. Chapter 2 covers the measurement of costs, and Chapter 3 outlines basic questions readers should ask when evaluating any pharmacoeconomic study. Chapters 4 through 7 expand on each of the four types of studies (CMA, CEA, CUA, and CBA) by reviewing the methods used to measure outcomes for each particular type. Chapter 8 provides an overview of health-related quality-of-life (HRQoL) measures. Chapter 8 was substantially expanded in this second edition, in large part due to the progress in methodology in this area. More in-depth contrasts and comparisons between utility measures (in Chapter 6) and quality-of-life measures were also added.

Part II: Advanced Topics

Chapter 9 outlines the use of decision analysis methods to model costs and outcomes that can be summarized in a single cycle. Chapter 10 explains Markov modeling, which is used for analyzing costs and outcomes that are estimated using multiple cycles. Chapter 11 discusses the advantages and disadvantages of using retrospective databases. Chapter 12 reviews the unique issues involved in evaluating the costs and outcomes associated with pharmacy services. The last two chapters address the use of pharmacoeconomic research in decision making. Chapter 13 summarizes the use of pharmacoeconomic evaluations by decision makers outside of the United States, and Chapter 14 outlines the extent to which pharmacoeconomic data are used to make decisions in the United States, includes barriers to its use, and discusses future issues. This second edition now includes preliminary information about the recent health care reform act in the United States.

✦ FEATURES

Essentials of Pharmacoeconomics contains the following elements that are geared toward the pharmacy student:

- **Composite research articles** that incorporate the positive and negative aspects found in a mix of published research articles. Most chapters contain at least one composite article. Depending on the classroom time allotted to pharmacoeconomics, these composite articles can be included as part of the didactic portion of the course, or they can be incorporated into small group discussion sections or assigned as homework. (Although topics are taken from actual articles, methods and data have been changed to illustrate points made in the chapter. Medication names in these composite articles are fictitious.) Due to positive feedback and reviewer requests, this second edition doubled the number of composite research examples throughout the text.
- **Key terms** are bolded throughout the textbook, and definitions of these terms are summarized in a glossary. Pharmacoeconomics research uses terminology derived from other disciplines, such as economics, that might not be familiar to all readers.
- **Examples** provide added information or instances from the literature about the chapter topic and reinforce chapter concepts. Most chapters have at least one example.
- **Equations** readers will need to know are explained using multiple example calculations.
- **Summaries** highlight and reinforce the main points of each chapter.
- **Questions/Exercises** appear at the end of each chapter so that readers can assess their understanding of key concepts. Instructors can find answers to these problems on the book's companion website.
- **References and Suggested Readings** at the end of each chapter provide resources available to the reader for further study on the chapter topic.

✦ STUDENT AND INSTRUCTOR RESOURCES

Student Resources

A Student Resource Center at http://thePoint.lww.com/rascati includes the following materials:

- **An Image Bank** that contains the figures and tables from the textbook
- **A sample worksheet** that includes the 14 questions you should use when critiquing a research article

Instructor Resources

In addition to the student resources just listed, an Instructor's Resource Center at http://thePoint.lww.com/rascati includes the following:

- **Answers to the questions/exercises found in the text**

Acknowledgments

Three of the chapters in the book are based on chapters published earlier cowritten with colleagues: Dr. James Wilson (Chapter 1), Dr. Jamie Barner (Chapter 7), and Dr. Gábor Vincze (Chapter 8). Another colleague and good friend, Dr. Carolyn Brown, served as my "sounding board" for some of the ideas for this book. Dr. Ken Lawson and Dr. Esmond Nwokeji proofread the first edition of the book. My major advisor, Dr. Carole Kimberlin, has long served as one of my role models. Her authorship of a textbook inspired me to consider this endeavor. My dean, M. Lynn Crismon, encouraged submission of the first edition of this book for The University of Texas 2009 Hamilton Book Award (textbook category)—it won. I would also like to thank my able administrative associate, Iris Jennings.

I would like to thank both the professional (PharmD) and graduate students at the University of Texas. Their intelligence and inquisitiveness, plus their insightful questions, keep me "on my toes" and current in the field. In particular, four students helped build new composite articles: Pooja Desai, Teresa Brucker, Grace Mbagwu, and Haesuk Park.

I would also like to thank the people I have met and worked with through the International Society for Pharmacoeconomics and Outcomes Research (ISPOR). Dr. Marilyn Dix-Smith has guided this organization to international prominence. When I participate on ISPOR committees or attend ISPOR meetings, I am reenergized by other people with an interest in and a passion for this field of study.

And last, but definitely not least, I am indebted to the reviewers for their excellent advice on ways to improve on the first edition and staff at Lippincott Williams & Wilkins/Wolters Kluwer, especially Sirkka Howes and Jennifer H. Verbiar.

Contents

PART II ✦ ADVANCED TOPICS

Chapter 1

Introduction

Objectives

Upon completing this chapter, the reader will be able to:

1. Define pharmacoeconomics.

2. Understand the importance and clinical relevancy of pharmacoeconomics.

3. Understand the relationship of pharmacoeconomics to other disciplines.

4. List and describe the differences between the four most common types of pharmacoeconomics studies.

✦ PHARMACOECONOMICS—WHAT IS IT?

Assessing the clinical effectiveness of any new health care intervention, including medications, is paramount in determining the role of the new intervention in clinical practice. But the new interventions may provide only a modest advantage (or no advantage) over existing treatment, usually at a higher cost. In the case of pharmaceutical interventions, pharmacoeconomics attempts to find whether the added benefit of one intervention is worth the added cost of that intervention. Pharmacoeconomics has been defined as the description and analysis of the costs of drug therapy to health care systems and society. It identifies, measures, and compares the costs and consequences of pharmaceutical products and services.[1] Clinicians and other decision makers can use these methods to evaluate and compare the total costs of treatment options and the outcomes associated with these options. To show this graphically, think of two sides of an equation (Fig. 1.1). The left-hand side of the equation represents the inputs (costs) used to obtain and use the pharmaceutical product or service. The right-hand side of the equation represents the health-related outcomes produced by the pharmaceutical product

---

*This chapter is adapted with the permission of The McGraw-Hill Companies from the following source: Wilson JP, Rascati KL. Chapter 8: Pharmacoeconomics. In Malone PM, Kier KL, Stanovich JE (eds). *Drug Information: A Guide for Pharmacists* (3rd ed.). New York: McGraw-Hill, 2006.

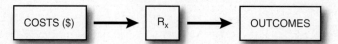

FIGURE 1.1.   Basic pharmacoeconomic equation. Pharmacoeconomic studies compare the costs (*left box*) associated with
providing a pharmacy product or service (represented as Rx)
to the outcome of the product or service.

or service. The center of the equation, the drug product or service being assessed,
is symbolized by R_x. If just the left-hand side of the equation is measured without
regard to outcomes, it is a **cost analysis** (or a partial economic analysis). If just the
right-hand side of the equation is measured without regard to costs, it is a clinical
or outcome study (not an economic analysis). To be a true pharmacoeconomic
analysis, both sides of the equation must be considered and compared. Theo-
retically, at least two options must be compared in pharmacoeconomics, but some
assessments consist of a "with or without" comparison, estimating what would occur if the product or service was provided (e.g., immunization or pharmacy clinic
services) compared with no provision of the product or service.

✦ WHY IS PHARMACOECONOMICS IMPORTANT?

The United States spent about $2.7 trillion on health care in 2010, for an average
of about $8,000 per person, or about 17% of the gross domestic product (GDP).
About 12% (over $900 per person) of health care expenditures were for medica-
tions.[2] Health care costs have been increasing each year more than the average rate
of inflation. This continued increase in costs has resulted in a need to understand
how limited resources can be used most efficiently and effectively. For example,
two medications that were approved by the U.S. Food and Drug Administration
(FDA) in 2012 (Kalydeco for cystic fibrosis and Gattex for short bowel syndrome)
are planned to be priced at about $300,000 per year.[3,4] It has been argued that these
medications save enough—by decreasing the number of hospital admissions or the
need for parental nutrition—to offset their high cost. Clinicians want their patients
to receive the best care and outcomes available, and payers want to manage rising
costs. Pharmacoeconomics combines these objectives by estimating the value of
patient outcomes received for the expenditures spent on medications and other
health care products and services.

This book provides examples of questions that can be addressed by using pharmacoeconomic analyses. Why should a health care professional (or a student in
a health care profession) learn about pharmacoeconomics? Some professionals
will incorporate this information on a patient-by-patient basis, while others may
specialize and make formulary and resource allocation decisions based on pharmacoeconomic analyses. The following examples are discussed in order of the number
of people affected—from an individual patient level to a societal level.

At the individual patient level, health care professionals can determine the best
medication (treatment) for each patient, depending on demographic, clinical, and
economic considerations. If a new branded medication is approved by the FDA that
has an advantage over another marketed medication that is less expensive, the professional can take this into account. For example, if the new treatment is $100 per
month ($40 patient co-pay, and $60 reimbursement by health insurance) compared

with a similar treatment that is available for $20 per month ($5 patient co-pay, and $15 reimbursement by health insurance), is the extra $35 per month out-of-pocket costs worth it to the patient? If the advantage is slight (e.g., more convenient once-a-day dosing compared with twice-a-day dosing of its competitor), the patient might not value the added convenience at $35 per month. But if the advantage is a reduction in side effects (e.g., no diarrhea or no daytime drowsiness), the added advantage may be worth the added cost (see **willingness to pay** in Chapter 7).

The next level would affect a group of patients locally. If a health care institution or community pharmacy wanted to implement a clinical pharmacy service, or hire a clinical pharmacist, they would look at the costs and compare them with the value of providing these services (see Chapter 12 on pharmacy services). The value of the services could be measured as profit (e.g., reimbursement minus costs for pharmacists to give vaccinations), as improved patient outcomes that decrease the need for other costly services (e.g., medication management of diabetes to reduce diabetes-related emergency room visits and hospitalizations), or as better quality of care (e.g., clinical pharmacist helps meet guidelines for accreditation, continued licensure, or legal mandates concerning quality measures).

The next level can affect a larger group of patients—for example, patients in a hospital system, managed care organization, or governmental plan (e.g., Veterans Administration). Each group is responsible for a specific patient population. Teams of professionals collaborate to determine the most effective and cost-effective options for their patient population. They develop drug use guidelines (e.g., more expensive medication not recommended for insurance coverage unless less expensive medication is tried first) and determine what medications will be listed on their **formulary** and at what co-payment level.

Chapter 13 discusses resource allocation decisions at a national, or societal, level. Governments that finance the majority of health care in their countries are particularly motivated to extract value in return for their health care spending. This may be accomplished by adding another level of control, which might include price negotiation, price setting, or formulary management at the national level.

Although health policy and health organization decision makers may use a more sophisticated level of pharmacoeconomics, all health care professionals (and aspiring professionals—i.e., students) are responsible for ensuring the appropriate use of scare resources. Therefore, it is important to understand the methods used by researchers and decision makers and be able to read and appraise the pharmacoeconomic literature.

✦ RELATIONSHIP OF PHARMACOECONOMICS TO OTHER RESEARCH

Unlike in other scientific fields, there is no standardized training for pharmacoeconomists, and it is a multidisciplinary field. The specific field of pharmacoeconomics is relatively new—the term first appeared in the literature in the mid-1980s—yet the concepts and methods are borrowed from other, more established disciplines and research areas. Pharmacoeconomics overlaps with both health care economics and pharmacy-related clinical or humanistic outcomes research, as illustrated in Figure 1.2. Health care economics encompasses a broad range of topics, including supply and demand for health care resources, the effects of health insurance, and manpower supply. Clinical or humanistic outcomes research is defined as the attempt to identify, measure, and evaluate the end results of health care services. It may include not only clinical and economic consequences

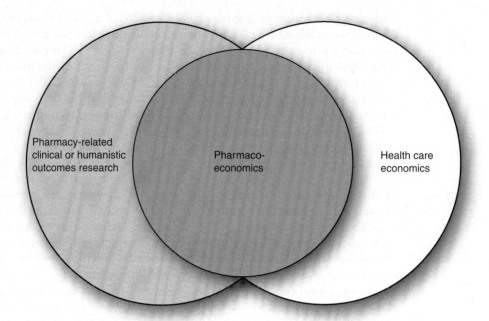

FIGURE 1.2.   Schematic of overlap between pharmacy-related clinical or humanistic outcomes research, health care economics, and pharmacoeconomics. This illustrates that pharmacoeconomics incorporates methodologies from outcomes research and the discipline of health care economics. (Adapted with permission from Rascati KL, Drummond MF, Annemans L, Davey PG. Education in pharmacoeconomics: An international multidisciplinary view. *Pharmacoeconomics* 22(3):139–147, 2004.)

but also outcomes such as patients' **health status** and satisfaction with their health care. Pharmacoeconomics is a type of outcomes research, but not all outcomes research is pharmacoeconomic research. If the research involves economic and clinical outcome evaluations and comparisons of pharmacy products or services, it can be termed a pharmacoeconomic study (overlapped area of Fig. 1.2).[5]

✦ TYPES OF PHARMACOECONOMIC STUDIES

There are four basic types of pharmacoeconomic studies (Table 1.1); **cost-minimization analysis** (CMA), **cost-effectiveness analysis** (CEA), **cost-utility analysis** (CUA), and **cost-benefit analysis** (CBA). Each method measures costs in dollars, but they differ regarding how health outcomes are measured and compared.

TABLE 1.1. THE FOUR BASIC TYPES OF PHARMACOECONOMIC ANALYSIS

Methodology	Cost Measurement Unit	Outcome Measurement Unit
Cost-minimization analysis (CMA)	Dollars or monetary units	Assumed to be equivalent in comparable groups
Cost-effectiveness analysis (CEA)	Dollars or monetary units	Natural units (life years gained, mm Hg blood pressure, mMol/L blood glucose)
Cost-benefit analysis (CBA)	Dollars or monetary units	Dollars or monetary units
Cost-utility analysis (CUA)	Dollars or monetary units	Quality-adjusted life year (QALY) or other utilities

Cost-Minimization Analysis

CMA has the advantage of being the simplest to conduct because the outcomes are assumed to be equivalent; thus, only the costs of the intervention are compared. The advantage of the CMA method is also its disadvantage: CMA cannot be used when outcomes of interventions are different. A common example of a CMA is comparing two generic medications that are rated as equivalent by the FDA. If the drugs are equivalent to each other (but manufactured and sold by different companies), only the differences in the cost of the medication are used to choose the one that provides the best value. Thus, the type of interventions that can be evaluated with CMA may be limited. It would not be appropriate to compare different classes of medications using cost-minimization analyses if there are noted differences in outcomes. For example, if a new antibiotic was available that had a higher rate of alleviating inner-ear infections (but a higher cost) than a currently marketed antibiotic, it would not be appropriate to choose the current antibiotic based solely on the basis that it cost less than the new product. The added value of the new product should be compared with its higher cost. Some contend that if outcomes are not "measured" but only assumed to be the same, the study is considered to be a cost analysis, and therefore not a full pharmacoeconomic analysis.

Cost-Effectiveness Analysis

CEA measures outcomes in natural units (e.g., mm Hg, cholesterol levels, symptom-free days [SFDs], years of life saved). The main advantage of this approach is that the outcomes are easier to quantify when compared with a CUA or a CBA, and clinicians are familiar with measuring these types of health outcomes because these outcomes are routinely collected in clinical trials and in clinical practice. One disadvantage of CEA is that programs with different types of outcomes cannot be compared. For example, it would not be possible to compare the cost-effectiveness of implementing an anticoagulation clinic with implementing a diabetes clinic because the clinical outcomes measured would be valued in different units (e.g., prothrombin time versus blood glucose measures).

Even if the primary clinical outcome unit is the same for the alternatives, if there are other major differences (e.g., side effects, impact on other diseases), it is difficult to combine the differences into a single effectiveness measure. For example, "first-generation" antihistamines (e.g., diphenhydramine) and "second-generation" antihistamines (e.g., fexofenadine) are both used to relieve allergy and cold symptoms, but first-generation antihistamines are more likely to cause patients to become drowsy. The main clinical unit of measure for both alternatives may be SFDs, or the number of days the patient did not suffer from allergy symptoms. However, this difference in the side effect of drowsiness is not incorporated into the comparison in a CEA.

Lastly, CEA may estimate the extra costs associated with each additional unit of outcome (cure, year of life, SFDs), but who is to say if the added costs are worth the added outcomes? Because no monetary amount is placed on the clinical outcomes to indicate the value of these outcomes, it is a judgment call by the patient, clinician, or decision maker as to whether the alternative is "cost-effective" in their view.

Cost-Utility Analysis

For some CEA comparisons, such as evaluations of chemotherapy agents, the primary clinical unit measure of effectiveness is the number of years of life gained because of treatment. But just measuring a patient's length of life because of treatment does not take into account the "quality" or **"utility"** of those years. **CUA** measures outcomes based on years of life that are adjusted by "utility" weights, which range from 1.0 for "perfect health" to 0.0 for "dead." These utility weights incorporate patient or society preferences for specific health states. When morbidity and mortality are both important outcomes of a treatment, CUA should be used to incorporate both into one unit of measure. The main disadvantage of CUA is that there is no consensus on how to measure these utility weights, and they are more of a "rough estimate" than a precise measure. Some researchers consider CUA as a subset of CEA.

Cost-Benefit Analysis

CBA is unique in that not only are costs valued in monetary terms, but also the benefits. Measuring both costs and benefits in monetary terms has two major advantages: First, clinicians and other decision makers can determine whether the benefits of a program or intervention exceed the costs of implementation. Second, clinicians and other decision makers can compare multiple programs or interventions with similar or unrelated outcomes. As mentioned previously, a disadvantage of the CEA method is that if one knows how much extra it costs to obtain added outcomes, it is a judgment call as to whether the added cost was worth the added benefit. With CBA, because dollar amount is estimated and used to place a value on the health outcomes, the answer to *Is the alternative cost-beneficial?* is less subjective. If the dollar value of the added outcomes exceeds the cost to obtain those outcomes, the answer is "yes." In addition, because all inputs and outcomes are converted to dollars, it is now possible to compare two alternatives that provide different types of outcomes (e.g., the implementation of an anticoagulation clinic versus the implementation of a diabetes clinic). The major disadvantage of CBA is that it is difficult to place a monetary value on health outcomes. There are different methods used to estimate the value of health outcomes, and similar to the measurement of **utilities**, different methods of measurement may elicit different estimates, and these estimates can be imprecise. Two articles that debate the use of CBA versus CEA highlight the issues related to these different methods of analysis.[6,7]

Other Types of Analyses

Although we have categorized studies into four distinct types, the differences may be less clear in practice, and more than one type of analysis (e.g., CEA and CBA) may be performed in a single study. Other types of analyses that involve the measurement of costs may be seen in the literature. For example, if only a list of costs and a list of various outcomes are presented, with no direct calculations or comparisons, this is termed a **cost-consequence analysis** (CCA).

Another type of economic analysis seen in the literature is the **cost-of-illness** (COI) analysis. In a COI study, the researchers attempt to determine the total economic burden (including prevention, treatment, losses caused by morbidity and mortality, and so on) of a particular disease on society. The costs included in this method are usually summarized into two categories: (1) **direct costs**, or the costs associated with providing treatment or prevention (e.g., medical services), and (2) **indirect costs**, or the costs attributable to loss of productivity of patients with that disease or condition. (See Chapter 2 for more in-depth explanation of direct versus indirect cost estimations.)

COI studies are used to indicate the magnitude of resources needed for a specific disease or condition, and they may be used to compare the economic impact of one disease versus another (e.g., costs of schizophrenia versus costs of asthma) or the economic impact of a disease on one country compared with another (e.g., costs of HIV in the United States versus costs of HIV in Zimbabwe). These estimates are sometimes used by pharmaceutical firms to determine the market potential for a new product or by payers to set priorities for reimbursement.

Table 1.2 shows examples of how COI study results are presented in the literature. The specific methods used to estimate COI are varied, and there is no agreement on a standard method for conducting COI studies. In addition, COI studies for the same diagnoses have found multifold cost variations.[8] The various methods and the debate surrounding them are beyond the scope of this book, but references are provided in the "Suggested Readings" section at the end of the chapter.

TABLE 1.2. **EXAMPLES OF COST-OF-ILLNESS STUDY OBJECTIVES AND RESULTS**

Objective	Results
To estimate the annual cost of illness of hyponatremia in the United States. (Hyponatremia is a disorder of fluid and electrolyte balance characterized by a relative excess of body water relative to body sodium content.)	The prevalence estimate for hyponatremia ranged from 3.2 million to 6.1 million persons in the United States on an annual basis. Approximately 1% of patients were classified as having acute and symptomatic hyponatremia, 4% acute and asymptomatic, 15%–20% chronic and symptomatic, and 75%–80% chronic and asymptomatic. Of patients treated for hyponatremia, 55%–63% are initially treated as inpatients, 25% are initially treated in the emergency room, and 13%–20% are treated solely in the office setting. The direct costs of treating hyponatremia in the United States on an annual basis were estimated to range between $1.6 billion and $3.6 billion.[a]
Cystic fibrosis (CF) is the most common life-shortening inherited disease in white people. The objective was to present an overview of COI studies of CF, identify deficits in the available analyses of CF, and discuss which specific factors are essential for the evaluation of CF.	Cost-of-illness studies of CF have predominantly been restricted to direct costs. According to the literature, direct costs amount to between $6,200 and $16,300 (1996 values) per patient per year. Because most studies likely underestimate the actual costs (e.g., by disregarding provision of certain health care services), real health care costs tend to be at the upper end of the cost range. Health care costs depend on the patient's age (for adults, costs are approximately twice as high as for children), the grade of severity (the cost relationship of severe to mild CF is between 4.5 and 7.1), and other factors. Lifetime direct costs of CF are estimated at $200,000–$300,000 (at 1996 values and a discount rate of 5%). The observation period must be long enough to identify long-term effects of interventions.[b]

[a]Adapted with permission from Boscoe A, Paramore C, Verbalis JG. Cost of Illness of Hyponatremia in the United States. Cost Effectiveness and Resource Allocation: C/E, 4:10, United States. [electronic publication] 2006.

[b]Adapted with permission from Krauth C, Jalilvand N, Welte T, Busse R. Cystic fibrosis: Cost of illness and considerations for the economic evaluation of potential therapies. Pharmacoeconomics 21(14):1001–1024, 2003.

SUMMARY

The United States spends almost $3 trillion per year on health care, and pharmacy products account for about 12% of this spending. To assess the value received for the resources expended, pharmacoeconomics is used to estimate and compare costs and health-related outcomes for pharmacy interventions (products or services). The methods used in pharmacoeconomic research are borrowed from other disciplines, such as health economics. These can be applied at the individual patient level, the local level, the organizational level, or even at the national, or societal level. Based on how health outcomes are measured, there are four basic types of pharmacoeconomic studies: **CMA**, **CEA**, **CUA**, and **CBA** (see Table 1.1). Each type has advantages and disadvantages, which are discussed in more detail in later chapters. Another type of economic research seen in health care literature is the **COI** analysis, which estimates the costs to society for a specific illness or disease category.

It is important to note that whatever type of analysis or combination of analyses is conducted, the economic comparisons are but *one part* of the decision-making process; social values and legal, ethical, and political considerations are also incorporated into the decision-making process.

QUESTIONS/EXERCISES

1. Find two pharmaceutical articles in the literature, one that has "cost-effectiveness" in the title and one that has "cost-benefit" in the title. Discuss why you think the researchers chose one type of analysis over the other.
2. Why do you think that governments from some other countries require pharmacoeconomic analyses of new medications but the US government does not?
3. List two specific questions that might be asked in clinical practice that could be answered, in part, using a pharmacoeconomic analysis.
4. Find two pharmacy research articles that discuss in their introduction section the cost of illness for a specific disease or condition. Did the authors include both direct (medical costs) and indirect (productivity) costs of the disease? If so, which were higher, the direct or indirect costs?

REFERENCES

1. Bootman JL, Townsend RJ, McGhan WF. *Principles of Pharmacoeconomics* (3rd ed.). Cincinnati, OH: Harvey Whitney Books Co., 2005.
2. Organisation for Economic Cooperation and Development. *OECD Health Data 2012*. Available at http://www.oecd.org/health/health-systems/oecdhealthdata2012-frequentlyrequesteddata.html; accessed February 2013.
3. *Inside the Pricing of a $300,000 Per Year Drug*. Available at http://www.forbes.com/sites/matthewherper/2013/01/03/inside-the-pricing-of-a-300000-a-year-drug/; accessed February 2013.
4. *Kalydeco, Drug that Treats Root Cause of Cystic Fibrosis, Approved by FDA*. Available at http://www.huffingtonpost.com/2012/01/31/kalydeco-cystic-fibrosis-cause-drug_n_1244218.html; accessed February 2013.
5. Rascati KL, Drummond MF, Annemans L, Davey PG. Education in pharmacoeconomics: An international multidisciplinary view. *Pharmacoeconomics* 22(3):139–147, 2004.
6. Johnson F. Why not real economics? *Pharmacoeconomics* 30(2):127–131, 2012.

7. Sculpher M, Claxton K. Real economics needs to reflect real decisions: A response to Johnson. *Pharmacoeconomics* 30(2):133–136, 2012.

8. Bloom BS, Bruno DJ, Maman DY, Jayadevappa R. Usefulness of cost-of-illness studies in healthcare decision making. *Pharmacoeconomics* 19(2):207–213, 2001.

SUGGESTED READINGS

Akobundu E, Ju J, Blatt L, Mullins CD. Cost-of-illness studies: A review of current methods. *Pharmacoeconomics* 24(9):869–890, 2006.

Drummond MF, Sculpher MJ, Torrance GW, O'Brien BJ, Stoddart GL. *Methods for the Economic Evaluation of Health Care Programmes* (3rd ed.). Oxford: Oxford University Press, 2005.

Grauer DW, Lee J, Odom TD, Osterhaus JT, Sanchez LA, Touchette DR (eds). *Pharmacoeconomics and Outcomes: Applications for Patient Care* (2nd ed.). Kansas City, MO: American College of Clinical Pharmacy, 2003.

Oliver A, Healey A, Donaldson C. Choosing the method to match the perspective: Economic assessment and its implications for health services efficiency. *Lancet* 359(931a):1771–1774, 2002.

Pizzi LT, Lofland JH. *Economic Evaluation in US Health Care.* Sudbury, MA: Jones and Bartlett Publishers Inc, 2005.

Polder JJ, Meerding WJ, Bonneux L, van der Mass PJ. A cross-national perspective on cost-of-illness: A comparison of studies from The Netherlands, Australia, Canada, Germany, United Kingdom, and Sweden. *European Journal of Health Economics: HEPAC: Health Economics in Prevention and Care* 6(3):223–232, 2005.

Tarricone R. Cost-of-illness analysis: What room in health economics? *Health Policy* 77(1):51–63, 2006.

Chapter 2

Measuring and Estimating Costs

Objectives

Upon completing this chapter, the reader will be able to:

1. Define different costing terms.

2. Categorize types of costs.

3. Determine the perspective of a study based on types of costs measured.

4. Understand when adjusting for timing of costs is appropriate.

5. Calculate net present value.

6. Compare average costs with marginal or incremental costs.

7. List common sources for obtaining cost data.

✦ COSTING TERMS

Costs are calculated to estimate the resources (or inputs) that are used in the production of a good or service. Resources used for one good or service are no longer available to be used for another. According to economic theory, the "true" cost of a resource is its **opportunity cost**—the value of the best-forgone option or the "next best option"—not necessarily the amount of money that changes hands. Resources committed to one product or service cannot be used for other products or services (opportunities). For example, if volunteers are used to help staff a new clinic, even though no money changes hands (i.e., volunteers are not paid), there is an opportunity cost associated with their help because they could be providing other services if they were not helping at the new clinic. Another example is if the new clinic required a part-time pharmacist and a currently employed pharmacist was asked to fill in at the clinic as part of his or her duties (instead of hiring a new part-time pharmacist for the clinic). The hourly rate of the pharmacist (plus fringe benefits) multiplied by the number of hours spent at the clinic would be used to estimate a portion of the costs of the new clinic even though no one new was added to the payroll. This is because if the pharmacist was not filling in at the clinic, he or she would have been providing other products or services—for example, filling prescriptions or providing clinical services to inpatients—"the next best option."

The "price" or the amount that is charged to a payer is not necessarily synonymous with the **cost** of the product or service. For example, if a hospital system wanted to calculate how much it cost to treat a patient with a specific diagnosis, there may be a substantial difference in what the total cost is to the hospital when compared with the amount the hospital charges the payer and what is actually collected from the payer after allowable amounts are factored in. Think of these differences as similar to the new car market. There is a cost to the car manufacturer to produce a car, a "sticker price," which is the suggested price of the car (higher than the cost to produce the car), and the amount paid by the average car buyer (usually lower than the sticker price, which is good news for the buyer, but is hopefully higher than the cost to produce the car, which is good news for the manufacturer). These, in turn, are similar to the actual cost of a hospital to provide a service, the charge billed to the payer (third-party insurance payer, patient payer, or a combination), and the **allowable charge** or **reimbursed** amount paid by the payer(s). Again, the reimbursed amount is hopefully higher than the cost of the hospital to provide the service (good news for the hospital) and lower than the standard charge listed by the hospital (good news for the payer[s]).

✦ COST CATEGORIZATION

In the 1980s and 1990s, most textbooks categorized pharmacoeconomic (PE)-related costs into four types: **direct medical costs, direct nonmedical costs, indirect costs**, and **intangible costs** (Table 2.1). These terms are not used consistently in the literature, and it has been noted that the economic term indirect costs, which refers to a loss of productivity, might be confused with the accounting definition of indirect costs, which is used to assign overhead. An alternative method of categorization has been recently proposed by Drummond et al.[1] that includes the following four categories: health care sector costs, costs to other sectors, patient and family costs, and productivity costs. Because of the variations that readers may find in research studies, both methods of categorization are presented and discussed.

Direct Medical Costs

Direct medical costs are the most obvious costs to measure. These are the medically related inputs used directly to provide the treatment. Examples of direct medical costs include the costs associated with the pharmaceuticals, diagnostic tests, physician visits, pharmacist visits, emergency department visits, and hospitalizations.

For chemotherapy treatment, for example, direct medical costs may include the chemotherapy products themselves, other medications given to reduce side effects of the chemotherapy, intravenous supplies, laboratory tests, clinic costs, and physician visits.

TABLE 2.1. **EXAMPLES OF TYPES OF COSTS**

Type of Cost Category	Examples
Direct medical costs	Medications Medication monitoring Medication administration Patient counseling and consultations Diagnostic tests Hospitalizations Clinic visits Emergency department visits Home medical visits Ambulance services Nursing services
Direct nonmedical costs	Travel costs to receive health care (bus, gas, taxi) Nonmedical assistance related to condition (e.g., Meals-on-Wheels, homemaking services) Hotel stays for patient or family for out-of-town care Child care services for children of patients
Indirect costs	Lost productivity for patient Lost productivity for unpaid caregiver (e.g., family member, neighbor, friend) Lost productivity because of premature mortality
Intangible costs	Pain and suffering Fatigue Anxiety

Direct Nonmedical Costs

Direct nonmedical costs are costs to patients and their families that are directly associated with treatment but are not medical in nature. Examples of direct nonmedical costs include the cost of traveling to and from the physician's office, clinic, or the hospital; child care services for the children of a patient; and food and lodging required for the patients and their families during out-of-town treatment.

For the chemotherapy treatment, patients may have increased travel costs related to traveling to the clinic or hospital. They may also have to hire a babysitter for the time they are undergoing treatment.

Indirect Costs

Indirect costs involve the costs that result from the loss of productivity because of illness or death. **Indirect benefits**, which are savings from avoiding indirect costs, are the increased earnings or productivity gains that occur because of the medical product or intervention. In the chemotherapy example, some indirect costs result from time the patient takes off from work to receive treatment or reduced productivity because of the effects of the disease or its treatment. On the other hand, some indirect benefits may accrue at a later time because of the increased productivity allowed by the success of the treatment in decreasing morbidity and prolonging life.

Intangible Costs

Intangible costs include the costs of pain, suffering, anxiety, or fatigue that occur because of an illness or the treatment of an illness. Intangible benefits, which are avoidance or alleviation of intangible costs, are benefits that result from a reduction in pain and suffering related to a product or intervention. It is difficult to measure or place a monetary value on these types of costs. In the example of chemotherapy, nausea and fatigue are common intangible costs of treatment. In Chapter 7 on **cost-benefit analysis**, an example of a method for incorporating intangible costs and benefits into PE equations—the **willingness-to-pay** technique—is discussed. In Chapter 6 on **cost-utility analysis**, the calculation of **utility** measures is meant to include intangible costs and benefits as well.

✦ ALTERNATIVE METHOD OF CATEGORIZATION

As mentioned, an alternative method of categorizing costs has recently been proposed by Drummond et al.[1] The first category is **health care sector costs**, which include medical resources consumed by health care entities. These types of costs are similar to the definition of direct medical costs but do not include direct medical costs paid for by the patient (e.g., deductibles, co-payments) or other non–health care entities. The second category is **other sector costs**. Some diseases and their treatment impact other non–health care sectors, such as housing, home-maker services, and educational services. One example often noted is that when measuring resources used and savings incurred by the treatment of patients with schizophrenia, researchers should consider the impact on other sectors, including public assistance and the prison system.

The third category is **patient and family costs**. This categorization includes costs to the patient and his or her family without regard to whether the costs are medical or nonmedical in nature. Thus, these costs include the patient's or family's share of direct medical as well as direct nonmedical costs.

The fourth category is termed **productivity costs** and is analogous to the economic term indirect costs but has the advantage of not being confused with the accounting term with the same name. Drummond et al.[1] advise against using the term intangible costs because they are "not costs (i.e., resources denied other uses)" and they are "not strictly intangible as they are often measured and valued, through the utility or willingness-to-pay approach." As mentioned above, these approaches are discussed in following chapters.

Treatment of an illness may include a combination of these types of costs and benefits. Many studies report only the direct medical (i.e., health care sector) costs. This may be appropriate depending on the objective of the study. For example, if the objective is to measure the costs to the hospital for two treatments that are expected to differ only in direct medical costs, measurement of the other types of costs may not be warranted.

✦ PERSPECTIVE

To determine what costs are important to measure, the **perspective** of the study must be determined. Perspective is an economic term that describes *whose costs* are relevant based on the purpose of the study. Conventional economic theory suggests that the most appropriate and comprehensive perspective is that of society. **Societal costs** include costs to the insurance company, costs to the patient, costs to the provider/institution, other sector costs, and indirect costs because of the loss of productivity. Although this may be the most appropriate perspective according to economic theory, it is not the most commonly seen in the PE literature because it is difficult and time-consuming to estimate all of these cost components. In many cases, researchers are not interested in the overall costs of each treatment alternative; instead, they are interested in the *differences* in costs between two alternatives, and if they do not expect differences in any costs except for direct medical costs, measurement of other types of costs would not be relevant. The most common perspectives used in PE studies are the perspective of the institution or provider (e.g., hospital or clinic) or the payer (e.g., Medicaid or private insurance plan) because these may be more pragmatic to answer the question at hand.

The payer perspective may include the costs to the third-party plan or the patient or a combination of the patient co-pay and the third-party plan costs. At the beginning of this chapter, the differentiation of actual costs versus charges versus the reimbursed amount was discussed. If the perspective of the analysis is the hospital, the actual cost to treat a patient should be estimated (similar to the cost to manufacture a product such as the example above about the cost to produce a car). If the perspective of the analysis is that of the payer, the amount that is reimbursed (similar to the actual amount paid for a car by the purchaser of the car) should be used when estimating costs. If the perspective is that of the patient, his or her out-of-pocket expenses, such as co-payments, deductibles, lost wages, and transportation costs, would be estimated. Example 2.1 provides a summary of perspectives and cost categories used in published research papers.

✦ TIMING ADJUSTMENTS FOR COSTS

Bringing Past Costs to the Present: Standardization of Costs

When costs are estimated from information collected for more than 1 year before the study, **adjustment of costs** is needed; this is also referred to as **standardization of costs**. If **retrospective data** are used to assess resources used over a number of years back, these costs should be adjusted, or *valued at one point in time*. If you compared costs for patients who received treatment in 2005 with those for patients who received treatment in 2010, the comparison of resources used would not be a fair comparison because treatment costs tend to go up each year; so patients who received the same treatment in 2005 would have lower costs than those who received the treatment in 2010. Adjustment of the 2005 costs to the amount they would have cost in 2010 is needed before a direct (fair) comparison can be made between these groups. For example, if the objective of the study is to estimate the difference in the costs of chemotherapy regimens, information on the past use of these two treatments might be collected from a review of medical records. If the retrospective review of these medical records dates back for more than 1 year, it may be necessary to standardize the cost of both medications by calculating the number of units (doses) used per case and multiplying this number by the current unit cost for each medication.

Table 2.2 illustrates an example of **adjustment** using this first method to estimate the treatment costs for a mild infection. These costs include two office visits, one laboratory service, and a prescription for an antibiotic. If retrospective data were collected over a number of years for patients who had received treatment for their

---

EXAMPLE 2.1   REVIEW OF COSTING PROCEDURES
IN PUBLISHED ARTICLES

Note: Summary of Neumann P. Costing and perspective in published cost-effectiveness
analysis. Medical Care 47(7 suppl 1):S28–S32, 2009.

The Tufts Medical Center Cost-Effectiveness Analysis (CEA) Registry contains information on over 3,000 published health economic studies in an online searchable
database (www.cearegistry.org). This paper considered the measurement of numerator of the economic equation—costs (rather than the denominator – outcomes). As
mentioned in this chapter, economic theory recommends assessing costs from a
"societal"—or all-encompassing—community perspective. But this perspective may
be impractical and/or conflict with that of the decision maker (payer). This paper
summarized the perspective used in 1,164 published cost-utility analysis (CUA)
studies conducted from 1976 to 2005. More recent studies were more likely to
include a clear study perspective (83% of those from 2002 to 2005, 52% from
1976 to 1997, and 74% from 1998 to 2001). Although about 41% of the authors
stated they used the societal perspective and about 33% of the authors stated they
used the payer's perspective (26% not stated or other), reviewers at the CEA Registry
categorized about 29% as societal and about 69% as the health care payer's
perspective (2% not stated or other). Some researchers considered the perspective
as societal if they included all types of medical costs (patient, third party, etc.), but
did not include nonmedical costs (parking, babysitting, loss of productivity, etc.),
while others may have reasoned that these nonmedical costs were captured by the
difference in outcomes measures—for example, it has been argued that patients'
preferences as measured by quality-adjusted life-years (QALYs) include the patients'
consideration of nonmedical costs and lost earnings. The author concluded that
researchers should be clearer about the perspective of their study.

---

infection, using unit costs from one point in time would achieve **standardization**
and allow for more uniform comparisons.

Another method used to **standardize** past costs is to multiply all of the costs
from the year the data were collected by the medical inflation rate for that year
(Table 2.3). Medical Consumer Price Index (MCPI) inflation rates can be found at
the Bureau of Labor Statistics's website (www.bls.gov) and have been between 3%
and 4% each year since 2005.[2]

**TABLE 2.2. EXAMPLE OF STANDARDIZATION: UNITS
MULTIPLIED BY COSTS**

Medical Resources Used to Treat Mild Infection	Units of Each Resource	Cost per Unit in 2005 ($)	Total Cost in 2005 ($)
Office visit	Two visits	62.00	124.00
Laboratory service to culture organism	One laboratory service	53.00	53.00
Antibiotic medication	28 capsules	1.03	28.84
Total			205.84

TABLE 2.3. **EXAMPLE OF STANDARDIZATION: USING MEDICAL CONSUMER PRICE INDEX (MCPI) INFLATION RATES**			
Medical Resources Used to Treat Mild Infection	Cost Estimate for Resource ($)	Year of Cost Estimate	Cost Adjusted to 2005 ($)
Office visits	115.00	2003	125.46[a]
Laboratory service to culture organism	50.00	2004	52.25[b]
Antibiotic medication	28.84	2005	28.84
Total			206.55

Medical CPI for 2004 = 4.4%; Medical CPI for 2005 = 4.5%
[a] $115 × 1.044 [1 + MCPI for 2004] × 1.045 [1 + MCPI for 2005]
[b] $50 × 1.045 [1 + MCPI for 2005]

Bringing Future Costs (Benefits) to the Present: Discounting

If costs are estimated based on dollars spent or saved in future years, another type of modification, called **discounting**, is needed. There is a time value associated with money. People (and businesses) prefer to receive money today rather than at a later time. Therefore, money received today is worth more than the same amount of money received next year. For example, if I asked to borrow $1,000 from you today and assured you I would pay you back the $1,000 in 3 years, you would not agree to lend me the money unless I paid you more than $1,000 in 3 years, even if I could guarantee there would be no inflation in the next 3 years. Money promised in the future, similar to health care savings promised in the future, is valued at a lower rate than money (savings) received today. Modifications for this time value are estimated using a **discount rate**. The discount rate approximates the cost of capital by taking into account the interest rates of borrowed money. From this parameter, the **present value** (PV) of future expenditures and savings can be calculated. The discount rate generally accepted for health care interventions is between 3% and 5%, but it is recommended that a comparison of results be conducted using high and low estimates of various discount rates. Varying these discount rates is an example of a **sensitivity analysis**, a term discussed in the next chapter.

The discount factor is equal to $1/(1 + r)^t$, where r is the discount rate and t is the number of years in the future that the cost or savings occur. For example, if the expenses of cancer treatment for the next 3 years are $5,000 for year 1, $3,000 for year 2, and $4,000 for year 3, discounting should be used to determine total expenses in PV terms. If one assumes that the expenses occur at the beginning of each year, then first-year costs are not discounted (see Table 2.4). It is equally

TABLE 2.4. **EXAMPLE OF DISCOUNTING: COSTS ASSESSED AT BEGINNING OF EACH YEAR**[a]			
Year Costs Are Incurred	Estimated Costs without Discounting($)	Calculation ($)	Present Value ($)
Year 1	5,000	5,000/1	5,000
Year 2	3,000	3,000/1.05	2,857
Year 3	4,000	$4,000/(1.05)^2$	3,628
Total	12,000		11,485

[a] Using a 5% discount rate.

TABLE 2.5. EXAMPLE OF DISCOUNTING: COSTS ASSESSED AT END OF EACH YEAR[a]

Year Costs Are Incurred	Estimated Costs without Discounting ($)	Calculation ($)	Present Value ($)
Year 1	5,000	5,000/1.05	4,762
Year 2	3,000	$3,000/(1.05)^2$	2,721
Year 3	4,000	$4,000/(1.05)^3$	3,455
Total	12,000		10,938

[a]Using a 5% discount rate.

acceptable to assume that expenses occur at the end of the first year (12 months later), and therefore, they are discounted (see Table 2.5). Example 2.2 looks at discounting both the estimated costs and estimated savings over 3 years of operating a new asthma clinic (using a 3% discount rate and no discounting for first-year costs and savings).

EXAMPLE 2.2 DISCOUNTING COSTS AND SAVINGS FOR AN ASTHMA CLINIC

This example shows why discounting (adjustment for the time value of money) is needed when extrapolating estimated costs and savings into the future. Start-up (first-year) costs of the clinic may be higher than in year 2 and year 3. The savings (attributable to fewer hospitalizations and emergency room visits) may not be seen until after the first year of operation of the clinic. All costs and savings must be valued at one point in time (year 1 or present value) to more accurately compare costs with savings.

	Year 1	Year 2	Year 3	Total
Costs of health clinic—not discounted ($)	200,000	150,000	150,000	500,000
Costs of health clinic—discounted[a] ($)	PV = 200,000	PV = 145,631	PV = 141,389	PV = 487,020
Savings from health clinic—not discounted ($)	100,000	200,000	250,000	550,000
Savings from health clinic—discounted[a] ($)	PV = 100,000	PV = 194,175	PV = 235,649	PV = 529,824
Net savings—not discounted ($)	(100,000)[b]	50,000	100,000	50,000
Net savings—discounted[a] ($)	PV = (100,000)[b]	PV = 48,544	PV = 94,260	PV = 42,804

PV, present value of future costs or future savings, assuming costs and savings occur at beginning of the year (i.e., first-year costs and savings not discounted).

[a]Discounting at 3% discount rate after year 1.

[b]Parentheses indicate a net cost, or negative monetary amount.

TABLE 2.6. **COMPARING AVERAGE AND INCREMENTAL COST RATIOS**		
	Treatment A	Treatment B
Total cost ($)	325	450
Effectiveness	87% successful	91% successful
Average cost-effectiveness ($)	325/0.87 = 373 per success	450/0.91 = 494 per success
Incremental cost-effectiveness[a] ($)	—	(450 − 325) / (0.91 − 0.87) = 3,125 for each additional success

[a]Difference in costs divided by difference in effectiveness.

Average versus Marginal or Incremental Costs

As mentioned, clinicians and other decision makers are trying to determine which alternative to select based on the costs and outcomes of the alternatives. When deciding between medication A and medication B, a clinician would find it useful to know the estimated *difference* in costs and the estimated *difference* in outcomes between the medications to determine whether *added* benefits outweigh the *added* costs. Therefore, when comparing the costs of options, it is important to look at the *change* in costs. The terms **marginal costs** and **incremental costs** are often used interchangeably to refer to this change or difference between alternatives. Others make the distinction that marginal costs refer to the cost of producing one extra unit of outcome or product, and incremental costs refer to the difference in cost between two competing options. In clinical practice, a realistic option may be to compare a new treatment with a standard treatment; thus, the *difference* in these costs is of interest to the decision maker. Therefore, the calculation of the *change* in costs divided by the *change* in outcomes should be used. The result of this calculation is termed the **incremental cost-effectiveness ratio** (ICER), and it can be very different from comparing the average costs of the options or alternatives, especially when the difference in outcomes is small. Table 2.6 shows an example of the disparity in results when calculating average costs per outcome compared with calculating incremental costs per outcome. Treatment B costs only $125 more per patient than treatment A ($450 versus $325, respectively), yet the cost per additional (incremental) success (the ICER) is $3,125. Some find it easier to understand this concept if they calculate this ratio another way. If a clinician is faced with the choice of treating 100 patients with treatment A (100 patients × $325 per patient = $32,500) or 100 patients with treatment B (100 patients × $450 = $45,000), it would cost $12,500 ($45,000 versus $32,500) more to treat 100 patients with treatment B. Of the 100 patients treated with treatment A, 87 would have a successful outcome, but 91 of the 100 patients treated with treatment B would have a successful outcome (four extra successes). Therefore, it is estimated that it costs $12,500 more to treat 100 patients with treatment B in order to achieve four extra successes (or as before $3,125 per extra success).

✦ RESOURCES FOR COST ESTIMATIONS

How does the researcher estimate common direct medical costs? Sometimes these costs are measured directly during a clinical study for each patient through record keeping and patient logs. The more similar a clinical study is to "real-world" practice, the better estimate this method provides. Sometimes costs are collected **retrospectively** from medical records or reimbursement **claims data**. Combing through medical records can be time-consuming and thus resource intensive. Claims data review is a relatively inexpensive way to collect cost data for patients but may be incomplete (see Chapter 11 on retrospective databases). Other times, these costs are estimated from various standard lists of costs. Sources of estimates for four types of common direct medical cost categories are addressed: medications, medical services, personnel costs, and hospitalizations.

Medications

The **average wholesale price** (AWP) is often used when calculating the cost of pharmaceutical products in the United States. This is considered the "list price" or "sticker price" of medications and can be found in readily available sources such as the Red book.[3] The AWP is higher than what pharmacies, institutions, or third-party payers actually pay for medications. Although the AWP has long been used as a benchmark for prescription prices, some argue that it has moved so far from the actual acquisition cost that it is no longer useful.[4] The wholesale acquisition cost (WAC) prices are estimates of costs to wholesalers from the manufacturer (some use the analogy of "catalog" prices), but these estimates do not include discounts. The **average manufacturer's price** (AMP), calculated to reflect the average amount paid to manufacturers by wholesalers after discounts are included, is a more precise estimate of what buyers (pharmacies) pay for medications, but the AMP calculations are proprietary and not available to the general public. Researchers should be clear about the source they use to estimate pharmacy costs, to enhance comparability of studies.[5]

Medical Services

Medical services, such as office or clinic visits and outpatient laboratory and surgical procedures, are frequently included in direct medical cost estimates. As mentioned, providers have a list of charges for these types of services, but payers usually pay less than this "list price." When the perspective is that of the purchaser (or payer), various sources are available to estimate these costs to the payers. A common source for US **reimbursement** rates (the amount reimbursed by payers to the providers of health services) is the *Physician's Fee Reference* (both a book and a searchable database are available).[6] Medicare reimbursement rates for these types of services are also provided by Centers for Medicare and Medicaid Services (CMS). Reimbursement figures from the *Physician's Fee Reference* are higher than those from the Medicare list.

Personnel

When the perspective of the study is that of the provider of health services (e.g., hospital, clinic, physician's office, pharmacy) and the provision of different health care alternatives involves a difference in the amount of time spent by medical personnel, attributing a cost to this difference is warranted. For example, if a hospital wanted to determine the cost-effectiveness of instituting a pharmacy discharge counseling service, an important cost estimate would include the time of the pharmacists who would provide this service. To estimate these costs, the amount of time spent in the activity would be multiplied by the salary plus fringe benefits of pharmacists. Estimating the time for the personnel may include the use of estimates based on similar services or may involve more precise **work measurement** methods. These work measurement methods may include using a stopwatch to time how long an activity takes on average (e.g., recording how long it takes for a nurse to hang an intravenous medication bag) or having the employees keep a log of when they are involved in certain activities (e.g., asking the pharmacist to write down how many hours are spent in the clinic and how many patients are counseled each day). Categorizations and examples of the various work measurement methods can be found elsewhere.[7,8]

Hospitalizations

The level of the precision of estimates varies widely for studies that include hospital costs as part of their evaluation. In order from least precise (gross or macro-costing) to most precise (micro-costing), four methods for estimating hospital costs are **per diem, disease-specific per diem, diagnosis-related group** (DRG), and **micro-costing**. The level used is determined by the importance of the hospital-related costs to the overall evaluation, the perspective of the study, the availability of cost data, and the resources available for conducting the study (more precision usually means more time intensive).

Per Diem

The least precise method of estimating hospital costs is the per diem method of costing. For each day that a patient is in a hospital setting, an average cost per day for all types of hospitalizations is used as a multiplier. For example, if the average cost reimbursement per day for hospitalizations of all patients was $2,000 per day, the cost estimate for a 3-day stay for appendicitis would be the same as the estimate for a 3-day stay for cardiac bypass surgery (3 days × $2,000/ day = $6,000).

Disease-Specific Per Diem

It would be more precise to use estimated costs per day for specific diseases, or a disease-specific per diem. Here the average reimbursement rate might be $1,500 per day for the appendicitis case ($4,500 for 3 days) and $10,000 per day ($30,000 for 3 days) for the cardiac bypass surgery case.

Diagnosis-Related Group

A relatively available and often-used method of estimating hospital costs to the payer is the payment rate for DRGs. This method is used to classify clinically cohesive diagnoses and procedures that use similar resources. These were first used by the federal government in the 1980s to contain the increase in Medicare costs. Each patient is assigned one of more than 500 DRGs based on factors such as principal diagnosis, specific procedures involved, secondary diagnoses, and age, and the average reimbursement for each DRG can be used to approximate the cost to the payer.

Micro-costing

The most precise method of estimating hospital costs is micro-costing. Micro-costing involves collecting information on resource use for each component of an intervention (in this example, each component of a hospitalization) to estimate and compare alternative interventions. For example, if the perspective of a study was a provider, such as a hospital, and the objective was to determine whether a new technology would save hospital resources for patients who had a specific DRG, then using the DRG reimbursement rate as a proxy for cost would not provide the information needed. In such situations, micro-costing would provide more useful information. This usually entails a review of patients' hospital records to determine what specific services (e.g., medications, laboratory services, procedures) were used and to assign a cost to each service. Records are kept for each service to determine how much to charge the payers (patient and third-party payers) for each hospital stay. As mentioned, charges are list prices, and most payers reimburse hospitals at a much lower rate, called the allowable charge, based on contractual agreements. To make a profit, the true costs of providing these services need to be lower than the amount of reimbursement from the payers. To simplify calculations, a cost-to-charge ratio for the entire hospital or for each department may be used to estimate true costs, which are difficult to determine, from charge data, which are easier to obtain. Refer to Example 2.3 for examples of the types of hospital costs measured using micro-costing and Example 2.4, which compares costs estimated using charges with costs estimated using cost-to-charge ratio calculations.

SUMMARY

This chapter summarized two schools of thought on categorizing different types of costs in PE analyses. The categories of costs that need to be measured depend on the perspective of the study (or *whose costs* is the study concerned about), which in turn depends on the objective of the study—in other words, what questions are the researchers trying to answer. After the categories of costs are decided upon, modifications of these costs based on timing issues might need to be addressed. If the data on costs are collected retrospectively for more than 1 year, adjustment calculations are used, or if the data on costs (or savings) are estimated into the future for more than 1 year, discounting methods are used. The need for incremental cost calculations was addressed, and some standard methods and sources used in estimating direct medical costs were outlined.

Now that readers have an understanding of the left hand of the PE equation (see Figure 1.1), Chapter 3 gives examples of questions to ask when reading or assessing a PE research article or report. Chapters 4 to 7 discuss how to measure the right-hand side of each type of PE study and then follow it up with a composite article that readers are encouraged to critique using the questions outlined in Chapter 3.

EXAMPLE 2.3 MICRO-COSTING

This is an example of micro-costing from the literature. Fentanyl and remifentanil are opiates used for patients undergoing surgery. It has been suggested that remifentanil speeds postoperative recovery because of its short duration of action (which can lead to the patients being disconnected from the breathing tube more quickly after surgery). One of the objectives of this study was to compare costs to the hospital between patients who received fentanyl and who received remifentanil for coronary bypass graft surgery without cardiopulmonary bypass. Charges listed on patient bills were multiplied by department-level **cost-to-charge ratios** to estimate the average cost to the hospital for each patient. Although some department-level costs were different between the two groups, the overall total costs for patients using fentanyl and remifentanil were not significantly different.

Cost Type	Fentanyl Costs ($) (n = 20)	Remifentanil Costs ($) (n = 39)
Ward	4,808	3,973
Operating room	2,216	2,284
Medical or surgical supplies	1,941	2,080
Intensive care unit	1,914	2,349
Cardiac catheterization laboratory	1,097	1,129
Laboratory	913	854
Pharmacy	611	575
Anesthesia	416	476
Intravenous therapy	414	470
Respiratory therapy	398	255
Transfusion	216	285
Emergency room	215	191
Radiology	176	147
Vascular laboratory	93	54
Recovery room	65	31
Electrocardiography	61	64
Pulmonary laboratory	34	0
Rehabilitation	21	7
Nuclear medicine	9	31
Computed tomography scan	0	17
Total Costs	15,616[a]	15,272

[a]Because of rounding, total does not equal addition of all costs listed.

Adapted from Reddy P, Feret BM, Kulicki L, Donahue S, Quercia RA. Cost analysis of fentanyl and remifentanil in coronary artery bypass graft surgery without cardiopulmonary bypass. *Journal of Clinical Pharmacy and Therapeutics* 27(2):127–132, 2002. Used with permission of Blackwell Publishing.

EXAMPLE 2.4	USE OF CHARGES VERSUS COST-TO-CHARGE RATIOS IN ECONOMIC COMPARISONS

This example summarizes some of the information found in Taira et al. (2003). The authors compared cost estimates of three multicenter clinical trials of patients with coronary artery disease. They used patient-level use of resources in these trials to compare various methods of measuring costs and cost differences between alternatives studied. Hospital charges included the itemized amount that was listed for the average patient. The hospital cost-to-charge ratios were calculated by dividing annual total hospital costs by annual total hospital charges. For example, in the first clinical trial, which compared angioplasty with atherectomy, the overall cost-to-charge ratio for the hospitals in this study was about 61%. The department-level cost-to-charge ratios were calculated by dividing each department's total annual costs (e.g., pharmacy, laboratory, surgery) by each department's total annual charges, multiplying each department's ratio by each department's charges, and then summing them together. For the first clinical trial, this resulted in a department-level cost-to-charge ratio of about 54%. This may seem like a large percent of profit, but readers should remember that hospitals' charges (remember the sticker price of a car example) do not equal hospital reimbursements or revenues (the amount actually paid to the hospital by payers). Also note that although there was a divergence in the magnitude of costs differences between alternative 1 and 2 depending on the method of cost estimation used, the answer to the question *Is there a statistical difference in these costs?* was the same for both methods.

	Mean Cost Estimates: Alternative 1 ($)	Mean Cost Estimates: Alternative 2 ($)	Statistical Difference in Means Using t-test
Clinical Trial 1	*Angioplasty*	*Atherectomy*	
Hospital charges	18,155	21,251	Yes; $p = 0.007$
Hospital-level cost-to-charge ratio	10,960	12,910	Yes; $p < 0.001$
Department-level cost-to-charge ratio	9,616	11,547	Yes; $p < 0.001$
Clinical Trial 2	*Palmaz-Schatz Stent*	*Multilink Stent*	
Hospital charges	21,706	21,594	No; $p = 0.92$
Hospital-level cost-to-charge ratio	11,693	11,487	No; $p = 0.68$
Department-level cost-to-charge ratio	8,865	8,841	No; $p = 0.96$
Clinical Trial 3	*Urokinase*	*AngioJet*	
Hospital charges	80,753	59,442	Yes; $p < 0.001$
Hospital-level cost-to-charge ratio	37,705	27,251	Yes; $p < 0.001$
Department-level cost-to-charge ratio	19,154	13,950	Yes; $p < 0.001$

Adapted from Taira DA, Seto TB, Siegrist R, et al. Comparison of analytic approaches for the economic evaluation of new technologies alongside multicenter clinical trials. *American Heart Journal* 145(3):452–458, 2003, with permission.

QUESTIONS/EXERCISES

1. For each situation, what type of cost is being measured?

   a. A patient must pay for a taxi ride to the clinic.
   b. A patient receives an influenza vaccination at the pharmacy.
   c. A patient is fatigued because of chemotherapy treatments.
   d. An adult daughter misses work to take care of her mother who recently had hip replacement surgery.

2. A new pharmaceutical product has just been developed for patients who are treatment-resistant to the current antipsychotic products on the market. Based on the following perspectives and objectives, what costs should be measured?

   a. An inpatient mental health hospital wants to estimate the effect of the new product on its budget.
   b. The state Medicaid program wants to estimate the effect of the new product on its budget.
   c. The governor of your state wants to estimate the effect of the new product on the state budget.

3. Based on the following costs from a *retrospective* analysis, what is the 2013 value for the three alternatives using a medical consumer price index (MCPI) inflation rate of 3.5% per year?

Year	2010	2011	2012	2013
Alternative 1 costs ($)	10,000	30,000	30,000	20,000
Alternative 2 costs ($)	15,000	15,000	25,000	25,000
Alternative 3 costs ($)	20,000	20,000	20,000	20,000

4. Based on a 3% discount rate, what is the 2013 present value of the costs of the three alternatives estimated to accrue over the next 4 years? Assume that costs are assessed (accrued) at the beginning of the year.

Year	2013	2014	2015	2016
Alternative 1 estimated costs ($)	10,000	30,000	30,000	20,000
Alternative 2 estimated costs ($)	15,000	15,000	25,000	25,000
Alternative 3 estimated costs ($)	20,000	20,000	20,000	20,000

REFERENCES

1. Drummond MF, Sculpher MJ, Torrance GW, et al. *Methods for the Economic Evaluation of Health Care Programmes* (3rd ed.). Oxford: Oxford University Press, 2005.
2. US Department of Labor Bureau of Labor Statistics. Available at www.bls.gov; accessed November 2012.
3. *RED BOOK: Pharmacy's Fundamental Reference*. Thomson Reuters. Available at http://www.redbook.com/redbook/online; accessed November 2012.
4. Gencarelli DM. Average wholesale price for prescription drugs: Is there a more appropriate pricing mechanism? *National Health Policy Forum Issue Brief*, No. 775, June 7, 2002.
5. Tunis S. A cost-effectiveness analysis to illustrate the impact of cost definitions on results, interpretations and comparability of pharmacoeconomic studies in the US. *Pharmacoeconomics* 27(9):735–744, 2009.
6. *Physicians' Fee Reference*. Wasserman Medical Publishers, Ltd., Milwaukee, MI, 2013 (ISBN 978-1-59891-080-3).

7. Rascati KL, Kimberlin CL, McCormick WC. Work measurement in pharmacy research. *American Journal of Hospital Pharmacy* 43:2445–2452, 1986.

8. Burke T, McKee J, Wilson H, Donahue R, Batenhorst A, Pathak D. A comparison of time-and-motion and self-reporting methods of work measurement. *The Journal of Nursing Administration* 30(3):118–125, 2000.

SUGGESTED READINGS

Freidman B, DeLaMare J, Andrews R, McKenzie DH. Practical options for estimating cost of hospital in patient stays. *Journal of Health Care Finance* 29(1):1–13, 2002.

Gold MR, Seigel JE, Russell LB, Weinstein MD (eds). *Cost-Effectiveness in Health and Medicine.* New York, NY: Oxford University Press, 1996.

Jacobs P, Ohinmaa A, Brady B. Providing systematic guidance in pharmacoeconomic guidelines for analysing costs. *Pharmacoeconomics* 23(2):143–153, 2005.

Jacobs P, Roos NP. Standard cost lists for healthcare in Canada. *Pharmacoeconomics* 15(6): 551–560, 1999.

Larson L. Cost determination and analysis. In Bootman JL, Townsend RJ, McGhan WF (eds). *Principles of Pharmacoeconomics* (3rd ed.). Cincinnati, OH: Harvey Whitney Books Co., 2005.

Ratery J. Economics notes: Costing in economic evaluation. *British Medical Journal* 320(7249): 1597, 2000.

Robertson J, Lang D, Hill S. Use of pharmacoeconomics in prescribing research. Part 1: Costs-Moving beyond the acquisition price for drugs. *Journal of Clinical Pharmacy and Therapeutics* 28(1):73–79, 2003.

Chapter 3

Critiquing Research Articles

Objectives

Upon completing this chapter, the reader will be able to:

1. List and give examples and explanations of 14 questions to consider when reviewing a pharmacoeconomic research article.

✦ APPROPRIATENESS OF METHODS OF ANALYSIS

There is no one standard, agreed-upon method used to conduct a pharmacoeconomic analysis; rather, there are many acceptable methods. The appropriateness of these methods depends on many factors, including the specific question or objective, the **perspective** of the study, the time period needed to determine outcomes of the alternatives, and the resources (e.g., time, money, databases) available to researchers. No study is perfect; thoroughness is balanced with the practicality of the research. However, several authors[1-3] do cite methodology to assist in systematically reviewing the pharmacoeconomic literature.

A summary of review articles that assessed the quality of health economic publications concluded that there has been a modest improvement in the quality of conducting and reporting economic evaluations in the past decade (1990 to 2001).[4] A review of economic evidence, in the form of dossiers, provided by manufacturers to a health plan also showed that about half did not comply with recommended economic practice standards (e.g., did not state the perspective—Question 5 in this chapter—or conduct any sensitivity analyses—Question 11 in this chapter).[5] If a study is carefully reviewed to ensure that the author(s) included all meaningful components of an economic evaluation, the likelihood of finding credible and useful results is higher.

✦ QUESTIONS TO USE WHEN CRITIQUING RESEARCH ARTICLES

The following 14 questions illustrate the types of questions that should be raised when reviewing pharmacoeconomic studies. Most of the following chapters contain a composite article that incorporates the positive and negative aspects found in a mix of real research articles. After each composite article, you will find answers to the list of 14 questions outlined here. (Although topics are taken from actual articles, methods and data have been changed to illustrate points made in the chapter. All medication names in these composite articles are fictitious.)

1. Complete Title: Is the Title Appropriate?

From reading the title, can it be determined what is being compared and what type of study is being conducted—**cost-minimization analysis** (CMA), **cost-effectiveness analysis** (CEA), **cost-utility analysis** (CUA), **cost-benefit analysis** (CBA), or a combination of them. Does the title sound biased?

For example, a title such as *Pharmacoeconomic Analysis of Glipizide versus Glyburide in the Veterans Administration* does not specify the type of study (CMA, CEA, CBA, or CUA) conducted. Although this is not wrong, readers may prefer to know what type of study was conducted when searching for articles that are relevant to their purpose. In addition, sometimes the title is vague about what is being compared. For example, the title *Cost-Effectiveness Analysis of Two Antibiotic Therapies in a Large Teaching Hospital* does indicate the type of study that was conducted but not the alternatives that were compared. When many therapies are compared, the title might get long if all of them were listed. In some cases, the title itself may seem biased. For example, a title (here using names of medications that do not exist) such as *Ultraceph Found Cost-Effective When Compared to Megaceph* sounds like advertising rather than a scientific-based research.

2. Clear Objective: Is a Clear Objective Stated?

Was a well-defined question posed in an answerable form? This should be clearly stated at the beginning of the article. Examples of clear objectives might be "The objective of this study was to calculate the **benefit-to-cost ratio** of pharmacist interventions in our hospital." or "Our purpose was to perform an incremental **cost-utility analysis** of standard chemotherapy compared with palliative treatment alone for patients with inoperable lung cancer." An example of an unclear statement would be "The objective of our study is to determine if Ultraceph is better than Megaceph." This statement leaves the reader wondering better in what way?

3. Appropriate Alternatives: Were the Appropriate Alternatives or Comparators Considered?

Ideally, the most effective treatments or alternatives should be compared. In pharmacotherapy evaluations, the manufacturers of innovative new products often compare or measure the new product against a standard current therapy. This selection should include the best clinical options or the options that are used most often in a particular setting at the time of the study. If a new treatment option is being considered, comparing it with an outdated treatment or a treatment with low efficacy rate is a waste of time and money. A new treatment should be compared with the next best alternative or the alternative it may replace. Keep in mind that the alternatives may include drug treatments and nondrug treatments (e.g., medication versus surgery). Head-to-head comparisons of the best alternatives provide more information than comparisons of a new product or service with an outdated or ineffective alternative. In many **cost-benefit analyses** (CBAs), the options may be thought of as a "with or without" option. The comparison of a service or a preventative therapy (e.g., a vaccination or immunization) is compared with the alternative of not implementing the service or providing the preventative therapy.

4. Alternatives Described: Was a Comprehensive Description of the Competing Alternatives Given?

Could another researcher replicate the study based on the information given? If pharmaceutical products are compared, the dosages and length of therapy should be included. It is not helpful for the researcher to compare a low dose of one drug with a high dose of a competing drug. In some cases, a range of doses is given based on the range given to a specific population of patients or based on a summary of more than one research study used to gather data on costs and effects. In chemotherapy research, sometimes researchers describe the doses as "equitoxic"—a dose based on the amount a patient can tolerate without severe side effects—because patients need to be individually dosed based on their body mass index, their immunity status, and their reactions to the medication.

If pharmacy services are compared, explicit details of the services make the paper more useful. For these services, a description of start-up and continuing resource needs should be addressed, if applicable. For example, additional training for pharmacists and other health care professionals and space, overhead, equipment, or software needs may be required to provide the service. A summary of the services provided should be outlined. For example, if a pharmacist in a diabetes clinic provides services, readers would want to know how patients are identified, what topics are covered with the patient, and what type of follow-up is provided. A large part of the expense of providing pharmacy services may be personnel costs. Information about the measurement of these costs is provided in Chapter 2.

5. Perspective Stated: Is the Perspective of the Study Addressed?

The **perspective** tells the readers *whose costs* are measured. It is important to identify from whose perspective the analysis will be conducted because this determines the costs to be evaluated. Is the analysis being conducted from the perspective of the patient, hospital, clinic, insurance company, or society? Depending on the perspective assigned to the analysis, different results and recommendations based on those results may be identified. Some articles are not clear about what type of costs or whose costs is used in the calculations, and it is up to the reader to guess the perspective. In more recent articles, editors and reviewers are more aware that readers look for a sentence that explicitly states, "The perspective of the study was. . ." Some articles may use acceptable phrases such as "total third-party reimbursements for prescription and medical services were measured and summed" or "costs to the Canadian health care system were assessed," indicating the perspective to the readers without using the specific term.

6. Type of Study: Is the Type of Study Stated?

Knowing up front the type of pharmacoeconomic study that is being conducted helps readers follow the rest of the research article. As mentioned, it is helpful if the type of study is mentioned in the title. Some articles contain more than one type of study. For example, an article comparing chemotherapy options may include both **cost-effectiveness** calculations (cost per year of life saved) and **cost-utility** calculations (cost per **quality-adjusted life year**) and may compare the results of both.

7. Relevant Costs: Were All the Important and Relevant Costs Included?

Based on the stated **perspective,** were the appropriate types of costs assessed? Were costs collected for an appropriate time period? If these costs were estimated from other research or source material, they should be referenced. The author's list should be compared with the reader's practice situation. Was there justification for any important costs or consequences that were not included? Sometimes the authors may admit that although certain costs or consequences are important, they were impractical (or impossible) to measure in their study. It is better that the authors state these limitations rather than ignore them. Other times, the costs are so small that it would not be worth the effort to measure them.

Protocol driven-costs should be excluded from calculations. Protocol-driven costs are costs that occur because of the research protocol of a randomized, controlled trial that would not occur in everyday practice. For example, randomized, controlled trials for medications to treat stomach ulcers may include endoscopy procedures at various intervals to determine the healing rate of the ulcers. In everyday practice, physicians commonly rely on patients' reports of symptoms (or lack of symptoms) to determine the effectiveness of the medication. Costs that are the same for all alternatives are also commonly excluded based on the argument that when conducting an **incremental cost-effectiveness analysis,** these costs would mathematically cancel out each other.

8. **Relevant Outcomes: Were the Important or Relevant Outcomes Measured?**

Are these the clinical outcomes that are important to clinicians? Were outcomes measured for an appropriate time period? For example, when comparing medications that reduce blood pressure, clinicians agree that the main outcomes are change in systolic and diastolic blood pressure. But when comparing medications that treat diabetes, is fasting blood glucose or hemoglobin A1C important (or are both important)? When comparing medications that treat asthma, there is more debate on what outcomes are most important to measure. Some clinicians may prefer to use forced expiratory volume (FEV) measurements, but it is common in pharmacoeconomic studies to use a measure called **symptom-free days (SFDs),** which are based on patient diaries or reports. When measuring outcomes, is the appropriate time period used? For acute medical problems, such as infections or influenza, following up patients until the problem is resolved (an episode of care) entails collecting information for every patient in a short time frame. Conversely, outcomes emanating from chronic conditions, such as high blood pressure and high cholesterol levels, may not be fully captured until many years have elapsed. It is important for the reader to evaluate whether the time period of data collection was appropriate for the clinical measures recorded. This is especially important when short-term clinical trial data are incorporated into pharmacoeconomic studies of chronic conditions.

9. **Adjustment or Discounting: Was Adjustment Appropriate? If So, Was It Conducted? Was Discounting Appropriate? If So, Was It Conducted?**

As mentioned in Chapter 2, if **retrospective data** were analyzed to assess resources used over a number of years, these costs should be **adjusted,** or standardized, to value resources at one point in time. In addition, if the costs or benefits were extrapolated more than 1 year out, the time-value of money must be incorporated into the cost estimates, using **discount rates** to calculate the **present value.** These are two different questions. It is possible that neither **adjustment** nor **discounting** is needed, that only adjustment is needed, that only discounting is needed, or that both are needed.

10. **Reasonable Assumptions: Are Assumptions Stated and Reasonable?**

Pharmacoeconomic studies frequently require researchers to use estimates of costs or outcomes. Whenever estimates are used, there is a possibility that these estimates may not be precise (or universally agreed upon by the readers). These estimates may be referred to as **assumptions.** For example, authors may assume the cost of a laboratory test is $50, that patient adherence with a regimen will be 100%, or that the **discount rate** is 3%. These types of assumptions should be stated explicitly. Authors may include estimates without using the term "assumption," although using this term helps the reader differentiate between the values that were directly measured and the values that were estimated. Readers should ask themselves whether these estimates seem reasonable in the context of their practice or decision-making processes.

11. Sensitivity Analyses: Were Sensitivity Analyses Conducted for Important Estimates or Assumptions?

Sensitivity analysis allows one to determine how the results of an analysis would change when "best guess" estimates, or **assumptions,** are varied over a relevant range of values. By using a plausible range of values for key assumptions, sensitivity analysis allows the researcher to examine the impact of these assumptions on the study conclusions. For example, if a researcher makes the assumption that the appropriate **discount rate** is 3%, this estimate might be varied from 0% to 6% to determine whether the same alternative would still be chosen within this range. This method helps determine whether the analysis is **robust.** Do small changes in estimates produce important differences in the results? If the same option or comparator were chosen for the full range of the sensitivity analyses, the analysis is said to be **insensitive,** or robust, to this range of values, thereby adding confidence in the study results. If the conclusions or choice of therapy changes on the basis of a plausible range of estimates, the results are deemed **sensitive** to this estimate, and readers should be aware of this when interpreting results.

In the previous chapter, Examples 2.3 and 2.4 estimates provided sensitivity analyses. In Example 2.2, the net savings of a clinic after 3 years was $42,804 if future costs and savings were **discounted** at 3%, and $50,000 if discounting was not conducted (0% discount rate). Either calculation resulted in positive net savings for the clinic; therefore, the choice of whether or not to implement the clinic was not affected by (insensitive to) the range of discount rates used (0% to 3%). Example 2.4 showed that for three multicenter trials of patients with coronary artery disease, the method of cost estimation (**charges** versus hospital-level **cost-to-charge ratios** versus department-level **cost-to-charge ratios**) did not change the answer to the question *Is there a significant difference in costs between alternatives studied?* Again, this indicates insensitivity to the cost estimation method used. More examples of sensitivity analyses are given in subsequent chapters of this book.

12. Limitations Addressed: Were Limitations Addressed?

Because of practical restrictions, no study is ideal; therefore, the authors should mention the most important limitations of their study. Using **retrospective databases** may increase the possibility of **selection bias.** Selection bias occurs when patients with certain characteristics are more likely to receive one treatment over another. Using a specific population may limit **generalizability** of results (see next critique question). Small sample sizes or missing data may limit statistical comparisons. There may be no data available on some cost or outcome values, which may require broad assumptions. It is better for the authors to address these limitations than to leave them unstated.

13. Appropriate Generalizations: Were Extrapolations Beyond the Population Studied Proper?

If the study is based on data from a specific population of patients who may be atypical (e.g., in age, socioeconomic status, resource use) compared with the general patient population, the researchers should caution readers against **generalizing,** or extrapolating the results beyond the population studied. For example, results based on patients of long-term care facilities, the Veterans Administration, or state Medicaid may be different (in both costs and outcomes) from the results based on a population of ambulatory patients with private health care insurance.

14. Unbiased Conclusions: Was an Unbiased Summary of the Results Presented?

Sometimes the conclusions seem to overstate or overextrapolate the data presented in the results section. Did the authors choose appropriate alternatives and use unbiased reasonable estimates when determining the results? In general, do you believe the results of the study? Does the study make sense? Rennie and Luft[6] make the case that although there is concern that some studies sponsored by drug manufactures may be biased to show that their medication is cost-effective (Example 3.1), health plans that conduct pharmacoeconomic research may have an inclination to show a new treatment is not cost-effective and therefore will not be covered by the health plan. Assessment of the level to which research is biased versus unbiased should be based on the questions outlined above, not the funding source.

EXAMPLE 3.1   REVIEW OF PHARMACOECONOMIC STUDY FUNDING AND FINDINGS

Lexchin et al. (2003) found and summarized previously published research articles that analyzed whether methodologic quality or outcomes differed by source of funding. Overall, 30 articles were summarized, and the authors concluded that although research funded by the pharmaceutical companies was more likely to find positive outcomes for their products, there was no difference in the quality of the research. Two of the theories as to why more positive outcomes were found for industry-sponsored projects included (1) that the industry is more likely to fund research when they believe their product has a distinct advantage and (2) **publication bias** is more prevalent for industry-sponsored research. (Publication bias is based on the premise that only research with positive results are submitted for publication.) Summary information for three of the articles reviewed is listed in the table.

Reference	Research Question	Results
Azimi	How often do cost-effectiveness analyses encourage a strategy requiring additional expenditures?	Industry-funded studies were more likely to support a strategy requiring additional expenditures than those without such funding
Friedberg	What is the relationship between drug company sponsorship and economic assessment of oncology drugs?	Drug company–sponsored studies were more likely to report favorable qualitative conclusions, but overstatement of quantitative results did not differ significantly
Sacristan	What is the relation between drug company sponsorship and results of cost-effectiveness studies?	For general medical journals, three of six cost-effectiveness studies with industry funding had positive results compared with 31 of 63 with no funding or other source of funding
		For pharmacoeconomic journals, all 18 cost-effectiveness studies with industry funding had positive results compared with four of six with no funding or other sources of funding

Adapted with permission from table 2 in Lexchin J, Bero LA, Djulbegovic N, Clark O. Pharmaceutical industry sponsorship and research outcome and quality: Systematic review. *British Medical Journal* 326(7400):1167–1176, 2003.

SUMMARY

In summary, when assessing the soundness and usefulness of a pharmacoeconomic research article, readers need to keep in mind questions such as:

- Were comparators appropriate?
- Was the correct type of analysis conducted?
- Were the costs and outcomes measured appropriately?
- Did the authors account for differences in costs across time?
- Were **assumptions** reasonable?
- Were **sensitivity analyses** conducted when needed?
- Were limitations addressed?
- Did the tone of the article seem unbiased?

This chapter has presented general questions to consider. If readers come across unfamiliar terms when evaluating articles, a good source to consult is the *Health Care Cost, Quality, and Outcomes: ISPOR Book of Terms.*[7]

QUESTIONS/EXERCISES

Based on the following abstract (condensed summary of a research article), please answer the following questions:

ABSTRACT

TITLE: Pharmacoeconomic Analysis of Ultraceph and Megaceph

BACKGROUND: Two new antibiotics, Ultraceph and Megaceph, were recently approved by the Food and Drug Administration. Both work equally well on the same spectrum of bacteria (i.e., their scope and efficacy have been shown to be equal), and the products are priced similarly. Ultraceph is dosed intravenously at 25 mg, three times per day. Ultraceph is affected by liver functioning, so monitoring is needed. Megaceph is dosed intravenously at 75 mg once per day and is associated with a 0.1% chance of hearing loss, which is reversible if caught within the first 2 days of treatment.

METHODS: The purpose of this study was to compare the costs to Mercy General Hospital between patients who received Ultraceph versus Megaceph. Patients admitted to the hospital during the first 6 months of 2012 who met study criteria were randomly given either Ultraceph or Megaceph. Medical and billing records for each patient were used to estimate costs. Costs were estimated using two methods: using billed charges and estimating costs using an overall hospital cost-to-charge ratio of 47%.

RESULTS: A total of 212 patients were included in the study (105 on Ultraceph and 107 on Megaceph). Effectiveness for these two groups of patients was similar. Total costs, on average per patient, for Ultraceph were $332 more than Megaceph when using cost estimates based on charges and $156 more when using cost-to-charge estimates.

CONCLUSION: Although the efficacy and product cost of the two antibiotics have been shown to be similar, differences in the costs of intravenous administration (once a day compared with three times a day) and additional monitoring for different adverse events increased the overall total cost of Ultraceph to the hospital.

1. Was the title appropriate? Why or why not?

_____

_____

_____

_____

2. Were you able to determine the perspective? If so, what was it?

_____

_____

_____

_____

3. Was either adjustment or discounting appropriate? If so, was it conducted?

_____

_____

_____

_____

4. Was a sensitivity analysis conducted? If so, on what estimate(s)?

_____

_____

_____

_____

5. Were limitations addressed? If so, what were they?

_____

_____

_____

_____

REFERENCES

1. Sanchez LA. Applied pharmacoeconomics: Evaluation and use of pharmacoeconomic data from the literature. *American Journal of Health System Pharmacy* 56(16):1630–1638, 1999.
2. Abarca J. Assessing pharmacoeconomic studies. In Bootman JL, Townsend RJ, McGhan WF (eds). *Principles of Pharmacoeconomics* (3rd ed.). Cincinnati, OH: Harvey Whitney Books Co., 2005.

3. Drummond MF, Sculpher MJ, Torrance GW, et al. *Methods for the Economic Evaluation of Health Care Programmes* (3rd ed.). Oxford: Oxford University Press, 2005.
4. Jefferson T, Demicheli V, Vale L. Quality of systematic reviews of economic evaluations in health care. *Journal of the American Medical Association* 287(21):2908–2812, 2002.
5. Colmenero F, Sullivan S, Palmer J, et al. Quality of clinical and economic evidence in dossier formulary submissions. *The American Journal of Managed Care*, 13(7):401–407, 2007.
6. Rennie D, Luft HS. Pharmacoeconomic analyses: Making them transparent, making them credible. *Journal of the American Medical Association* 283(16):2158–2160, 2000.
7. Berger ML, Bingefors K, Hedblom EC, et al. *Health Care Cost, Quality, and Outcomes: ISPOR Book of Terms*. International Society for Pharmacoeconomics and Outcomes Research, 2003.

SUGGESTED READINGS

Drummond M, Brown R, Fendrick AM, et al. Use of pharmacoeconomics information: Report of the ISPOR Task Force on Use of Pharmacoeconomic/Health Economic Information in Health Care Decision Making. *Value in Health* 6(4):407–416, 2003.

Drummond M, Sculpher M. Common methodological flaws in economic evaluations. *Medical Care* 43(7 suppl):II-5–II-14, 2005.

Evers S, Goossens M, de Vet H, van Tulder M. Criteria list for assessment of methodological quality of economic evaluations: Consensus on health economic criteria. *International Journal of Technology Assessment in Health Care* 21(2):240–245, 2005.

McGhan W, Al M, Doshi J, Kamae I, Marx S, Rindress D. The ISPOR Good Practices for Quality Improvement of Cost-Effectiveness Research Task Force Report. *Value In Health: The Journal of The International Society for Pharmacoeconomics and Outcomes Research*, 12(8):1086–1099, 2009.

Ofman JJ, Sullivan SD, Neumann PJ, et al. Examining the value and quality of health economic analyses: Implications of utilizing the QHES. *Journal of Managed Care Pharmacy* 9(1):53–61, 2003.

Schumock GT, Butler MG, et al. Evidence of the economic benefit of clinical pharmacy services: 1996–2000. *Pharmacotherapy* 23(1):113–132, 2003.

Husereau D, Drummond M, Loder E, et al. Consolidated Health Economic Evaluation Reporting Standards (CHEERS)—explanation and elaboration: A report of the ISPOR Health Economic Evaluation Publication Guidelines Good Reporting Practices Task Force. *Value In Health: The Journal of The International Society for Pharmacoeconomics and Outcomes Research*, 16(2):231–250, 2013.

Chapter 4

Cost-Minimization Analysis

Objectives

Upon completing this chapter, the reader will be able to:

1. Define and describe cost-minimization analysis (CMA).

2. Address advantages and disadvantages of CMA.

3. Critique a CMA composite article.

✦ OVERVIEW

As mentioned in Chapter 1, **cost-minimization analysis** (CMA) measures and compares input costs, and assumes outcomes to be equivalent. Thus, the types of interventions that can be evaluated with this method are limited. The strength of each CMA lies in the acceptability by the readers or evaluators that outcomes are indeed equivalent. As mentioned in Chapter 1, a common example of a CMA is the comparison of generic equivalents of the same drug entity. For a generic medication to be approved for market, the manufacturer must demonstrate to the Food and Drug Administration (FDA) that its product is bioequivalent to the initially branded medication. Therefore, when comparing medications that are the same chemical entity and the same dose, and have the same pharmaceutical properties as each other (brand versus generic or generic made by one company compared with a generic made by another company), only the cost of the medication itself needs to be compared because outcomes should be the same.

Another example of a CMA analysis includes measuring the costs of receiving the same medication in different settings. For example, researchers could measure the costs of receiving intravenous antibiotics in a hospital and compare this with receiving the same antibiotics (at the same doses) at home via a home health care service. Example 4.1 provides a summary of an article that compared inpatient with outpatient care.

There is some debate about the use of the term CMA. Some contend that if outcomes are *not measured*, the study is considered to be a partial economic analysis that is termed a **cost analysis** and not a full pharmacoeconomic analysis. In addition, when both costs and clinical outcomes are *measured*, yet clinical outcomes are found to be *equivalent*, some categorize the study as a CMA because outcomes were equivalent,[1,2] but others categorize the study as a **cost-effectiveness study,** or

| EXAMPLE 4.1 | COST-MINIMIZATION ANALYSIS (CMA) THAT COMPARES OUTPATIENT AND INPATIENT COSTS |

The costs in the following table are based on a study, by Farmer et al., that estimated the costs associated with administering prostaglandin E2 gel intracervically to expectant mothers on the day before labor was to be induced (to help ripen the cervix). They compared the costs of (1) application of the gel, followed by a 2-hour monitoring period and then sending the expectant mother home for the night compared with (2) application of the gel followed by a 2-hour monitoring period and then sending the expectant mother to the maternity unit overnight. Both groups received oxytocin the next day at the hospital to augment or induce labor.

The perspective was that of the payer, so only direct medical costs were included. The authors used "usual and customary charges" from one hospital as a proxy for costs because they were readily obtainable. The authors collected and compared the costs associated with labor and delivery but specifically did not include the cost of infant care because newborn outcomes (e.g., Apgar scores) were the same between the two groups. Because the same drug was being administered in the same dose, the authors expected the outcomes for both groups to be the same. In addition, they measured maternal outcomes (e.g., percent of cesarean sections performed, amount of oxytocin needed) and found that there were no statistical differences between the groups. The authors said they conducted a CMA because outcomes were expected to be the same, but others (including me) might have labeled it a cost-effectiveness analysis because outcomes were measured but found to be the same.

Type of Costs	Costs for Outpatients Mean (n = 40) (SD)	Costs for Inpatients Mean (n = 36) (SD)	Statistical Difference
Labor costs	$575 (366)	$902 (482)	Yes; $p = 0.002$
Delivery costs	$471 (247)	$453 (236)	No; $p = 0.754$
Pharmacy costs	$150 (102)	$175 (139)	No; $p = 0.384$
Hospital costs	$3,835 (2,172)	$5,049 (2,060)	Yes; $p = 0.015$

Adapted with permission from Farmer KC, Schwartz WJ, Rayburn WF, Turnbull G. A cost-minimization analysis of intracervical PGE2 for cervical ripening in an outpatient versus inpatient setting. *Clinical Therapeutics* 18(4):747–756, 1996.

CEA, (see Chapter 5) because clinical outcomes were measured. (If outcomes were measured and found to be equivalent, I would tend to refer to the study as a CEA.)

Publications that use CMA are less common than other types of pharmacoeconomic studies. One theory for the small number of CMA publications is that there may be resistance to publish studies that only claim that a new intervention (e.g., medication) is no better than the existing option.[3] Also, many CMAs may be conducted in-house by institutions or health plans to determine the least costly option for their specific situation (e.g., based on makeup of their patient bases, policies on inpatient versus outpatient care, and discounts available on various medications) and were never intended for publication.

SUMMARY

Cost-minimization analysis is the simplest of the four types of pharmacoeconomics analyses because the focus is on measuring the left-hand side of the pharmacoeconomic equation (see Fig. 1.1)—costs—and the right hand side of the equation—outcomes—is assumed to be the same (or is found to be the same). But this method has limited use because it can only compare alternatives with the same outcomes.

COMPOSITE ARTICLE: CMA—ANTI-NAUSEA

Title: ECONOMIC ANALYSIS OF ONCOPLATIN ALONE (A CHEMOTHERAPY AGENT) COMPARED WITH ONCOPLATIN COMBINED WITH NONAUSEA (AN ANTINAUSEA AGENT)

BACKGROUND: A relatively new chemotherapy agent, Oncoplatin, is administered intravenously in physician offices and clinics. Originally, because of problems with chemotherapy-induced nausea, the recommended administration directions were to split the monthly dose needed for each cycle in half and administer each half 5 days apart. Follow-up studies found that if patients were given NoNausea, an antinausea medication, at the same visit, the full monthly dose of Oncoplatin could be given at one visit. Clinical effectiveness measures of the chemotherapy treatment were shown to be the same for the two methods of administration (previous clinical literature should be cited in a real article).

OBJECTIVE: The objective of the study was to perform a cost-minimization analysis (CMA) comparing the cost of Oncoplatin given in two doses with Oncoplatin combined with NoNausea administered in one dose. The perspective of the study is the third-party payer.

METHODS: Over a 6-month period (February 2007 to July 2007), patients from two oncology clinics were enrolled in this study and randomized to receive either the split dose of Oncoplatin (25 mg/m^2 on days 1 and 5) or the single dose of Oncoplatin (50 mg/m^2) plus the oral antinausea medication (35 mg of NoNausea). Adverse drug events (ADEs) of the treatment were recorded. The average wholesale prices (AWP) of Oncoplatin and NoNausea from the 2007 Red book were used to estimate prescription costs. Costs for intravenous infusions and physician or clinic visits were estimated using the 2007 *Physicians' Fee Reference.* Other costs

were assumed to be equivalent between the two groups. It was assumed that the physician or clinic visits to receive chemotherapy were in addition to regular visits. Only the first cycle of chemotherapy for each patient was included in the analysis because it was thought that follow-up cycles would produce similar results.

RESULTS: Demographic and clinical characteristics in Exhibit 4.1 indicate that patients in each group were similar and that there were no statistical differences in adverse effects reported. A summary of costs for the first cycle of chemotherapy is listed in Exhibit 4.2. Although the medication costs are higher in the group with NoNausea, this increase is offset by a decrease in administration and office visit costs. The savings for the once-per-cycle dose was approximately $88. Sensitivity analyses (Exhibit 4.3) were conducted by varying the medication costs (both chemotherapy and NoNausea costs), office visit costs, and administration costs by 25% above and below baseline estimates. Results were similar to the base analysis, and savings for the once-per-cycle option ranged from $68 to $108.

CONCLUSIONS: Direct medical costs associated with the once-per-cycle dose of Oncoplatin plus NoNausea were lower than when the monthly dose was split. Although only direct medical costs to the third-party payer were assessed, if cost savings to the patient (decreased travel costs) and to society (increased patient productivity is possible if less time is spent at the physician's office or clinic) were included, this would further increase the economic advantage of the once-per-cycle option.

EXHIBIT 4.1

Patient Comparisons

	Split Dosing of Oncoplatin (n = 293)	Full Dose of Oncoplatin Plus NoNausea (n = 295)
Gender (% women)	54.6	52.5
Mean age (SD)	58.3 (10.0)	59.2 (11.0)
Ethnicity (% white)	79.9	80.7
Adverse Events [N (%)]		
Nausea	13 (4.4)	12 (4.1)
Fever	14 (4.8)	13 (4.4)
Fatigue	10 (3.4)	8 (2.7)
Pain	6 (2.0)	7 (2.4)
Other	8 (2.7)	9 (3.0)

EXHIBIT 4.2

Costs for First Cycle of Treatment

	Split Dosing of Oncoplatin (n = 293)	Full Dose of Oncoplatin Plus NoNausea (n = 295)
Average cost of Oncoplatina	$2,964	$2,980
Average cost of NoNausea (35 mg)[a]	N/A	$40
Cost of IV administration[b]	$160	$80
Cost of physician or clinic visit[b]	$128	$64
Total cost per patient	$3,252	$3,164

[a]2007 AWP costs were 25 mg/m^2 for two doses versus 50 mg/m^2 in one dose.

[b]2007 Physician Fee Reference, 50th percentile.

EXHIBIT 4.3

Sensitivity Analyses

	Split Dosing of Oncoplatin: Total Cost	Full Dose of Oncoplatin Plus NoNausea: Total Cost
Baseline costs	$3,252	$3,164
Cost of medications increased by 25%	$3,993	$3,919
Cost of medications decreased by 25%	$2,511	$2,409
Cost of IV administration increased by 25%	$3,292	$3,184
Cost of IV administration decreased by 25%	$3,212	$3,144
Cost of physician or clinic visit increased by 25%	$3,284	$3,180
Cost of physician or clinic visit decreased by 25%	$3,220	$3,148

WORKSHEET FOR CRITIQUE OF CMA COMPOSITE ARTICLE

1. Complete Title?

    _____

    _____

    _____

    _____

2. Clear Objective?

    _____

    _____

    _____

    _____

3. Appropriate Alternatives?

    _____

    _____

    _____

    _____

4. Alternatives Described?

    _____

    _____

    _____

    _____

5. Perspective Stated?

    _____

    _____

    _____

    _____

6. Type of Study?

    _____

    _____

    _____

    _____

7. Relevant Costs?

_____

_____

_____

_____

8. Relevant Outcomes?

_____

_____

_____

_____

9. Adjustment or Discounting?

_____

_____

_____

_____

10. Reasonable Assumptions?

_____

_____

_____

_____

11. Sensitivity Analyses?

_____

_____

_____

_____

12. Limitations Addressed?

_____

_____

_____

_____

13. Generalizations Appropriate?

_____

_____

_____

_____

14. Unbiased Conclusions?

_____

_____

_____

_____

CRITIQUE OF CMA COMPOSITE ARTICLE

1. **Complete Title:** The title did identify the two therapeutic options that were being compared. The title did not indicate that the type of study was a CMA.

2. **Clear Objective:** The objective "was to perform a cost-minimization analysis comparing the cost of Oncoplatin given in two doses versus Oncoplatin combined with NoNausea administered in one dose." This was clear.

3. **Appropriate Alternatives:** The authors explained why the alternatives were important and referenced clinical literature to back up the similarity of outcomes.

4. **Alternatives Described:** The dosing and days of dosing were listed.

5. **Perspective Stated:** The perspective of the study was explicitly stated as the third-party payer, which would entail measuring direct medical costs only.

6. **Type of Study:** The study was correctly identified as a CMA because the outcomes were assumed to be the same based on past clinical research.

7. **Relevant Costs:** Based on the perspective, only direct medical costs to a third-party provider were assessed. Other costs, such as patient or family costs, direct nonmedical costs (e.g., other sector costs), and productivity (indirect) costs, were not measured. Although these were not measured, if they were included, they would have likely increased the amount of cost savings estimated for the once-per-cycle dose.

8. **Relevant Outcomes:** Because this study was a CMA, the effectiveness of the two methods of dosing was not directly measured, but was assumed to be the same based on previous clinical studies. However, because the avoidance of nausea was an important factor in this treatment, the prevalence of adverse events in both groups was evaluated and was found to be similar. The time period of one cycle may have been too short to determine overall differences for all cycles.

9. **Adjustment or Discounting:** All costs were valued in 2007 US dollars. Costs and outcomes were assessed for less than 1 year, so discounting was not needed.

10. **Reasonable Assumptions:** It was assumed that the office visit for each administration of chemotherapy was in addition to the usual physician visits. If, in fact, administration of some cycles were on the same day as a usual visit, the extra costs of the visit might be slightly lower. It was also assumed that patients would continue to have similar adverse events in future cycles of chemotherapy. Clinicians might not know if this was a reasonable assumption until patients received more cycles of chemotherapy.

11. **Sensitivity Analyses:** Sensitivity analyses were based on all third-party direct medical costs (medicine, administration, and visits), and the results were found to be robust. Practically, as long as the cost of the antinausea drug was less than a visit that included administration of chemotherapy, the once-per-cycle dosing would be cost saving.

12. **Limitations Addressed:** The authors did not directly address any limitations. Readers might ask, "If some patients are more susceptible to nausea, should they automatically be placed on once-per-cycle dosing?" Costs were measured for only one cycle of treatment. Did any patients ask to switch to twice-a-cycle dosing on subsequent administration because of adverse events?

13. **Generalizations Appropriate:** Although the authors did not directly address generalizations of the findings, costs were taken from standard US price lists, so generalization to general US third-party payers is reasonable. Because of the simplicity and transparency of the calculations, readers could substitute their costs and recalculate estimated cost savings.

14. **Unbiased Conclusions:** As with most CMAs, believability of the findings hinge on one important question: Does the reader accept that the clinical outcomes of the options are the same? If so, as long as the cost of the extra antinausea medication is lower than the cost of the extra administration or visit, the choice of once-a-cycle dosing is cost saving.

QUESTIONS/EXERCISES

Based on the following abstract, which is a condensed summary of a research article, please answer the following questions:

ABSTRACT

TITLE: Cost Analysis of Outpatient Treatment of Deep Vein Thrombosis

BACKGROUND: When patients have the complication of deep vein thrombosis (DVT) after surgery, the standard anticoagulation treatment includes heparin—either intravenous unfractionated heparin (UFH) or a subcutaneous low-molecular-weight heparin (LMWH) product—in combination with warfarin. After the patient's international normalized ratio (INR) is greater than 2.0, the patient discontinues the heparin product but continues on oral warfarin for 3 to 6 months. LMWH products have been approved for outpatient use.

OBJECTIVE: The objective of this study was to retrospectively measure the costs of treating patients with uncomplicated DVT discharged with either oral warfarin alone or a combination of oral warfarin and LMWH.

METHODS: Medical and prescription claims for Health Plan X were assessed. Costs to the health plan for hospitalized patients discharged in 2006 with a diagnosis of uncomplicated DVT were included in the analysis, and their claims history was followed for 1 year after initial hospital discharge date.

RESULTS: Compared with patients discharged on warfarin alone, the outpatient pharmacy costs were, on average, $750 higher for the patients discharged on the LMWH and warfarin combination, but the average hospital length of stay was 2 days less, resulting in a savings, on average of $2,300 in hospitalization costs. Therefore, mean total costs to the health plan per patient were $1,550 less for patients discharged on combination therapy. One-year follow-up showed no differences in readmission rates due to DVT for the two groups of patients, indicating similar effectiveness.

CONCLUSIONS: Outpatient anticoagulation therapy for uncomplicated DVT with a combination of LMWH and warfarin had higher outpatient pharmacy costs but lower hospitalization costs compared with warfarin alone, which resulted in overall savings to Health Plan X.

1. Was the title appropriate? Why or why not?

_____

_____

_____

_____

2. What was the objective of the study? Was this clear?

_____

_____

_____

_____

3. Were you able to determine the perspective? If so, what was it?

_____

_____

_____

_____

4. What type of pharmacoeconomic analysis was conducted? Why?

_____

_____

_____

_____

5. Was a sensitivity analysis conducted? If so, on what estimate(s)?

_____

_____

_____

_____

REFERENCES

1. Shireman T, Almehmi A, Wetmore J, Lu J, Pregenzer M, Quarles L. Economic analysis of cinacalcet in combination with low-dose vitamin D versus flexible-dose vitamin D in treating secondary hyperparathyroidism in hemodialysis patients. *American Journal of Kidney Diseases: The Official Journal of The National Kidney Foundation* 56(6):1108–1116, 2010.
2. Patel GW, Duquaine SM, McKinnon PS. Clinical outcomes and cost minimization with an alternative dosing regimen for meropenem in a community hospital. *Pharmacotherapy* 27(12):1637–1643, 2007.
3. Newby D, Hill S. Use of pharmacoeconomics in prescribing research. Part 2: Cost-minimization analysis—When are two therapies equal? *Journal of Clinical Pharmacy and Therapeutics* 28(2): 145–150, 2003.

SUGGESTED READINGS

Basskin L. Using cost-minimization analysis to select from equally effective alternatives. *Formulary* 33(12):1209–1214, 1998.
Briggs AH, O'Brien BJ. The death of cost-minimization analysis? *Health Economics* 10(2):179–184, 2001.

Chapter 5

Cost-Effectiveness Analysis

Objectives

Upon completing this chapter, the reader will be able to:

1. Define and describe cost-effectiveness analysis (CEA).

2. Address the advantages and disadvantages of CEA.

3. Discuss the different methods of presenting cost-effectiveness results.

4. Illustrate the use of a cost-effectiveness grid and a cost-effectiveness plane.

5. Compare intermediate- with final-outcome measurements.

6. Compare the terms "efficacy" and "effectiveness."

7. Critique a CEA composite article.

✦ OVERVIEW

Cost-effectiveness analysis (CEA) measures costs in dollars and outcomes in natural health units, which indicate an improvement in health such as cures, lives saved, or blood pressure reductions. This is the most common type of pharmaco-economic analysis found in the pharmacy literature. An advantage of using a CEA is that health units are common outcomes that are routinely measured in clinical trials, so they are familiar to practitioners. These outcomes do not need to be converted to monetary values. A disadvantage to CEA is that the alternatives used in the comparison must have outcomes that are measured in the same clinical units. You cannot use CEA to directly compare the outcomes of an antihypertensive product (which may measure mm Hg changes to determine the outcome) with the outcomes of an asthma product (which may measure forced expiratory volume [FEV] to determine the outcome). In addition, even if products for similar diseases or conditions are compared, more than one type of clinical outcome may be important. For example, when measuring the effects of hormone-replacement therapies, the effect on menopausal symptoms as well as bone mineral density measures may be salient. This may justify the calculation of multiple cost-effectiveness ratios for the comparison.

For many medications, both the effectiveness in treating the disease and the side effects of treatment may differ significantly between alternative treatments. For example, one chemotherapy regimen may be more effective in lengthening the time until the disease progresses than another chemotherapy regimen, but the more effective regimen may also cause more toxic side effects. With the CEA method, it is difficult to collapse different outcomes into one unit of measurement.

Some researchers consider **cost-utility analysis** (CUA) to be a special subset of CEA that uses units such as **quality-adjusted life years** (QALYs) to collapse different types of outcomes into one unit of measure. But there are also disadvantages to CUA, which are discussed in Chapter 6.

✦ PRESENTATION OF COSTS AND EFFECTIVENESS

Table 5.1 illustrates various ways that costs and effectiveness are presented in the literature. When patients have symptoms indicating a stomach ulcer, the health care provider may make a diagnosis based on the interview with the patient or based on the results of an endoscopy (during which a scope is used to look for evidence of ulcerations in the stomach lining).

Correspondingly, measuring the results or outcomes of medications used to treat stomach ulcers may be based on the patient's reports of symptom reductions or based on follow-up endoscopies. Data in the table correspond to the costs and outcomes of treating stomach ulcers using three therapy options (drugs A, B, or C) and using two outcome measures, **symptom-free days** (SFDs, or how many days,

TABLE 5.1. **EXAMPLES OF WAYS TO PRESENT COST AND EFFECTIVENESS RESULTS**			
	Drug A	Drug B	Drug C
Method 1: Cost-Consequence Analysis			
Cost	$600 per year	$210 per year	$530 per year
Outcomes			
GI SFDs	130	200	250
% Healed	50	70	80
Method 2: Average Cost-Effectiveness Ratios			
	$600 / 130 = $4.61 per SFD	$210 / 200 = $1.05 per SFD	$530 / 250 = $2.12 per SFD
	$600 / 0.5 = $1,200 per cure	$210 / 0.7 = $300 per cure	$530 / 0.8 = $662 per cure
Method 3: Incremental Cost-Effectiveness Ratios			
	B compared with A = Dominant for both GI SFDs and % healed		
	C compared with A = Dominant for both GI SFDs and % healed		
	C compared with B = ($530 − $210) / (250 − 200 GI SFDs) = $6.40 per extra GI SFD		
	C compared with B = ($530 − $210) / (0.8 − 0.7) = $3,200 per extra healed ulcer		

GI = gastrointestinal; SFD = symptom-free day.

on average, patients did not have gastrointestinal symptoms during the year) and percent healed (patients in whom endoscopy indicated that the ulcer was healed). As mentioned in Chapter 1, sometimes, for each alternative the costs and various outcomes are listed but no ratios are conducted; this is termed a **cost-consequence analysis** (CCA).

The second method of presenting results includes calculating the average **cost-effectiveness ratio** (CER) for each alternative. The CER is the ratio of resources used per unit of clinical benefit, and it implies that this calculation has been made in relation to "doing nothing" or no treatment. Table 5.1 shows these calculations as cost per SFD and cost per healed ulcer. In clinical practice, the question is infrequently, "Should we treat the patient or not?" or "What are the costs and outcomes of this intervention versus no intervention?" More often, the question is, "How does one treatment compare with another treatment in costs and outcomes?" To answer this more common question, an **incremental cost-effectiveness ratio** (ICER) is calculated. As mentioned in Chapter 2, the ICER is the ratio of the *difference* in costs divided by the *difference* in outcomes. If incremental calculations produce negative numbers, this indicates that one treatment, the **dominant** option, is both more effective and less expensive than the other, **dominated** option. The magnitude of the negative ratio is difficult to interpret, so it is suggested that authors instead indicate which treatment is the dominant one. When one of the alternatives is both more expensive and more effective than another, the ICER is used to determine the magnitude of the added cost for each unit in health improvement.

✦ COST-EFFECTIVENESS GRID

A **cost-effectiveness grid** can be used to illustrate the definition of "cost-effectiveness" (Fig. 5.1). To determine whether a therapy or service is cost-effective, both the costs and the effectiveness must be considered. Think of comparing a new drug with the current standard treatment. If the new treatment (1) is both more effective and less costly *(cell G)*, (2) is more effective at the same price *(cell H)*, or (3) has the same effectiveness at a lower price *(cell D)*, then it is considered cost-effective *(darkly shaded cells* in Fig. 5.1). On the other hand, if the new drug (1) is less effective and more costly *(cell C)*, (2) has the same effectiveness but costs more *(cell F)*, or (3) has lower effectiveness for the same costs *(cell B)*, then it is not cost-effective *(lightly shaded cells* in Fig. 5.1). There are three other possibilities *(cells with no shading* in Fig. 5.1); the new drug (1) is more expensive and more effective *(cell I)* (a very common finding), (2) is less expensive but less effective *(cell A)*, or (3) has the same price and the same effectiveness as the standard product *(cell E)*. For the middle *cell E*, other factors may be considered to determine which medication might be best. For the other two cells, ICER is calculated to determine the extra cost for each extra unit of outcome. It is left up to the readers to determine whether they think the new product is "cost-effective" on the basis of value judgment. The underlying subjectivity as to whether the added benefit is worth the added cost is a disadvantage of CEA.

From the previous example of ulcer treatment, when comparing drug B with drug A, and when comparing drug C with drug A, these comparisons would fall into *cell G* of the grid, indicating dominant cost-effectiveness for both drug B and drug C compared with drug A. On the other hand, when comparing drug C with

COST-EFFECTIVENESS	Lower Cost	Same Cost	Higher Cost
Lower effectiveness	A Conduct ICER	B Dominated	C Dominated
Same effectiveness	D Dominant	E Arbitrary	F Dominated
Higher effectiveness	G Dominant	H Dominant	I Conduct ICER

FIGURE 5.1. **Cost-effectiveness grid.** The cells represent possible results when comparing two alternatives with regard to costs and effectiveness. If one compares a new alternative with a standard alternative, the *lightly shaded cells* (B, C, or F) represent when the new alternative would not be considered cost-effective (i.e., would be dominated by the standard alternative), and the *darkly shaded cells* (D, G, or H) represent when the new alternative would be considered cost-effective (i.e., the dominant choice). If the comparison falls in the *nonshaded cells* A or I, more information is needed (e.g., how much extra cost per extra unit of outcome, which is determined by conducting an incremental cost-effectiveness ratio). If the comparison shows similar effectiveness and similar costs (*cell E*), other factors may be considered.

drug B, this comparison would fall into *cell I* of the grid, indicating that ICER should be calculated (Fig. 5.2). In this example, using drug C compared with using drug B would cost $6.10 more for every extra SFD, or $3,200 more for every extra healed ulcer (Table 5.1). Is drug C cost-effective compared with drug B? That depends if the evaluator believes the extra cost is worth the extra health benefit.

COST-EFFECTIVENESS	Lower Cost	Same Cost	Higher Cost
Lower effectiveness	A	B	C
Same effectiveness	D	E	F
Higher effectiveness	G Drug B - Drug A Drug C - Drug A	H	I Drug C - Drug B

FIGURE 5.2. **Cost-effectiveness grid for ulcer example.** In the ulcer example, when comparing drug B or drug C with drug A, drug B and drug C are both dominant over drug A (*cell G*) because they are more effective at a lower cost. On the other hand, when comparing drug C with drug B, drug C is more effective but at a higher cost, so an incremental cost-effectiveness ratio should be calculated.

✦ COST-EFFECTIVENESS PLANE

A graphical depiction of cost-effectiveness comparisons is also sometimes seen in the literature. Figure 5.3 is a **cost-effectiveness plane.** The point on the plane where the *x* and *y* axes cross indicates the starting point of costs and effectiveness for the standard comparator. A point is placed on the plane for each alternative to the standard comparator by indicating how much more or less it costs than the starting point (*y*-axis) and how much more or less effective it is than the starting point (*x*-axis). If an alternative is more expensive and more effective than the standard comparator, this point will fall in quadrant I, and the tradeoff of the increase in costs for the increase in benefits would need to be considered. If an alternative is less expensive and more effective, the point would fall in quadrant II, and the alternative would **dominate** the standard comparator. If the alternative was less costly and less effective, the point would fall in quadrant III, and again a tradeoff would have to be considered. (Do the cost savings of the alternative outweigh its decrease in effectiveness?) If an alternative was more expensive and less effective, the point would fall in quadrant IV, and the alternative would be dominated by the standard comparator.

Following up on the ulcer example, points in the cost-effectiveness plane would fall into quadrant II (dominant) for both drug B compared with drug A and drug C

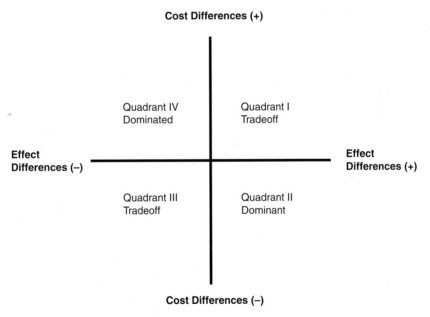

FIGURE 5.3. Cost-effectiveness plane. This cost-effectiveness plane is a visual method for representing the comparison of alternatives. For example, when comparing a new alternative with the standard alternative, if the new alternative is more effective but at a higher cost, this comparison will fall into quadrant I, which indicates that the decision maker must decide if the higher effectiveness is worth the higher cost. If the new alternative is less effective, but at a lower price (quadrant III), the decision maker must again make a decision: Is the lower price enough to outweigh the lower effectiveness? If the new alternative is more effective at a lower cost (quadrant II), then it "dominates" the standard and is considered cost-effective. If the new alternative is less effective at a higher cost (quadrant IV), it is "dominated" by the standard and is not considered cost-effective.

compared with drug A. If we change the comparator to drug B (now represented as [0,0] in the graph), because drug C is both more expensive and more effective than drug B, the cost-effectiveness point would appear in quadrant I (tradeoff).

A more complicated depiction of cost-effectiveness comparisons that is used when many treatment options are compared is called the "cost-effectiveness frontier." An explanation of this type of illustrative technique and its usefulness to decision makers can be found in the article by Bala and Zarkin.[1]

As mentioned previously, there are some limitations associated with the calculation and interpretation of CERs. It has been suggested that a newer technique, **incremental net benefit** (INB) analysis, may overcome some of these restrictions. Example 5.1 summarizes the advantages and disadvantages of the INB technique, and Example 5.2 illustrates how to use this method to calculate results using the composite article data.

✦ INTERMEDIATE OUTCOMES VERSUS PRIMARY OUTCOMES

Although it would be ideal to capture the complete effects on morbidity and mortality when comparing alternative therapies, it is not always practical to do so. Primary or final outcomes, such as the cure of a disease, the eradication of an infection, or life years saved are preferred units of measurement. When it is not feasible to collect primary outcomes because of time or monetary resources,

---

EXAMPLE 5.1   INCREMENTAL NET BENEFIT ANALYSIS

As mentioned previously, there are disadvantages to using cost-effectiveness analyses. A newer technique termed incremental net benefit (INB) analysis has been suggested to overcome some of these limitations. This method may also be seen in the literature under the terms "net benefit framework" or **net monetary benefit** (NMB). Results of cost-effectiveness (and cost-utility) analyses are usually presented as incremental cost-effectiveness ratios (ICERs), which are calculated by dividing the difference in costs by the difference in health benefits (outcomes). There are interpretation and statistical concerns when using these ratios. This example mainly discusses the interpretation concerns.

An ICER used alone for decision making can be ambiguous. Results occurring in different quadrants of the cost-effectiveness plane can have identical numerical ICERs, although the conclusions of the analysis would be opposite (see figure that follows). When the ICER is positive and in quadrant I (see *unshaded square*; the most common result in published articles), it indicates that the intervention of interest is both more effective and more expensive than the comparator. Yet it does not answer whether the intervention is more cost-effective, that is, is the added benefit worth the added cost? When the ICER is negative and in quadrant II (see *shaded square*), a large magnitude is desirable for both the numerator (large decrease in costs) and denominator (large increase in effects). However, these two desirable features drive the ICER in opposite directions, so a negative ICER does not lend itself to meaningful interpretation. These ratios do not have linear properties. A small change in the denominator (measuring change in health outcome) can make a large impact on the ratio, especially when the difference in outcomes nears zero.

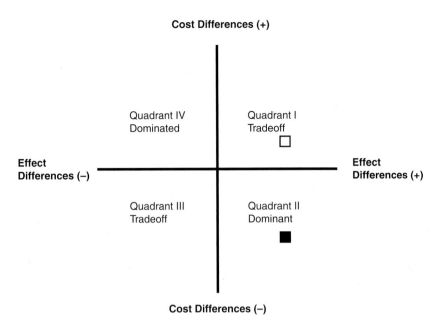

Cost-effectiveness plane example.

An alternative to using ICERs is the INB technique. Basically, an estimate of the value for health benefits (outcomes) is substituted into the incremental analysis. This estimated value, or maximum acceptable **willingness to pay,** is represented by lambda (λ), and a range around λ is used to conduct sensitivity analyses. The INB is calculated by multiplying λ by the additional units of health benefit from the intervention and then subtracting the additional cost of the intervention. See the equation below:

$$\text{INB} = (\lambda \times \Delta \text{ Effects}) - \Delta \text{ Costs}$$

If the INB is above zero, the intervention is deemed cost-effective. If it is below zero, it is not cost-effective. This is similar to the calculations provided in cost-benefit analyses (CBAs), except that instead of measuring the value of the precise intervention by the group of patients being studied, the λ is assumed to represent society's willingness to pay for a unit of health (e.g., a symptom-free day or quality-adjusted life-year) that is constant across disease categories and patient populations. Although this framework was created to reduce statistical restrictions of ICERs (e.g., the difficulty in assessing uncertainty estimates or confidence intervals for these ratios), it has other advantages as well. Results from INB calculations are less ambiguous than those of ICERs. A positive INB result is favorable for the intervention, and a negative INB result is not. Values of the INB become continuously more favorable in a linear manor as the INB results increase and less favorable as the number decreases. The major disadvantage to the INB framework (similar to CBA calculations) is that a monetary value must be placed on a health benefit (in this case, by using λ). Some researchers do not consider this a major drawback because it forces the explicit consideration of this value, and they recommend conducting sensitivity analyses for a range of λ values.

(continues)

EXAMPLE 5.1	INCREMENTAL NET BENEFIT ANALYSIS (*Continued*)

Suggested Readings

Hoch JS, Briggs AH, Willan AR. Something old, something new, something borrowed, something blue: A framework for the marriage of health econometrics and cost-effectiveness analysis. *Health Economics* 11(5):415–430, 2002.

Laska EM, Meisner M, Siegel C, Stinnett AA. Ratio-based and net benefit-based approaches to health care resource allocation: Proofs of optimality and equivalence. *Health Economics* 8(2):171–174, 1999.

Sculpher MJ, Price M. Measuring costs and consequences in economic evaluation in asthma. *Respiratory Medicine* 97(5):508–520, 2003.

Stinnett AA, Mullahy J. Net health benefits: A new framework for the analysis of uncertainty in cost-effectiveness analysis. *Medical Decision Making* 18(suppl):S68–S80, 1998.

Willan AR. Analysis, sample size, and power for estimating incremental net health benefit from clinical trial data. *Controlled Clinical Trials* 22(3):228–237, 2001.

Willan AR, Chen EB, Cook RJ, Lin DY. Incremental net benefit in randomized clinical trials with quality-adjusted survival. *Statistics in Medicine* 22(3):353–362, 2003.

Willan AR, Yin DY. Incremental net benefit in randomized clinical trials. *Statistics in Medicine* 20(11):1563–1574, 2001.

Zethraeus N, Johannesson M, Jonsson B, et al. Advantages of using the net-benefit approach for analyzing uncertainty in economic evaluation studies. *Pharmacoeconomics* 21(1): 39–48, 2003.

EXAMPLE 5.2	INCREMENTAL NET BENEFIT CALCULATIONS AND INTERPRETATION

In Exhibit 5.4, costs and outcomes for BreatheAgain were compared with inhaled corticosteroids. BreatheAgain had total costs of $537 and provided 90 symptom-free days (SFDs) compared with $320 and 45 SFDs for ICS. The incremental cost-effectiveness ratio (ICER) was $4.82 per extra SFD [($537 − $320 = $217) / (90 SFDs − 45 SFDs = 45 SFDs)]. Is BreatheAgain cost-effective? It depends on the value placed on a SFD. It has been suggested that a day without asthma symptoms is worth at least $5 (Rutten-van Molken et al.[1]) If we use the $5.00 as the baseline λ, the calculations are as follows:

$$\text{INB} = (\lambda \times \Delta \text{ SFDs}) - \Delta \text{ Costs}$$
$$\text{INB}_{\lambda=\$5} = (\$5 \times 45 \text{ SFDs}) - \$217$$
$$\text{INB}_{\lambda=\$5} = +\$8$$

Because the INB is greater than zero, BreatheAgain is more cost-effective than ICS when λ = $5.00. Some would point out that the $5.00 per SFD was estimated more than 10 years ago and that because of inflation, it would be higher. (As a side note, more recent research estimated the value of relieving depression at $10 per SFD [Katon et al.[2]].) The figure that follows shows that for a range of λ from $1 to $10, the range for the INB is −$172 to +$233, indicating that the results are sensitive to this range used to place a value on a SFD (λ). Although the advantage of this method may not be readily apparent from this graph (if the value of a SFD is above $4.82, BreatheAgain is cost-effective, which is the same conclusion as with the ICER), there are other advantages. If BreatheAgain had instead cost $217 less and provided 45 fewer SFDs than ICS, the ICER (−$217 /−45 SFD) would have been mathematically identical ($4.82 per SFD), but the INB would have been below zero (INB = [$5 × −45] − [−217] = −$8), indicating that BreatheAgain is not cost-effective compared with ICS.

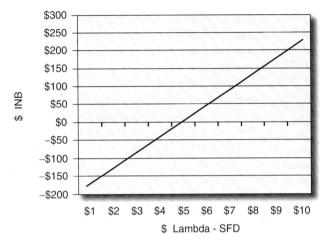

Calculation of incremental net benefit for range of lambda values for symptom-free days

References
1. Rutten-van Molken M, Van Doorslaer E, Jansen MC, Kerstjens HA, Rutten FF. Costs and effects of inhaled corticosteroids and bronchodilators in asthma and chronic pulmonary disease. *American Journal of Respiratory Critical Care Medicine* 151:975–982, 1995.
2. Katon W, Unutzer J, Fan M, et al. Cost-effectiveness and net benefit of enhanced treatment of depression for older adults with diabetes and depression. *Diabetes Care* 29(2):265–270, 2006.

intermediate or surrogate outcomes, such as laboratory measures or disease markers (e.g., cholesterol levels or blood pressure measurements) are used as proxies or surrogate endpoints. The limitation of using intermediate outcomes is reduced as the strength of the association between the intermediate and primary outcome measures increases.

✦ EFFICACY VERSUS EFFECTIVENESS

Many pharmacoeconomic studies use data from **randomized clinical trials**. These studies are sometimes referred to as cost-efficacy analyses. RCTs are the gold standard for determining if a medication is efficacious, and they are required by the Food and Drug Administration (FDA) before a medication can be approved for use in the United States. RCTs are used to establish **efficacy**—"if a drug can work"—under relatively ideal conditions. Pharmacoeconomic studies are more interested in the assessment of **effectiveness**—"if a drug does work"—in real-world practice. Although RCTs are essential to drug development, results from RCTs should be used with caution in pharmacoeconomic analyses. Both costs and outcomes may be different under RCT conditions compared with when used in the general population. In RCTs, specific groups of patients are recruited for the studies. Patient recruitment criteria may exclude patients outside of a specific age range and those with confounding comorbidities. Patients in RCTs are routinely monitored more closely than in general medical practice (which can increase monitoring costs), and they are likely to be more adherent to medications because they know they are being monitored (which can increase the cost of the drug and the magnitude of the outcomes). As mentioned in the Chapter 3, RCTs capture data for a short time period, even for chronic conditions. In addition, although a drug is approved by the FDA for a specific diagnosis that was used to recruit RCT participants, it is oftentimes used for other diagnoses and conditions (off-label use) after it becomes available to patients.

When RCT data are used to estimate costs and outcomes in the general patient population, the above limitations should be addressed. Researchers should be sure to exclude **protocol-driven costs,** such as frequent monitoring of patients or laboratory tests that are conducted more often than in usual practice. They should also conduct **sensitivity analyses** to account for possible differences between RCT results and results that may be seen in a broader array of patients. The differences between efficacy and effectiveness are referred to again in Chapter 11, which discusses the use of **retrospective databases**.

✦ CONSENSUS AND DEBATE

Although there is general agreement by researchers on many aspects of performing CEAs (e.g., **discounting** of costs and sensitivity analysis should be conducted when appropriate), there is no agreement on other aspects (e.g., what **discount rate** should be selected, what method should be used to value productivity). In 1995, an article by Luce and Simpson[2] addressed these areas of consensus and debate. For example, although there is agreement on the need for discounting when it comes to measuring costs or outcomes in dollar values, there is no universal agreement on whether or not to discount nonmonetary outcomes. One side contends that, as with monetary gains, people would rather receive health gains today instead of in the future, so future health gains should be discounted to their present value. Others point out that with some health outcomes (i.e., years of life), you cannot trade future gains (being alive in 10 years) with present gains (being alive today). In addition, if researchers decide to discount health gains, there is further debate about whether to discount health gains at the same rate as monetary costs. Because of this ongoing debate, many researchers provide results using a sensitivity analysis that uses various rates of discounting (including 0% to reflect no discounting).

Because of the use of various methods, and lack of agreement on some issues, it has been said, "If you've seen one CEA, you've seen one CEA."[2] Although some call for using a standard set of rules and procedures when conducting CEA studies, others are concerned that this may stifle new research on better methods in an evolving field. In 1993, the US Public Health Service (PHS) commissioned the Panel on Cost-Effectiveness in Health and Medicine. The panel was composed of a multidisciplinary group of experts and charged with developing a consensus on appropriate methods for conducting health-related to cost-effectiveness analyses. A book by Gold et al.[3] was published in 1996 as a result of this endeavor, and included a "reference case" example using suggested standard methods outlined by the panel. Chapters 13 and 14 further discuss the use of guidelines by researchers and decision makers.

SUMMARY

CEA is the most common type of pharmacoeconomic research seen in the literature. The advantage of using CEA is that outcomes are measured in clinical units, which are familiar and acceptable to clinicians. The disadvantages are that only one outcome at a time can be compared and that although an ICER can provide an estimate of the additional cost for the additional clinical benefit, readers must make a judgment call as to whether the additional cost is worth the additional benefit. Costs and outcomes can be presented independently without calculating ratios using CCA, by calculating the average cost per outcome using a CER or by calculating the incremental cost per incremental outcome using an ICER. To graphically illustrate the results of a CEA, a cost-effectiveness grid, cost-effectiveness plane, or cost-effectiveness frontier may be used. Although the measurement of final or primary outcomes is preferred, intermediate outcomes may be a more practical measure for some diseases or conditions. If data from **randomized controlled trials** (RCTs) are used, the term **cost-efficacy** analysis may be more appropriate because results may not be similar to those of everyday clinical practice. Although there is consensus on many of the methods used for CEA, there is still debate on others, leading to a lack of standard rules for CEA research.

COMPOSITE ARTICLE 1: CEA—ASTHMA

Note: The composite article compares treatments for asthma. Three reviews of published articles that look at the economics of asthma treatment are listed below:
Persson U, Ghatnekar O. Cost-effectiveness analysis of inhaled corticosteroids in asthma: A review of the analytical standards. Respiratory Medicine *97(1):1–11, 2003.*
Sculpher MJ, Price M. Measuring costs and consequences in economic evaluation in asthma. Respiratory Medicine *97(5): 508–520, 2003.*
Akazawa M, Stempel, D. Single-inhaler combination therapy for asthma: a review of cost-effectiveness. Pharmacoeconomics *24(10):971–988, 2006.*

Title: COST-EFFECTIVENESS ANALYSIS OF ADDING A SECOND AGENT TO INHALED CORTICOSTEROIDS FOR PATIENTS WITH ASTHMA

INTRODUCTION: Asthma is a chronic disorder characterized by bronchoconstriction and airway inflammation. Inhaled corticosteroids (ICSs) are used routinely in patients with asthma, but sometimes the use of ICS alone is not enough to effectively control asthma symptoms. Two new medications have become available that can be used in addition to ICSs, BreatheAgain and AsthmaBeGone [clinical references on the efficacy of these medications would be included here if these were real medications]. The objective of this study was to compare the costs and efficacy of two new adjunctive therapies, BreatheAgain and AsthmaBeGone, with ICS use alone.

METHODS: Adult asthma patients (age > 18 years) were enrolled and randomized into three groups: ICS + placebo, ICS + BreatheAgain, and ICS + AsthmaBeGone for 6 months. Both of the new medications were administered by inhalation once in the morning and once in the evening. ICS use was allowed as needed throughout the day. Per protocol, patients returned to the clinic once per month for 6 months. At these visits, FEV_1 (forced expiratory volume in 1 second) was measured 2 to 4 hours after the morning doses of asthma medication. Patients kept diaries and recorded their use of all asthma medications, any asthma-related emergency room visits, hospitalizations or nonprotocol office or clinic visits, evening peak expiratory flow (PEF) measurements, and asthma-related symptoms (e.g., wheezing, shortness of breath, chest tightening, or night-time awakening caused by their asthma).

Costs were estimated based on all asthma-related nonprotocol-driven direct medical resources used. This included the study medications and any nonprotocol medical visits (office, clinic, emergency department, or hospitalization) related to asthma. Usual charges (in 2013 US dollars) by the study clinic were used to estimate the costs of each of these visits.

Two clinical outcomes were assessed: an improvement at 6 months in FEV_1 of at least 12% from baseline and the number of SFDs during the 6-month study, defined as any day in which the patient recorded in a diary that he or she had none of the following symptoms: chest tightness, wheezing, shortness of breath, or nighttime awakening.

RESULTS: Exhibit 5.1 shows the baseline comparisons of the three groups of patients. Exhibit 5.2 lists the costs and outcomes for each group. Only one person was hospitalized because of asthma exacerbations during the 6-month trial. Most of the costs of treatment were medication costs. Exhibit 5.3 shows the average costs per clinical outcome, and Exhibit 5.4 shows the ICERs for the three comparisons. Based on the analysis, although the ICS + placebo group was the least costly, it was also the least effective. The ICS + AsthmaBe-Gone group was comparable to the ICS + BreatheAgain in effectiveness but was less costly.

CONCLUSIONS: Adding either of these new adjunctive treatments to ICS was associated with clinical improvement as shown by both the improvement in FEV_1 measures and the increase in SFDs recorded by this population of asthma patients at a relatively low increase in cost (<$5 per additional SFD; <$900 per additional successful treatment). AsthmaBeGone had similar effectiveness to BreatheAgain but at a lower cost.

EXHIBIT 5.1

Baseline Comparisons

Baseline Variable	ICS + Placebo (n = 220)	ICS + BreatheAgain (n = 210)	ICS + AsthmaBeGone (n = 213)
Age (range), years	40 (18–69)	39 (18–64)	38 (18–66)
Gender (% female)	50	49	51
Race (% white)	81	80	78
Baseline predicted FEV_1 (%)	66	68	67
Average use of ICS inhalers 6 months before enrollment (canisters/month)	1.5	1.6	1.4

EXHIBIT 5.2

Efficacy and Cost Comparisons

Outcome	ICS + Placebo (n = 220)	ICS + BreatheAgain (n = 210)	ICS + AsthmaBeGone (n = 213)
Clinical Outcomes			
Number (%) with FEV$_1$ increase ≥12%	77 (35%)	126 (60%)	130 (61%)
Number (%) of SFDs in 6 months per patient [N (%)]	9,900	18,900	19,170
	45 (25%)	90 (50%)	90 (50%)
6-Month Costs			
Medication costs	$64,900 ($295 per patient)	$112,140 ($534 per patient)	$80,514 ($378 per patient)
Unscheduled office visits	23 visits = $1,380 ($6 per patient)	7 visits = $420 ($2 per patient)	6 visits = $360 ($2 per patient)
Emergency room visits	Four visits = $1,100 ($5 per patient)	One visit = $275 ($1 per patient)	One visit = $275 ($1 per patient)
Hospitalizations	1 = $3,080 ($14 per patient)	0	0
Total costs	$70,460 ($320 per patient)	$112,835 ($537 per patient)	$81,149 ($381 per patient)

ICS = inhaled corticosteroid; FEV$_1$ = forced expiratory volume in 1 second; SFD = symptom-free day; pt = patient.

EXHIBIT 5.3

Average Cost-Effectiveness Ratios

Medication(s)	Success[a] (%)	SFDs per Patient	Cost per Patient ($)	Average Cost per Success ($)	Average Cost per SFD ($)
ICS + Placebo (I)	35	45	320	914	7.11
ICS + BreatheAgain (B)	60	90	537	895	5.97
ICS + AsthmaBeGone (A)	61	90	381	625	4.23

[a]Success is ≥12% improvement in FEV$_1$.

ICS = inhaled corticosteroid; FEV$_1$ = forced expiratory volume in 1 second; SFD = symptom-free day.

EXHIBIT 5.4

Cost-Effectiveness Ratios

Comparison	ICER—Success[a]	ICER—SFDs
BreatheAgain versus ICS (B–I)	($537 – $320) / (0.60 – 0.35) = $868 per extra success	($537 – $320) / (90 d – 45 d) = $4.82 per extra SFD
AsthmaBeGone versus ICS (A–I)	($381 – $320) / (0.61 – 0.35) = $235 per extra success	($381 – $320) / (90 d – 45 d) = $1.35 per extra SFD
AsthmaBeGone versus BreatheAgain (A–B)	A dominates B	A dominates B

[a]Success is ≥12% improvement in FEV1.

ICS = inhaled corticosteroid; FEV$_1$ = forced expiratory volume in 1 second; SFD = symptom-free day.

WORKSHEET FOR CRITIQUE OF CEA COMPOSITE ARTICLE 1

1. Complete Title?

    _____

    _____

    _____

    _____

2. Clear Objective?

    _____

    _____

    _____

    _____

3. Appropriate Alternatives?

    _____

    _____

    _____

    _____

4. Alternatives Described?

    _____

    _____

    _____

    _____

5. Perspective Stated?

    _____

    _____

    _____

    _____

6. Type of Study?

    _____

    _____

    _____

    _____

7. Relevant Costs?

_____

_____

_____

_____

8. Relevant Outcomes?

_____

_____

_____

_____

9. Adjustment or Discounting?

_____

_____

_____

_____

10. Reasonable Assumptions?

_____

_____

_____

_____

11. Sensitivity Analyses?

_____

_____

_____

12. Limitations Addressed?

_____

_____

_____

_____

13. Generalizations Appropriate?

_____

_____

_____

_____

14. Unbiased Conclusions?

_____

_____

_____

_____

Cost-Effectiveness Grid

Which cells represent the following comparisons?

a) BreatheAgain + ICS compared with ICS + Placebo
b) AsthmaBeGone + ICS compared with ICS + Placebo
c) AsthmaBeGone + ICS compared with BreatheAgain + ICS

COST-EFFECTIVENESS	Lower Cost	Same Cost	Higher Cost
Lower effectiveness	A	B	C
Same effectiveness	D	E	F
Higher effectiveness	G	H	I

CRITIQUE OF CEA COMPOSITE ARTICLE 1

1. **Complete Title:** The title did identify the type of study (CEA) but not the study drugs.

2. **Clear Objective:** The objective of this study was "to compare the costs and efficacy of two new adjunctive therapies, BreatheAgain and AsthmaBeGone to ICS use alone." This was clear.

3. **Appropriate Alternatives:** There were three alternatives: ICS + placebo, ICS + BreatheAgain, and ICS + AsthmaBeGone. Based on the clinical literature cited, the readers would determine if these were appropriate clinical alternatives.

4. **Alternatives Described:** The scheduling of the new products and placebo (one puff twice a day) was mentioned, but the dose of the new inhalers was not included—there may be more than one dose available. Also, the use of ICSs was vague. Which ICS was used, what dosage was used? Persson and Ghatnekar caution that dosing can be important in determining the economic effects of asthma medications. They maintain that if the researcher doubles the recommended dose of an asthma medication, costs of the medication double, while clinical effectiveness may not increase much.

5. **Perspective Stated:** The perspective of the study was not explicitly stated. Because the researchers only report measuring direct medical costs, we assume the perspective is that of the payer. Because patients were already keeping a diary, the researchers could have had them keep a record of productivity lost because of asthma exacerbations and treatment (e.g., time to go to an unscheduled medical visit).

6. **Type of Study:** The study was correctly identified as a CEA because outcomes were valued in clinical units (patients with $\geq 12\%$ improvement in FEV_1 and SFDs). A more precise term for this study might be a *cost-efficacy analysis* because data from a clinical trial were used. Although the researchers were careful not to include protocol-driven costs into the calculations, patient behavior (e.g., medication adherence) and subsequently outcomes may differ when patients are not being monitored monthly (as per protocol).

7. **Relevant Costs:** If the perspective was of the payer of medical costs, then the relevant costs were measured, that is, nonprotocol-driven asthma-related direct medical costs. Sometimes whether costs are fully related to the disease state is questioned. For example, if a patient gets a cold or the flu and this exacerbates the person's asthma, should all costs of treatment for this episode be included as asthma-related costs? "Charges" to the clinic were used as a proxy for "costs" to the average payer. The actual reimbursement for these services is usually lower than the charges, so these cost estimates may be inflated.

8. **Relevant Outcomes:** Outcomes of the treatment were measured in two ways: improvement in FEV_1 of at least 12% and number of SFDs. Is a 12% change the relevant cutoff for successful versus unsuccessful treatment? The authors need to explain why this cutoff was used. There are various definitions of SFDs; the authors listed the four symptoms that needed to be absent (wheezing, shortness of breath, chest tightness, and nighttime awakening because of asthma) for a patient to have an SFD. Although PEF was measured by patients, it was not used in the analysis. No side effects of treatment were measured, and any dropouts or discontinuations by patients were not addressed. Although asthma is a chronic disease, changes in health outcomes can be seen shortly after changing treatment plans. If practical, it would have been better to capture a full year's worth of data because the severity of asthma differs by season.

9. **Adjustment or Discounting:** All costs were valued in 2013 US dollars. Data were collected for 6 months, so discounting was not needed.

10. **Reasonable Assumptions:** There were some implicit assumptions made. One was the assumption that a 12% improvement in FEV_1 is the correct cutoff for defining success of treatment, and another is that the charges from one clinic were representative of the costs of treatment.

11. **Sensitivity Analyses:** Sensitivity analyses were not conducted. A range of FEV_1 cutoffs could have been used to test if findings were robust to this assumption. Also, cost estimates generated from standard price lists could have been substituted for clinic charges as another sensitivity analysis.

12. **Limitations Addressed:** The authors did not directly address any limitations, although some have already been discussed in this critique (e.g., use of cutoff, charges versus costs).

13. **Generalizations Appropriate:** Because data on both costs and outcomes were collected from only one clinic under study protocol rules, caution should be used when extrapolating to other populations who are treated in other settings and who are not bound by study restrictions.

14. **Unbiased Conclusions:** The authors summarize that adjunctive treatment to ICS use improves outcomes but also increases costs (see cost-effectiveness grid below). Although the differences in outcomes between the two new treatments are minimal, the differences between the combination treatments versus ICS alone are striking. The authors indicate that the increase in costs is worth the increase in outcomes (and therefore is cost-effective). The problem with any CEA is that when one option is better but more costly, it is a judgment call as to whether the added benefit is worth the added cost.

Cost-Effectiveness Grid

COST-EFFECTIVENESS	Lower Cost	Same Cost	Higher Cost
Lower effectiveness	A	B	C
Same effectiveness	D Drug A - Drug B	E	F
Higher effectiveness	G	H	I Drug B - Drug I Drug A - Drug I

Drug I = ICS + Placebo
Drug B = BreatheAgain + ICS
Drug A = AsthmaBeGone + ICS

Both active drugs (AsthmaBeGone and BreatheAgain) in combination with ICS are more effective that ICS + placebo but also more expensive (*cell I*), indicating the need to calculate an ICER. AsthmaBeGone and BreatheAgain have the same effectiveness, but AsthmaBeGone is less expensive (*cell D*), so it would be a cost-effective alternative compared with BreatheAgain.

COMPOSITE ARTICLE 2: CEA—POST–MYOCARDIAL INFARCTION HEART FAILURE

Note: Grace Mbagwu, a PharmD student, helped develop this composite article.
Three articles comparing the cost-effectiveness of adding an aldosterone antagonist to standard therapy in the treatment of post-myocardial infarction (MI) heart failure are referenced below:
McKenna C, Walker S, Lorgelly P, et al. Cost-effectiveness of aldosterone antagonists for the treatment of post-myocardial infarction heart failure. Value Health 15(3):420–428, 2012.
Szucs TD, Holm MV, Schwenkglenks M, et al. Cost-effectiveness of eplerenone in patients with left ventricular dysfunction after myocardial infarction—An analysis of the EPHESUS study from a Swiss perspective. Cardiovasc Drugs Ther 20(3):193–204, 2006.
Weintraub WS, Zhang Z, Mahoney EM, et al. Cost-effectiveness of eplerenone compared with placebo in patients with myocardial infarction complicated by left ventricular dysfunction and heart failure. Circulation 111(9):1106–1113, 2005.

Title: COST-EFFECTIVENESS ANALYSIS OF ADDING AN ALDOSTERONE ANTAGONIST TO STANDARD THERAPY IN HEART FAILURE PATIENTS POST-MYOCARDIAL INFARCTION

INTRODUCTION: Heart failure is a chronic disease characterized by physical symptoms such as fatigue and shortness of breath on exertion; its incidence increases with age. Heart failure has a projected annual treatment cost of $26 billion. The most common precipitating event in the development of heart failure is ischemic heart disease, which often presents acutely as a MI or "heart attack." The underlying pathophysiology involves the activation of neurohormones, including aldosterone, which increase the strain on the heart causing it to work harder, enlarge and become less efficient in pumping blood. Evidence-based practice guidelines have identified ACE inhibitors (ACEI) and beta-blockers (β-blockers) as integral components of the heart failure medication regimen; more recent clinical trials have indicated that aldosterone antagonists reduce mortality in post-MI heart failure patients. An aldosterone antagonist, Notyrd (not a real medication name), became available in 2010 for the treatment of post-MI heart failure. This study aimed to compare the cost-effectiveness of Notyrd, in addition to standard therapy (i.e., an ACEI and a β-blocker), versus standard therapy alone from the perspective of a large health insurance company, HealthMed.

METHODS: A total of 400 patients with left ventricular systolic dysfunction and symptoms of heart failure post-MI were identified retrospectively from a HealthMed database. Half (200 patients) were identified as having received standard therapy after the index event of the heart attack, or MI; while the other half (200 patients) were identified as having received standard therapy plus Notyrd. Data were collected and analyzed for 36 months following the index event.

Costs were estimated from HealthMed reimbursement rates. Costs included were: cardiovascular-related medical utilization (rehospitalizations, emergency room visits, labs, and clinic services) in addition to heart failure medications (ACEIs, β-blockers, and Notyrd). Indirect and intangible costs were not included in the analysis based on the perspective. Resource utilization was calculated on an intent-to-treat basis and **adjusted** to 2013 costs. Outcomes measured were cardiovascular-related rehospitalization and cardiovascular-related mortality.

Using the following costs: cardiovascular-related rehospitalization, clinic services, emergency room visits, labs, medication acquisition, and the outcome of CV-related mortality, an ICER was calculated. An ICER was also calculated using the above mentioned costs, and the outcome of cardiovascular-related rehospitalization.

A sensitivity analysis was conducted, to test the robustness of our results, by varying rehospitalization costs and the cost of Notyrd by ±20% (Note: costs of standard therapy were similar in both arms so sensitivity analysis on this input cost was not conducted).

RESULTS: Baseline characteristics are summarized in Exhibit 5.5. The combined costs of cardiovascular-related rehospitalizations, clinic services, labs, and emergency room visits were less in the active treatment arm compared with the standard therapy cohort while cardiovascular medication costs were greater in the active treatment arm as expected (Exhibit 5.6). Average survival rates for 36 months were 79%

(158 / 200) and 70% (140 / 200) for Notyrd and standard therapy respectively (Exhibit 5.7). The ICER for Notyrd plus standard therapy, compared with standard therapy alone, per cardiovascular-related death prevented was −$6,053 (Exhibit 5.8). The ICER for Notyrd plus standard therapy, compared with standard therapy alone, per cardiovascular-related rehospitalization prevented was −$14,527 (Exhibit 5.8). The Notyrd intervention was more effective compared with standard therapy alone in decreasing rehospitalizations and all-cause mortality and was also less costly. Sensitivity analysis confirms that Notyrd is dominant compared with standard therapy (Exhibit 5.9).

CONCLUSIONS: Adding Notyrd to standard therapy with ACEI and β-blockers post-MI has been shown to decrease mortality as well as the combined costs of rehospitalization and clinic visits. Notyrd was shown to have greater effectiveness at a decreased total cost. This new aldosterone antagonist should be included as part of the current combination of therapies indicated in post-MI heart failure patients.

EXHIBIT 5.5

Baseline Patient Characteristics

Comparison of Treatment Arms	Notyrd + Standard Therapy (n = 200)	Standard Therapy (n = 200)	p-value
Baseline Characteristics			
Age (mean years)(SD)	64.2 (14.0)	64.7 (14.5)	0.75
Women	55.0%	56.0%	0.84
Diabetes	31.4%	35.0%	0.46
Hypertension	59.3%	60.0%	0.92
History of stroke	32.0%	32.0%	0.66

EXHIBIT 5.6

Costs Over 3 Years Adjusted to 2013

Utilization and Costs Over 36 Months	Notyrd + Standard Therapy (n = 200)		Standard Therapy (n = 200)		Difference	
Resources Used						
CV emergency room visits[a]	N = 400	$1,200,000	N = 600	$1,800,000	N = +200	+$600,000
CV hospitalizations[b]	N = 150	$1,500,000	N = 170	$1,700,000	N = +20	+$200,000
CV clinic visits[c]	N = 1,524	$381,000	N = 1,380	$345,000	N = −144	$−36,000
CV labs[d]	N = 410	$32,800	N = 580	$46,400	N = +170	+$ 13,600
Total non-RX costs		$3,113,800		$3,891,400		+$ 777,600
Medications[e]	Patient days of Rxs = 148,336	$890,016	Patient days of Rxs = 134,320	$402,960		−$487,056
Total cost		$4,003,816		$4,294,360		+$290,544

[a]2013 CV-related Emergency Room cost (per visit) = $3,000
[b]2013 CV-related Hospitalization cost (per DRG) = $10,000
[c]2013 CV-related Clinic cost (per visit) = $250
[d]2013 CV-related Lab cost (per lab) = $80
[e]2013 CV-related medications: Standard therapy cost (per patient per day) = $3.00; Notyrd plus standard therapy cost (per patient per day) = $3.00 + $3.00; 80% adherence assumed for each year if patients are alive (see following Exhibit).

EXHIBIT 5.7

Mortality—Number of Patients Alive at End of Each Year

	Year 1 End	Year 2 End	Year 3 End	Life Years
Notyrd + standard therapy (N = 200)	180	170	158	508
Standard therapy (N = 200)	170	150	140	460
		Life years saved		48

EXHIBIT 5.8

Incremental Cost-Effectiveness Ratios

Total Cost Difference (Notyrd/ST − ST)	$ 290,544
Life years saved	48
Rehospitalizations avoided	20
ICER (per cardiovascular-related death prevented)	−$6,053 (dominant)
ICER (per cardiovascular-related rehospitalization prevented)	−$1,452 (dominant)

ST = standard therapy.

EXHIBIT 5.9

Sensitivity Analyses

Variable	Range L = Low Estimate H = High Estimate	Notyrd + ST (Overall Costs)	ST Alone (Overall Costs)	Δ Costs
Base case		$4,003,816	$4,294,360	$290,544
Cost of Notyrd per day (Base: $3.00)	L = $2.40 H = $3.60	L = $3,914,814 H = $4,092,818	L = $4,294,360 H = $4,294,360	L = −$379,546 H = −$201,542
Cost of Hospitalization (Base: $10,000)	L = $8,000 H = $12,000	L = $3,703,816 H = $4,303,816	L = $3,954,360 H = $4,634,360	L = −$250,544 H = −$330,544

WORKSHEET FOR CRITIQUE OF CEA COMPOSITE ARTICLE 2

1. Complete Title?

2. Clear Objective?

3. Appropriate Alternatives?

4. Alternatives Described?

5. Perspective Stated?

_____

_____

_____

_____

6. Type of Study?

_____

_____

_____

_____

7. Relevant Costs?

_____

_____

_____

_____

8. Relevant Outcomes?

_____

_____

_____

_____

9. Adjustment or Discounting?

_____

_____

_____

_____

10. Reasonable Assumptions?

_____

_____

_____

_____

11. Sensitivity Analyses?

_____

_____

_____

_____

12. Limitations Addressed?

_____

_____

_____

_____

13. Generalizations Appropriate?

_____

_____

_____

_____

14. Unbiased Conclusions?

_____

_____

_____

_____

CRITIQUE OF CEA COMPOSITE ARTICLE 2

1. **Complete Title:** The title identified the type of study being conducted but not the study drugs being compared.

2. **Clear Objective:** The objective of the study was explicitly stated "this study aimed to compare the cost-effectiveness of Notyrd, in addition to standard therapy (i.e., an ACEI and β-blocker), versus standard therapy alone." However, the objective did not include the names of all medications involved in the study, the specific medication doses being compared, and the anticipated effect of these medications "i.e., this study aimed to compare the cost-effectiveness of Notyrd 20 mg, in addition to standard therapy with Tamipril (not a real drug) and Seolol (not a real drug), versus standard therapy alone in preventing cardiovascular-related hospitalization and cardiovascular-related death."

3. **Appropriate Alternatives:** The treatment alternative in this study (standard therapy alone) may not have been complete. Other aldosterone antagonists

have been approved for the treatment of post–heart failure MI; it may have been more appropriate to determine if this medication is superior to the existing standard of therapy with other aldosterone antagonists.

4. **Alternatives Described:** Alternatives were not described in sufficient detail. The names and doses of the medications included in standard therapy were not explicitly stated; the Notyrd dose was not stated. Differences in these variables, between the two groups being compared, could confound the study results and decrease the validity of the study results.

5. **Perspective Stated:** The perspective of the study was clearly stated " ... from the perspective of a large health insurance company, HealthMed."

6. **Type of Study:** This study was a true cost-effectiveness analysis; both costs and outcomes were measured. Costs were measured in dollars. The relevant outcomes were "clinical" in nature—cardiovascular-related rehospitalizations prevented and cardiovascular-related deaths prevented.

7. **Relevant Costs:** Costs included were medications, CV-related emergency room visits, CV-related hospitalizations, CV-related clinic visits, and CV-related labs. All of these costs are relevant from the perspective of a third-party payer, including health plans such as HealthMed. "Charges" to the health plan from clinics and hospitals were used as proxies for actual costs. This may have overestimated costs; reimbursement rates are typically lower than charges.

8. **Relevant Outcomes:** Outcomes included were cardiovascular-related rehospitalization and cardiovascular-related mortality. These outcomes are relevant to a health plan as hospitalization represents a significant proportion of costs to the health plan and mortality is a significant predictor of effective management of patients' health. "Patient reported symptoms of heart failure" would have also been an appropriate outcome measurement. Since heart failure is a disease characterized by signs and patient reported symptoms, many of which persist chronically in the outpatient setting, it would have been appropriate to measure the effect of Notyrd on physical symptoms of heart failure.

9. **Adjustment or Discounting:** Costs, estimated from HealthMed reimbursements rates, were adjusted to 2013 rates. This study was a retrospective analysis and cost savings were not projected to future years; discounting was therefore unnecessary.

10. **Reasonable Assumptions:** A major assumption of this study was that standard therapy would be equivalent in both study groups. Depending on the types and doses of ACEIs and β-blockers used, the observed treatment effect may have been due to differences in standard therapy, not the inclusion of Notyrd. Secondly, this study was conducted on an intent-to-treat basis and assumed that individuals who had at least one prescription for Notyrd recorded in the HealthMed prescription database remained on the medication for the duration of the study. This assumption may have under estimated both the positive and any potential negative effects of Notyrd on the investigated outcomes.

11. **Sensitivity Analyses:** A sensitivity analysis was conducted by varying medication (Notyrd) and hospitalization cost estimates by 20%.

12. **Limitations Addressed:** The authors did not directly address any limitations; some have been addressed in this critique (i.e., charges used as proxies for costs, intent-to-treat protocol etc.)

13. **Generalizations Appropriate:** This study was based on data from a single third-party payer, HealthMed. Therefore, the study results can only be generalized to a limited population; one that is demographically similar to the HealthMed patient population.

14. **Unbiased Conclusions:** The study results suggest that adding Notyrd to standard therapy with ACEI and β-blocker post-MI decreases mortality as well as the combined costs of rehospitalization and clinic visits. The authors conclude that Notyrd should be included as part of the current combination of therapies indicated in post-MI heart failure. This conclusion may be considered an over-generalization of study results seeing as this study did not aim to determine the place of Notyrd in the current post-MI heart failure treatment protocol. This study sought solely to determine the effectiveness of Notyrd in decreasing cardiovascular-related mortality and rehospitalization, when combined with standard therapy.

QUESTIONS/EXERCISES

There are three 3-month-long options to treat studentitis, a depression-like condition in which a student thinks he or she will be in college forever with no option for parole. Results (effectiveness) cannot be determined until students have been exposed to the treatments for a period of 3 months. Option I is the standard option, which consists of group counseling. Option II consists of a new studentitis medication that has no side effects. Option III consists of a combination of the new medication and group counseling.

The costs of the standard option, Option I (counseling), are $100 per month. This treatment alone is measured to be effective in 40% of the cases.

The costs of Option II (medication) are $50 per month for the medication. This treatment alone is measured to be effective in 60% of the cases.

The costs of Option III (counseling and medication) are the combined costs of Options I and II. The effectiveness of this combination treatment is measured to be 90%.

Each option includes 3 months of therapy for these 3 months:

1. Calculate a CER for:
   a. Option I
   b. Option II
   c. Option III

2. Calculate an ICER comparing Option I (the standard) with Option II.

3. Calculate an ICER comparing Option I (the standard) with Option III.

4. Place a "II" in the cell that represents comparing Option II with the standard (Option I).

Cost or Outcome	Lower Cost	Same Cost	Higher Cost
Less effective			
Same effectiveness			
More effective			

5. Place a "III" in the cell that represents comparing Option III with the standard (Option I).

Cost or Outcome	Lower Cost	Same Cost	Higher Cost
Less effective			
Same effectiveness			
More effective			

REFERENCES

1. Bala MV, Zarkin GA. Application of cost-effectiveness analysis to multiple products: A practical guide. *American Journal of Managed Care* 8(3):211–218, 2002.
2. Luce BR, Simpson K. Methods of cost-effectiveness analysis: Areas of consensus and debate. *Clinical Therapeutics* 17(1):109–125, 1995.
3. Gold MR, Seigel JE, Russell LB, Weinstein MD (eds). *Cost-Effectiveness in Health and Medicine.* Oxford: Oxford University Press, 1996.

SUGGESTED READINGS

Lopert R, Lang DL, Hill SR. Use of pharmacoeconomics in prescribing research. Part 3: Cost-effectiveness analysis—A technique for decision-making at the margin. *Journal of Clinical Pharmacy and Therapeutics* 28(3):243–249, 2003.

Willan AR, Briggs AH. *Statistical Analysis of Cost-Effectiveness Data.* Chichester, UK: John Wiley and Son, 2006.

Higgins A, Harris A. Health economic methods: cost-minimization, cost-effectiveness, cost-utility, and cost-benefit evaluations. *Critical Care Clinics* 28(1):11–24, 2012.

Chapter 6

Cost-Utility Analysis

Objectives

Upon completing this chapter, the reader will be able to:

1. Define and describe cost-utility analysis (CUA).

2. Address advantages and disadvantages of CUA.

3. List the steps involved in measuring and calculating utility-based outcomes.

4. Compare the different methods used in estimating utilities.

5. Compare the different types of populations used to elicit utility estimates.

6. Compute quality-adjusted life-year (QALY) calculations.

7. Critique a CUA composite article.

✦ OVERVIEW

As mentioned in Chapter 5 on cost-effectiveness analysis (CEA), some consider **cost-utility analysis** (CUA) a subset of CEA because the outcomes are assessed using a special type of clinical outcome measure, usually the **quality-adjusted life-year** (QALY). A CUA takes patient preferences, also referred to as **utilities,** into account when measuring health consequences.[1] While the term *utility* has a more precise meaning in the field of economics, it is used in a general way in other disciplines to indicate personal or group preferences. Some authors prefer to use other terms, such as *preference weight* or *preference value*, in place of the word *utility*. As mentioned above, the most common outcome unit used in CUA is the QALY, which incorporates both the quality (morbidity) and quantity (mortality) of life. Other outcome units that are seen less frequently include disability-adjusted life-years (DALYs) and healthy-year equivalents (HYEs), among others.[2-5]

The advantage of a CUA is that different types of health outcomes and diseases with multiple outcomes of interest can be compared (unlike in CEA) using one common unit such as the QALY. CUA incorporates morbidity and mortality into this one common unit without having to determine or estimate the monetary value of these health outcomes (unlike CBA). The disadvantage of this method is that it is difficult to determine an accurate utility or preference weight value. Therefore, although the number of CUA research articles in the literature is increasing yearly, the methods for estimating utilities/QALYs may not be fully understood or embraced yet by many US providers or decision makers.[6,7]

For some research questions, utility adjustments may not be warranted. For example, if two pharmaceutical products have different outcomes based on the number of life-years saved (LYS), but the quality of each year of life for those on the two treatments are thought to be the very similar (see Fig. 6.1A), quality adjustment may not be as crucial. However, in many cases—for example, cancer treatment—both the length of life and the quality of life are different, depending on the therapy selected. Sometimes the treatments that extend life the longest are also the most toxic, so a measure that incorporates both length of life and quality of life is needed in these cases (see Fig. 6.1B). Many health conditions do not have an impact on patients' length of life, but *only* on the quality of their life, and CUA may be a good choice for comparing treatments for these conditions (see Fig. 6.1C). Examples include conditions such as hearing loss, seasonal allergies, and erectile dysfunction. CUAs may also be useful when comparing treatments and outcomes that are very different (e.g., when comparing the treatment of heart disease with prenatal care) because outcomes for both treatments can be summarized into one common unit, such as QALYs.

By convention, perfect health is assigned a value of 1.0 utility (μ) per year, and death is assigned a value of 0.0. If a person's health is diminished by disease or treatment, 1 year of life in this state is valued somewhere between 0 and 1. Some researches point out that there are disease states worse than death, so negative utility weights may be needed to depict these values. This debate is beyond the scope of this book, and in the vast majority of studies, this is not an issue, and the values for each year are estimated to be between 0.0 and 1.0.

To estimate utility weights for various conditions or "health states" between perfect health and death, two broad methods are used to elicit, or generate, these scores: direct elicitation and indirect elicitation.[8] Direct elicitation methods (**rating scale**, **standard gamble**, and **time tradeoff**) are described in this chapter. Indirect elicitation methods, using standardized weightings (e.g., EQ-5D and SF-6D surveys), will be covered in Chapter 8.

✦ STEPS IN CALCULATING QALYS

To calculate QALYs, the following steps apply:

1. Develop a description of each disease state or condition of interest.
2. Choose a method for determining utilities.
3. Choose subjects who will determine utilities.
4. Sum the product of utility scores by the length of life for each option to obtain QALYs.

Each of these steps is explained below.

Step 1: Develop a Description of Each Disease State or Condition of Interest

The description should concisely depict the usual health effects expected from the disease state or condition. It should include the amount of pain or discomfort, any restrictions on activities, the time it may take for treatment, possible

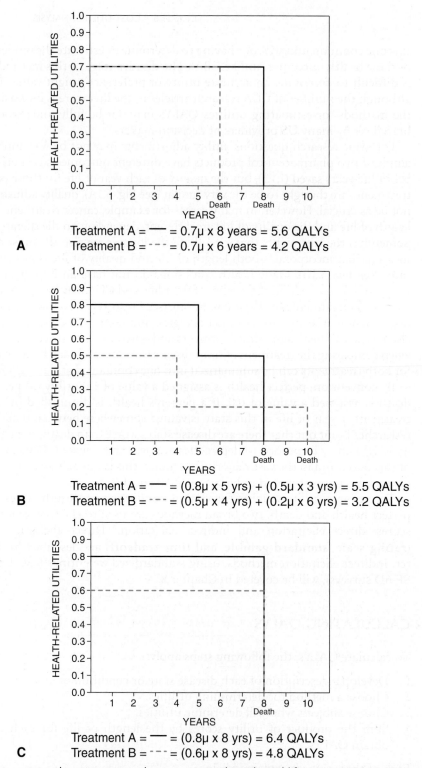

FIGURE 6.1. Examples estimating and comparing quality-adjusted life years (QALYs). **A:** Example illustrating when two treatment options produce different outcomes on the basis of the number of life years saved (LYS), but the quality of each year of life for those on the two treatments are thought to be the very similar (quality adjustment not needed). **B:** Example illustrating when both the length of life and the quality of life are different depending on the therapy selected (quality adjustment appropriate). **C:** Example illustrating options that do not have an impact on patients' length of life but only on the quality of their life (quality adjustment appropriate).

changes in health perceptions (worry or concern), and any mental changes. Examples describing hospital-based kidney dialysis and diabetic retinopathy are presented below:

Description of Hospital-Based Kidney Dialysis

You often feel tired and sluggish. A piece of tubing has been inserted into your arm or leg, which may restrict your movement. There is no severe pain but rather chronic discomfort. You must go to the hospital twice a week for 6 hours per visit. You must follow a strict diet (low salt, little meat, no alcohol). Many people become depressed because of the nuisances and restrictions, and some feel they are being kept alive by a machine.

Description of Diabetic Retinopathy

You have an illness that affects your blood sugar levels. You need to take medication every day and test your blood. If your blood sugar level drops below a certain level, you are in danger of becoming seriously ill. You sometimes experience blurry vision, and you have some problems with your central vision. You have trouble reading, especially fine or small print and sometimes have trouble seeing things clearly at night. You feel anxious that your sight will get worse in the future. You feel somewhat depressed about your level of vision and the risk that you might develop further complications.

Step 2: Choose Method for Determining Utilities

The three most common methods for determining preference, or utility, weights are rating scales (RS), standard gamble (SG), and time tradeoff (TTO). For each of these methods, a disease state or condition or multiple disease states or conditions are described to subjects who help determine where these disease states or conditions fall between 0.0 (dead) and 1.0 (perfect health).

Rating Scale

An RS consists of a line on a page with scaled markings, somewhat like a thermometer with perfect health at the top (100) and death at bottom (0). An instrument called the Visual Analog Scale (VAS) is similar to the RS, but it does not have any markings between the best and worst scores, and subjects are told to mark an "X" somewhere between the two extremes to indicate their preferences. Different disease states or conditions are described to subjects (see the two examples above for dialysis and retinopathy), who are asked to place their estimated preferences for the different disease states or conditions somewhere on the RS, indicating values relative to all diseases described. As an example, if they place a disease state at 70 on the scale, the disease state is given a utility score of 0.7. Most people would agree that mild seasonal allergies would not decrease a person's quality of life as much as being in a coma for the year. Therefore, the preference score for mild allergies would be near the 1.0 (or 100) mark at the top of the RS, and the value for being in a coma would be near 0, or the bottom of the scale. Figure 6.2 shows an example of how a subject might estimate some values from various conditions using an RS. Notice that how long a person will be in the disease state may influence the score.

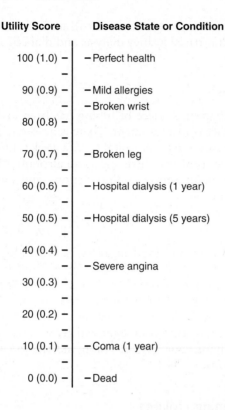

Utility Score   **Disease State or Condition**

100 (1.0) — — Perfect health

90 (0.9) — — Mild allergies
— — Broken wrist
80 (0.8) —

70 (0.7) — — Broken leg

60 (0.6) — — Hospital dialysis (1 year)

50 (0.5) — — Hospital dialysis (5 years)

40 (0.4) —
— — Severe angina
30 (0.3) —

20 (0.2) —

10 (0.1) — — Coma (1 year)

0 (0.0) — — Dead

FIGURE 6.2.   Rating scale (RS) with example estimates for various disease states or conditions. The RS uses a thermometer-like illustration to ask respondents to estimate the utility of different health states ranging from 0 (dead) to 1.0 (or 100; perfect health). In this example, the respondent estimated that being in a coma for 1 year has a lower utility (0.1) than having hospital dialysis for 1 year (0.6). Both are lower than the utility estimate for mild allergies (0.9).

Standard Gamble

The second method for determining patient preference (or utility) scores is the SG method. For this method, each subject is offered two alternatives. Alternative 1 is treatment with two possible outcomes: either the return to normal health or immediate death. Alternative 2 is the certain outcome of a chronic disease state for life based on a person's life expectancy (Fig. 6.3). The probability, or p, of normal health

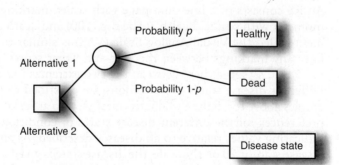

FIGURE 6.3.   Standard gamble (SG). Using the SG approach, the respondent is asked to think about being in a chronic health state and then told that he or she could gamble on an intervention (e.g., an operation) that could either cure the condition (probability = p), although he or she might die from the intervention (probability = $1- p$). A base probability is given and the respondent is asked whether he or she would have the intervention or live with the chronic condition. This probability is varied until the respondent is indifferent (the two options are difficult to chose between). The probability at this indifference point is the utility associated with the condition.

(versus immediate death, or $1-p$) for Alternative 1 is varied until the subject is indifferent between Alternatives 1 and 2 (living with the disease state or condition).

As an example, a person considers two options: a kidney transplant with a 20% probability of dying (80% chance of returning to normal health) during the operation (Alternative 1) or certain dialysis for the rest of his or her life (Alternative 2). If the person says he or she would have the operation if the chance of the successful operation p is 80% (chance of immediate death, 20%), the percent chance of success is *decreased* until the person reaches his or her point of indifference (the point where the two options are nearly equal and the person cannot decide between the two). If the person says he or she would not have the operation if the percent chance for success was 80% (chance of dying, 20%), the percent chance of success is *increased* until the person reaches his or her point of indifference. Let us say that the first person chooses a 70% chance (p) of a successful operation (with a 30% chance [$1-p$] of immediate death) as the point of indifference between having a kidney transplant and living with kidney dialysis for life. The utility score for this person for this disease state or condition (kidney dialysis) would be calculated as the probability (p) of living a normal life after the operation, or 0.7. These calculations hold for a disease state or condition that is chronic. Using the second example—diabetic retinopathy, the respondent might be asked to choose between eye surgery and living with poor sight. Most would not accept a very high probability of death during surgery to gain better sight, so the utility score for this condition (p) would be higher for the average respondent compared with that corresponding to surgery (transplant) to alleviate kidney dialysis. The calculations for a temporary health state are more complex and can be found elsewhere.[9]

Time Tradeoff

The third technique for measuring health preferences, or utilities, is the TTO method (Fig. 6.4). Again, the subject is offered two alternatives. Alternative 1 is a certain disease state for a specific length of time (t), the life expectancy for a person with the disease, and then death. Alternative 2 is being healthy for time x, which is less than t. Time x is varied until the respondent is indifferent between the two alternatives. The utility score for the health state is calculated as x divided by t. For example, a person with a life expectancy of 40 years is given two options:

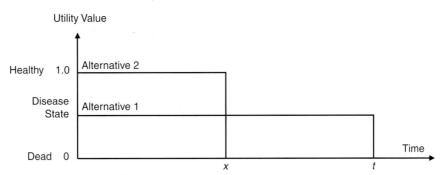

FIGURE 6.4. Time tradeoff (TTO). This TTO schematic represents the choice a respondent makes about trading off years of life for better health for a shorter period of time. The respondent is given the choice of living a full life (to time t) with a specific condition or living fewer years (to time x) without the condition (being healthy). The time of living healthy is varied until the respondent is indifferent between living in full health x years and living with the condition for t years. The utility calculated for the condition is x/t.

Alternative 1 is having a chronic condition (e.g., kidney disease or diabetes) for 40 years, and Alternative 2 is being healthy (no disease) for 20 years followed by death. If the person says he or she would rather have the disease for 40 years (t) than be healthy for 20 years, the number of years (x) in the healthy state is *increased* until the person is indifferent between the two alternatives. If the person would rather be healthy for 20 years than have the disease for 40 years, the number of years (x) in the healthy state is *decreased* until the person is indifferent between the two alternatives. Let us say that for a person who expects to live 40 more years, the person's point of indifference is 30 years of health versus 40 years of kidney disease. The utility score would be $x/t = 30/40$ or 0.75. As with the SG method illustrated above, these calculations are for chronic diseases or conditions, and calculations for a temporary health state are more complex and can be found elsewhere.[9]

Comparisons of the Three Methods

The advantage of using the RS method to determine utilities is that many disease states or conditions can be described to each subject, and this method can be conducted via a questionnaire without face-to-face interaction. People are familiar with indicating preferences on these types of scales, and it is less cognitively demanding than the other two methods. One disadvantage of using the RS method is that it does not incorporate time into the utility score as easily as the other two methods. It also may be biased in that people do not tend to cluster their values at the extreme ends of the scale but spread them throughout the range given, even if some health states are very similar in their values. In addition, respondents are not asked to make preference choices between options.

The advantage of using the SG method is that it is the "gold standard" and based on economic theory. It is more difficult for the participants, and few disease states or conditions can be "cured" by an intervention that brings a person back to "normal health." Because subjects need to be asked repeated questions (increasing or decreasing the probabilities, depending on their previous answer), this is better administered in a face-to-face setting, or through an iterative process, which takes more resources than a self-administered questionnaire.

Some advantages of the TTO method are that it is more adaptable to diseases states than the SG, and it incorporates the time in the disease state or condition more easily than the RS. As with the SG, subjects need to answer repeated questions because the time in a healthy state varies depending on the subject's previous answer. Therefore, again, face-to-face administration or an iterative process is needed.

Unfortunately, the average utility scores for each disease state or condition may differ depending on which method is used. RS scores have been shown to be consistently lower than either SG or TTO scores, and TTO scores are sometimes lower than SG scores.[10] Some work has been done on creating algorithms that transform scores from one method to approximate scores collected from another method.[11] In addition, interactive computer programs have been used to decrease the need for face-to-face questioning for the SG method.[12]

Step 3: Choose Subjects Who Will Determine Utilities

In the previous examples of the three methods, the term *subject* was used to describe the person who would be questioned to determine the utility, or preference scores. Who is this subject? Who should determine utilities, the patient with the disease, the health care professional, the caregiver, or people from the general public?

An advantage of eliciting utility scores from patients with the disease or condition of interest is that these patients may understand the effects of the disease better than the general public. However, some believe these patients provide a biased view of their disease compared with other diseases. In many cases, a patient with the specific disease state or condition reports higher utility scores than others (e.g., general population, caregivers). It has been hypothesized that this may be because of the patient's adapting or adjusting to the disease state or condition. If the patient is not able to determine utilities (e.g., a young child or person with dementia), the parent or caregiver may need to estimate values on behalf of the patient.

Some contend that health care professionals could provide good estimates because they understand various diseases. Others argue that these professionals may not rate discomfort and disability as seriously as patients or the general public. For example, researchers found that when patients were asked about side effects of medications to treat hepatitis C, patients were more concerned (gave lower utility scores) than the providers about the side effects of treatment.[13]

Health economists reason that if the viewpoint of the analysis is that of society, the utility scores should be determined by the general population or the community (society). The disadvantage of using this group is that they may not be familiar with the complex outcomes associated with each disease state or outcome, and short descriptions may not encompass all of the issues related to the disease state or condition. If researchers attempt to include all of the issues related to the health state, it may become too time intensive or cognitively demanding for the general population.[14]

In the literature, health care professionals are often asked to determine utility scores. This may be based on practicality because these professionals have had experience with the disease states and are easily accessible for interviews.

Step 4: Multiply Utilities by the Length of Life for Each Option to Obtain QALYs

When comparing the options, the difference in the length of life permitted by each option is multiplied by the utility scores obtained above. For example, in Table 6.1, we will assume that the utility score for each year of additional life is constant. In actuality, for many conditions, the utilities would change over time as the condition improves or worsens (see Fig. 6.1B).

In Table 6.1, we compare two treatment options, drug A and drug B. Although drug B extends the person's life for more years, the quality of life for those years is lower than with drug A. If a CEA were conducted, option B would be relatively

TABLE 6.1. **QALY CALCULATIONS**

	Cost for Treatment (dollars)	Years of Life Saved	Utility for Each Year of Life Saved	QALYs
Drug A	$10,000	5	0.8	4.0
Drug B	$20,000	7	0.5	3.5
	Calculation		Result	
CEA	($20,000 − $10,000) / (7 years − 5 years)		$5,000 per extra year of life	
CUA	($20,000 − $10,000) / (3.5 QALYs − 4.0 QALYs)		Drug A dominant	

CEA = cost-effectiveness analysis; CUA = cost-utility analysis; QALYs = quality-adjusted life-years.

cost-effective at an incremental cost per year of life of $5,000. If the quality of those years is incorporated into the equation by calculating QALYs, option A becomes **dominant** in that it costs less and provides a better outcome (more QALYs).

When cost-utility ratios are calculated, there is still some debate about the **discounting** of QALYS. As mentioned in Chapter 2, there is agreement that discounting of monetary benefits is needed in economic analyses if monetary costs or benefits are extrapolated more than 1 year into the future. Discounting takes into account the time-preference for money—it is preferable to receive monetary benefits today than in the future—so future benefits are discounted to account for this preference. The debate centers around the question "Is it preferable to receive health benefits today compared with receiving them in the future?" If so, should the same discount rate apply to both QALYs and monetary benefits? Most studies use the same discount rate for both monetary and health benefits, but, additionally conduct sensitivity analyses using a range of discount rates.[15]

✦ TRENDS IN CUA ANALYSES

Researchers have evaluated trends in published CUAs. CUA articles (for both pharmaceutical and other health interventions) published between 1998 and 2001 ($n = 1,210$) were evaluated. Over one-third of the studies (36%) used direct elicitation methods (standard gamble, time tradeoff, or rating scales) to estimate utility weights, 26% used indirect generic health status instruments (e.g., EQ-5D) that are discussed in Chapter 8, while others used judgments from authors or clinicians (19%). Utility weights were elicited from the general public (30%), patients (23%), clinicians (21%), and/or the author (19%). These percentages do not total 100% for two reasons; (1) Some studies generated weights using more than one method or obtained responses from more than one of these groups, and (2) some authors did not clearly report how these weights were estimated.[16]

CUAs articles, published between 1976 and 2006, that assessed pharmaceutical products ($n = 640$) were reviewed. The pharmaceutical industry sponsored 41% of the studies, 33% reported funding from other organizations, and 26% did not disclose their funding source. The percent of studies that used appropriate methods (e.g., clearly stating the study perspective, discounting costs and QALYs, and conducting incremental analysis) was similar between studies with industry and non-industry funding, and the quality of CUA studies increased over this time period.[17]

Information from 70 CUA articles was analyzed to determine the extent of sensitivity analyses (SA) reported. Authors specifically assessed if sensitivity analyses were conducted for estimates of (1) costs, (2) discount rates, and (3) health-related quality-of-life (HRQoL) assessments. Each article could contribute up to two SAs for each of the variables tested. The authors also reported if different conclusions would be reached based on the sensitivity analyses (i.e., were the results sensitive to these ranges). Of the total number of sensitivity analyses extracted, 133 tested a range of costs, 99 tested a range of discount rates, and 128 tested HRQoL ranges. Sensitivity to the estimated ranges was reported for 20% of the cost estimates, 15% of the discount rate estimates, and 31% for the HRQoL estimates. [18]

As with CEA, an incremental cost-utility ratio can estimate the added costs for the added benefit of a treatment. But, as with CEA, it does not quantify if the added cost is worth paying for the added benefit. In other words, what is a QALY worth? Example 6.1 addresses past literature and comments about placing a monetary value on a QALY. Continuing with the idea of placing a monetary value (or range of monetary values) on a QALY, as mentioned in Example 5.1, **incremental net benefit** (INB) calculations can be useful to decision makers. Example 6.2 illustrates the use of INB for the CUA data provided in the first composite article. Example 6.3 summarizes the range and magnitude of CUA ratios reported in the literature.

EXAMPLE 6.1	WHAT IS A QALY WORTH?

Note: *This summary is adapted from the editorial Rascati KL. The $64,000 question: What is a quality-adjusted life-year worth? Clinical Therapeutics 28(7):1042–1043, 2006 updated with newer key findings.*

Many studies assessing and comparing health outcomes use the QALY measure to incorporate both the difference in length of life (life-years saved) and the quality of life of various options into one summary unit. Although the validity of using QALYs as a health outcomes summary measure is still debated, it is commonly recommended (e.g., US Public Health Service Panel[1]) and used (e.g., United Kingdom's National Institute for Clinical Effectiveness [NICE][2]) to assess health care options. If there is reasonable agreement that the QALY is an adequate measure of health care outcomes, the next questions are *What value should be placed on a QALY? How much is it worth? What should policymakers and society be willing to pay for this additional (or incremental) unit of health gain?*

Eichler et al.[3] provide a comprehensive summary of "thresholds," or limits that have appeared in the literature that pertain to the value of a QALY or similar measure. The authors provide a table that compares various methods and sources that have been used to determine this value and adjusts the results to 2002 US dollars. Four of these sources include: (1) an often-quoted "rule of thumb" of US$50,000 per QALY; (2) estimates by the World Health Organization (WHO) of three times the nation's gross domestic product (GDP) per capita (which would be about US$108,000 in 2002) for a DALY averted; (3) literature that used past decisions by health care policymaking bodies to infer an implicit threshold or limit; and (4) literature that estimated the value society places on this outcome. The last two sources are expanded on in the next two paragraphs.

Some researchers have used past decisions by health care policy groups to estimate an implicit value or range of values for a year of life or QALY. George et al.[4] assessed decisions made by the Pharmacy Benefits Advisory Committee (PBAC) in Australia. The authors concluded that the PBAC was unlikely to add a pharmaceutical product to the formulary if the cost per year of life saved was over 76,000 1998/99 AU$ (48,000 1998–1999 US$), and it was unlikely to reject the addition if the cost were less than 42,000 1998–1999 AU$ (27,000 1998–1999 US$).

Devlin and Parkin[5] looked retrospectively at 33 health technology decisions made by UK's NICE by May 2002. Although NICE had stated its range of acceptable cost-effectiveness was £20,000 to £30,000 per QALY (about 36,000 to 55,000 US$), the authors found two negative decisions below this range and five positive decisions above it. Other factors in addition to cost per QALY (e.g., uncertainty of estimates and burden of disease) helped explain the probability of acceptance by NICE. As summarized by Eichler et al.,[3] there is no "hard threshold" that would lead these

(continues)

EXAMPLE 6.1   WHAT IS A QALY WORTH? (Continued)

decision makers to automatically accept or reject a health care option. Instead, there is a "soft threshold," or range, that would allow other factors to be considered. If the cost per QALY was below this range, its acceptance would be more likely; above this range, its acceptance would be less likely; but within the range, other factors would be critically analyzed.[3]

Other researchers have attempted to incorporate preference methods such as **willingness to pay** or **contingent valuation** techniques to address the question of how the public or society values a QALY. For example, King et al.[6] measured the values that three patient populations ($n = 391$ patients) would place on a QALY. The authors reported these patients would be willing to spend between \$12,500 and \$32,200, in US \$2,003 an additional QALY. Although some insist that public preference should play a role in distributing health care resources, others maintain that there are mathematical and theoretical obstacles to using preference methods to determine one unique value for a QALY.[7–11] One issue to consider is that public preferences for an increased unit of health may differ depending on patient demographics (e.g., higher preference for younger people) or by health effect (improvement in health versus a prevented decline in health). Public valuation of QALYs may not only be different from policymakers, but there are wide differences depending on the method used to estimate them.

There is also the overarching issue that even if a specific body of decision makers or the public could agree on a specific value or limit they would pay for a QALY, implementation of all options below that limit could be impossible because of budget constraints. Buxton[12] also points out that if adhering to this threshold would lead to the discontinuation of current treatments, policymakers would be placed in a difficult political position.

Back to the question: What is a QALY worth? Although no policymaking body has offered an explicit answer to this question, the literature shows a wide range of implicit answers. So the answer to the question is "it depends" (an answer that some of my students do not particularly like to hear). It depends on whom you ask. More wealthy countries (and more wealthy patients) put a higher value on a QALY. It also depends on other political, equity, and budgetary factors and considerations. In the United States, the most often-cited estimate is 50,000 US\$ as a base case, with a large range (usually \$20,000 to \$100,000) for **sensitivity analyses.** Ironically, this figure has been cited since the 1980s, and would be nearly double if adjusted for inflation. Even though there is no one unique answer to this question, the calculation of the additional cost per additional QALY is an important ingredient to consider in the mix, so it should continue to be calculated, and decisions that are made, in part, using this value should continue to be monitored. In an article published in 2008, the author predicted that it is likely that the \$50,000 baseline threshold, while not based on empirical theory or testing, will continue to be appealing for the next 5 years as it is a round number that is often cited as a point of comparison. He also speculated that the \$100,000 per QALY threshold will increasingly be applied, especially in the United States.[13]

References

1. Gold MR, Siegel JE, Russell LB, Weinstein MC. *Cost-Effectiveness in Health and Medicine.* Oxford: Oxford University Press, 1996.
2. National Institute for Clinical Excellence. Available at http://www.nice.org; accessed June 23, 2006.

3. Eichler HG, Kong SX, Gerth WC, et al. Use of cost-effectiveness analysis in health-care resource allocation decision-making: How are cost-effectiveness thresholds expected to emerge? *Value in Health* 7(5):518–528, 2004.

4. George B, Harris A, Mitchell A. Cost-effectiveness analysis and the consistency of decision making: Evidence from pharmaceutical reimbursement in Australia (1991 to 1996). *Pharmacoeconomics* 19(11):1103–1109, 2001.

5. Devlin N, Parkin D. Does NICE have a cost-effectiveness threshold and what other factors influence its decisions? A binary choice analysis. *Health Economics* 13(5):437–452, 2004.

6. King JT, Tsevat J, Lave JR, Roberts MS. Willingness-to-pay for a quality-adjusted life-year: Implications for societal health care resource allocation. *Medical Decision Making* 25(6):667–677, 2005.

7. Schwappach DLB. Resource allocation, social values and the QALY: A review of the debate and empirical evidence. *Health Expectations* 5(3):210–222, 2002.

8. Gyrd-Hansen D. Willingness to pay for a QALY: Theoretical and methodological issues. *Pharmacoeconomics* 23(5):423–432, 2005.

9. Johnson FR. Einstein on willingness to pay per QALY: Is there a better way? *Medical Decision Making* 25(6):607–608, 2005.

10. O'Brien BJ, Gertsen K, Willan AR, Faulkner LA. Is there a kink in consumers' threshold value for cost-effectiveness in health care? *Health Economics* 11:175–180, 2002.

11. Hirth RA, Chernew ME, Miller E, et al. Willingness to pay for a quality-adjusted life year: In search of a standard. *Medical Decision Making* 20(3):332–342, 2000.

12. Buxton MJ. How much are health-care systems prepared to pay to produce a QALY? *The European Journal of Health Economics* 6(4):285–287, 2005.

13. Grosse SD. Assessing cost-effectiveness in healthcare: History of the $50,000 per QALY threshold. *Expert Review of Pharmacoeconomics & Outcomes Research* 8(2):165–178, 2008.

EXAMPLE 6.2 INCREMENTAL NET BENEFIT ANALYSIS USING CUA COMPOSITE DATA

In Exhibits 6.1 and 6.2, data on the cost-utility analysis of Oncoplatin compared with Oncotaxel are presented. Oncoplatin cost $3,000 more than Oncotaxel ($10,000 versus $7,000, respectively) and produced an additional 0.04 QALY (0.19–0.15); therefore, the incremental ratio was $75,000 per extra QALY. Is Oncoplatin more cost-effective than Oncotaxel? It depends on the value of a QALY. There has been debate on the value of a QALY, and broad ranges of estimates have appeared in the literature (see Example 6.1). The most often-cited value from the US literature is $50,000 per QALY. Below are incremental net benefit calculations using a λ of $50,000 as an estimate of the value of the health benefit of one QALY.

$$INB = (\lambda \times \Delta \ QALYs) - \Delta \ Costs$$
$$INB_{\lambda=\$50,000} = (\$50,000 \times 0.04 \ QALY) - \$3,000$$
$$INB_{\lambda=\$50,000} = -\$1,000$$

Because the INB is less than zero, Oncoplatin is not cost-effective compared with Oncotaxel when $\lambda = \$50,000$. As mentioned in Example 6.1, the $50,000 per QALY estimate has been cited since the 1980s without adjustment for inflation and would be approximately double if inflated to 2012 dollars. The figure that follows indicates that if the λ were varied from $20,000 to $100,000 per QALY, the INB of Oncoplatin compared with Oncotaxel would range from –$2,200 to more than $1,000, indicating that the answer to "Is Oncoplatin cost-effective compared with Oncotaxel?" would depend on (i.e., be sensitive to) the value placed on a QALY (λ).

(continues)

Calculation of INB for range of lambda values for QALYs.

EXAMPLE 6.3 SUMMARY OF CUA RATIOS IN THE LITERATURE

Note: This summary is based on two articles:

1. Bell C, Urbach DR, Ray JG, et al. Bias in published cost-effectiveness studies. *British Medical Journal* 332(7543):699–703, 2006. Used with permission from BMJ Publishing Group, Ltd.
2. Greenberg D, Earle C, Fang C, Eldar-Lissai A, Neumann P. When is cancer care cost-effective? A systematic overview of cost-utility analyses in oncology. *Journal of the National Cancer Institute* 102(2):82–88, 2010.

The objective of the article by Bell et al. was to investigate published studies that reported cost-effectiveness ratios using quality-adjusted life-years as an outcome measure. They found 1,433 ratios reported in 494 articles that met their criteria for inclusion into their study. Of these ratios, 82% ($n = 1,179$) reported that the intervention of interest was both more effective and more costly, 9% ($n = 130$) were dominant (i.e., cost saving), and 9% ($n = 124$) were dominated. About 50% ($n = 712$) reported cost-effectiveness ratios below $20,000 per QALY, about 18% ($n = 262$) reported ratios between $20,000 and $50,000, 11% ($n = 155$) between $50,000 and $100,000, and the remaining 21% ($n = 304$) reported ratios above $100,000 per QALY. If ratios below $50,000 per QALY are used to indicate "positive" results and ratios above $100,000 per QALY are used to indicate "negative" results, the authors point out that positive and negative results tend to be reported more often than "intermediate" results (ratios between $50,000 and $100,000 per QALY). The median cost per QALY for studies sponsored by industry was about half ($13,083) of those with nonindustry sponsors ($27,400).

A more recent study by Greenberg et al. evaluated published cost-utility analyses for cancer-related interventions through 2007. Of the 636 incremental cost-utility ratios calculated in 242 articles (120 articles presented more than one ratio), the median ratios, categorized by type of cancer, ranged from $22,000 for colorectal cancer to $48,000 for hematological cancer for an additional QALY. About 60% of the ratios fell below the $50,000 threshold or were dominant, 15% fell between $50,000 and $100,000, while the rest (25%) fell above $100,000 or were dominated. More than two-thirds did not directly elicit utility weights, using published estimates instead. In addition, the authors scored the quality of these CUA studies, and found industry-sponsored studies scores were similar to those of studies sponsored by other organizations.

SUMMARY

CUA is considered by some researchers to be a special type of CEA analysis. CUA has the advantage of using one outcome measure (usually QALYs) to incorporate various morbidity- and mortality-related health outcomes. On the other hand, utility measurement is not regarded as being as precise or "scientific" as natural health unit measurements (e.g., blood pressure, cholesterol levels, years of life) used in CEAs. Utility measures have been criticized for not being sensitive to small, but clinically meaningful, changes in **health status.** For the direct elicitation measures of utilities discussed in this chapter—rating scales, standard gamble, and time trade off methods—there is no consensus on which type of instrument to use or which group of people (e.g., patients, clinicians, or the general population) to interview to determine utility scores, and different results may be generated depending on which instrument and which group is chosen.

Although estimating and weighting utilities or health preferences is not without problems, in many cases ignoring quality-of-life differences between options would provide less than complete data to clinicians and other decision makers.

COMPOSITE ARTICLE 1: CUA—ONCOLOGY

Note: The composite article compares treatments for oncology patients. One review of oncology articles that use CUA is: Earle CC, Chapman RH, Baker CS, et al. Systematic overview of cost-utility assessments in oncology. Journal of Clinical Oncology 18(18):3302–3317, 2000.

Title: COST-UTILITY ANALYSIS OF BEST SUPPORTIVE CARE VERSUS ONCOPLATIN AND ONCOTAXEL IN THE TREATMENT OF RECURRENT METASTATIC BREAST CANCER

BACKGROUND: For patients diagnosed with recurrent metastatic breast cancer, the prognosis is grim. Two agents, Oncoplatin and Oncotaxel, have been used to help prolong the lives of these patients (authors would cite clinical literature here for real pharmaceutical products). As with other chemotherapy treatments, the toxic effects of the medications can be severe and vastly decrease the patient's quality of life. Some would argue that the small increase in life expectancy from these agents might not be worth the tradeoff in suffering from the adverse effects of the agents during the treatment period. Instead of chemotherapy, palliative treatments, such as best supportive care (BSC), have been suggested as an option. BSC includes measures to keep the patient comfortable. These may include medications to alleviate pain, antibiotics, or radiotherapy to reduce tumor size.

The objective of this study was to compare the costs and utility of two chemotherapy treatments, Oncoplatin and Oncotaxel, with those of BSC in patients with recurrent metastatic breast cancer.

METHODS: The practice sites for data collection included three oncology clinics that are part of a multihospital, multiclinic health care system. Utility scores were collected via the time tradeoff (TTO) method. A panel of experts helped create descriptions of the health states of patients undergoing the different treatment options. Based on these descriptions, utility scores were elicited from two sources: oncology nurses at the three clinics and a random sample of patients from general (nononcology) clinics associated with the health care system.

Data on treatment and survival time were collected for the past 3 years from a retrospective analysis of charts at three oncology clinics. Medical services and procedures associated with these treatment options were recorded. Treatment data included medications and their administration, as well as laboratory, radiology, and various types of medical visits (physician, clinic, emergency room, and hospital). Charges listed by the health care system in 2013 were used to estimate current costs for each service or procedure.

RESULTS: Exhibit 6.1 lists the costs and survival times found by the review of charts. Using the TTO method, treatment utility scores were estimated by nurses from the oncology clinics and a random sample of patients who did not have cancer. Although the chemotherapy regimens provided a longer survival (Oncoplatin, 200 days; Oncotaxel, 160 days) than BSC (130 days), the utility score was higher for BSC (0.60–0.61) compared with the chemotherapy regimens (0.32–0.35). Oncology nurses gave similar estimates compared with the group of nononcology patients.

If the difference in quality of life is not incorporated into the analysis, cost-effectiveness calculations based on survival time alone (Life years saves - LYS) indicate that chemotherapy is more effective but at a higher cost (Exhibit 6.2). When survival time is adjusted for the differences in utilities (preferences) for treatment, the use of BSC is dominant over both chemotherapy treatments because of its lower cost and higher QALY estimate.

Sensitivity analyses were conducted by reducing cost estimates using the clinic's cost-to-charge ratio of 0.83:1 and by varying the days of survival by their 95% confidence intervals. As with the comparison of oncology nurses versus patient utility estimates, the results were robust.

CONCLUSION: There are some limitations to this study. The data were collected from a small sample of patients. Although data were collected from three clinics, these clinics were all part of the same health care system. Oncology treatment in other clinics may vary in both costs and outcomes. Although utility scores were collected from health care professionals and general patients, they were not collected from patients with metastatic breast cancer. We believed that administering the instrument to these women might have placed an undue burden on patients with a poor prognosis. Actual cost data were not available, so charge data were used as a proxy, and a sensitivity analysis was conducted on this variable.

As with previous research, using BSC was found to be less expensive than using chemotherapy agents to treat advanced cancer. Although best supportive care may not be as effective as chemotherapy in traditional measures of effectiveness (e.g., survival time, progression-free survival time), when preferences for a less toxic treatment are factored into the decision, BSC may become the preferred treatment, and it should be considered as an option.

EXHIBIT 6.1

Data – Oncology Study

	BSC (n = 29)	Oncoplatin (n = 36)	Oncotaxel (n = 35)
Treatment charges: Mean (SD)	$5,000 ($1,000)	$10,000 ($2,000)	$7,000 ($2,000)
Survival (days): Mean (range)	130 (110–140)	200 (180–215)	160 (110–190)
Utility scores: Oncology nurses	0.60	0.35	0.35
Utility scores: Nononcology patients	0.61	0.32	0.32

BSC = best supportive care; SD = standard deviation.

EXHIBIT 6.2

Calculations – Oncology Study

Cost-Effectiveness	BSC (n = 29)	Oncoplatin (n = 36)	Oncotaxel (n = 35)
Cost per LYS = (cost/days) × 365 days/year	$14,038	$18,250	$15,969
Incremental cost per LYS = (Δ Costs/Δ days) × 365 days/year		Oncoplatin vs. BSC = $26,071 per additional LYS	Oncotaxel vs. BSC = $24,333 per additional LYS
Cost-Utility			
QALY = Days × utility/ 365 days	O = 0.21 QALY P = 0.22 QALY	O = 0.19 QALY P = 0.17 QALY	O = 0.15 QALY P = 0.14 QALY
Average cost per QALY	O = $23,809 P = $22,727	O = $52,631 P = $58,823	O = $46,667 P = $50,000
Incremental cost per QALY = Δ Costs/Δ QALYs	Both Oncoplatin and Oncotaxel dominated by BSC for both O and P estimates	Oncoplatin vs. Oncotaxel O = $75,000 per additional QALY P = $100,000 per additional QALY	

BSC = best supportive care; LYS = life-years saved; O = based on utility scores from oncology nurses; P = based on utility scores from nononcology patients; QALY = quality-adjusted life-year.

WORKSHEET FOR CRITIQUE OF CUA COMPOSITE ARTICLE 1

1. Complete Title?

    _____

    _____

    _____

    _____

2. Clear Objective?

    _____

    _____

    _____

    _____

3. Appropriate Alternatives?

_____

_____

_____

_____

4. Alternatives Described?

_____

_____

_____

_____

5. Perspective Stated?

_____

_____

_____

_____

6. Type of Study?

_____

_____

_____

_____

7. Relevant Costs?

_____

_____

_____

_____

8. Relevant Outcomes?

_____

_____

_____

_____

9. Adjustment or Discounting?

_____

_____

_____

_____

10. Reasonable Assumptions?

_____

_____

_____

_____

11. Sensitivity Analyses?

_____

_____

_____

_____

12. Limitations Addressed?

_____

_____

_____

_____

13. Generalizations Appropriate?

_____

_____

_____

_____

14. Unbiased Conclusions?

_____

_____

_____

_____

Cost-Effectiveness Grid – Oncology Study

Which cells represent the following comparisons for LYS and QALYs?

a) Oncoplatin compared with BSC
b) Oncotaxel compared with BSC
c) Oncoplatin compared with Oncotaxel

COST-EFFECTIVENESS	Lower Cost	Same Cost	Higher Cost
Lower effectiveness	A	B	C
Same effectiveness	D	E	F
Higher effectiveness	G	H	I

CRITIQUE OF CUA COMPOSITE ARTICLE 1

1. **Complete Title:** The title identified the type of study (CUA), the treatments that were being compared (BSC, Oncoplatin, and Oncotaxel), and the disease state (metastatic breast cancer).

2. **Clear Objective:** The objective of this study was "to compare the costs and utility of two chemotherapy treatments, Oncoplatin and Oncotaxel, with those of best supportive care." This was clear.

3. **Appropriate Alternatives:** The three alternatives were BSC, Oncoplatin, and Oncotaxel. A case was made that BSC is sometimes overlooked as a valid option. Based on the clinical literature cited, the readers would determine if the two chemotherapy options were appropriate.

4. **Alternatives Described:** Chemotherapy dosing is very individualized, and data were collected from three clinics; average doses of agents were not included. BSC was defined as keeping the patient comfortable, including providing pain medications, antibiotics, and radiotherapy, if needed.

5. **Perspective Stated:** The perspective of the study was not explicitly stated. Because the researchers only report measuring direct medical costs, the perspective could have been that of the payer or that of the health care system that included the three oncology clinics. Charges were measured, so the perspective is still unclear. If actual costs to the health system were estimated, the perspective could have been the health care system. If reimbursed costs were used, the perspective could have been that of the average third-party payer.

6. **Type of Study:** The study was correctly identified as a CUA because outcomes were valued in QALYs. For comparison purposes, incremental **cost-effectiveness ratios** were also calculated based on length of survival for the three options, so the answer could be that both a CUA and a CEA were conducted.

7. **Relevant Costs:** Because we are unsure of the perspective of the study, it is difficult to determine if relevant costs were measured. It seems as if all relevant direct medical costs were measured. Patient costs, such as time traveling to and from the clinic, might be different for BSC than for chemotherapy, but these costs were not measured.

8. **Relevant Outcomes:** Outcomes of the treatment were measured by determining the length of life from chart reviews and utilities via two groups, oncology nurses, and general patients. The TTO technique was used to elicit utility scores. A description of the health states used in eliciting these responses would have been a helpful addition to the article.

9. **Adjustment or Discounting:** Data were collected from charts that spanned a 3-year period. To adjust for this, units of service were multiplied by current charges for each service. Discounting was not needed because neither costs nor outcomes were extrapolated into the future.

10. **Reasonable Assumptions:** One assumption was that utility scores from the oncology staff would be accurate. To test this assumption, scores were also obtained from another group (a random sample of nononcology patients). Another assumption was that charges were a valid substitute for actual costs.

11. **Sensitivity Analyses:** Sensitivity analyses were conducted. Utility scores from two groups were compared, and costs and survival time were varied. Although the authors indicated that results were insensitive to these analyses, a table with the numbers based on these new calculations would have been useful.

12. **Limitations Addressed:** The authors did address some of their limitations at the beginning of the conclusion section. One limitation that was not addressed is that patients were not randomized to the three treatment options. It is possible that patients who received BSC were different from those who received chemotherapy. They may have been older or may have been in a more advanced stage of the disease. This problem is called selection bias, and it is discussed further in Chapter 11.

13. **Generalizations Appropriate:** Because data on both costs and outcomes were collected from only one health care system (albeit from three clinics within the system), caution should be used when extrapolating to other populations who are treated in other settings.

14. **Unbiased Conclusions:** The authors state that when survival is adjusted for patient preferences, BSC is a valid option for treating patients with recurrent metastatic breast cancer. BSC costs less than chemotherapy treatments and provides a higher QALY score. Sensitivity analyses found the results to be robust (i.e., not sensitive to changes in estimates).

Cost-Effectiveness Grid – Oncology Study

COST-EFFECTIVENESS	Lower Cost	Same Cost	Higher Cost
Lower effectiveness	A	B	C QALY: OP - BSC QALY: OT - BSC
Same effectiveness	D	E	F
Higher effectiveness	G	H	I LYS: OP - BSC LYS: OT - BSC LYS: OP - OT QALY: OP - OT

BSC = best supportive care
LYS = life years saved
OP = Oncoplatin
OT = Oncotaxel
QALY = quality-adjusted life year

When assessing comparisons of LYS, both chemotherapy treatments are more effective but more costly than BSC (*cell I*). When comparing the two chemotherapy treatments, Oncoplatin is more effective (in both LYS and QALY) and more costly than Oncotaxel (*cell I*). When assessing comparisons using QALYs, both chemotherapy treatments are less effective and more costly than BSC (*cell C*), indicating BSC is a cost-effective option compared with chemotherapy when taking quality-of-life preferences into consideration.

COMPOSITE ARTICLE 2: CUA—IMMUNOSUPPRESSION

Note: Teresa Brucker, a PharmD student, helped develop this composite article.
The composite article compares cost-utility of three different maintenance immunosuppression regimens in patients who have undergone kidney transplants. A review of utility assessments for patients with kidney disease is:
Wyld M, Morton RL, Hayen A, Howard K, Webster AC. A Systematic Review and Meta-Analysis of Utility-Based Quality of Life in Chronic Kidney Disease Treatments. PLoS Medicine (9):e1001307. Accessed September 27, 2012. www.plosmedicine.org/article/info%3Adoi%2F10.1371%2Fjournal.pmed.1001307

Title: COST-UTILITY ANALYSIS OF THREE MEDICATIONS AS MAINTENANCE IMMUNOSUPPRESSION THERAPY IN PATIENTS POST KIDNEY TRANSPLANT

INTRODUCTION: Kidney transplantation is an option for many patients who have progressed to stage 5 of chronic kidney disease, or end-stage renal disease (ESRD). Studies show that a successful kidney transplant offers enhanced quality and duration of life and is more effective than long-term dialysis therapy. For kidney transplants in particular, survival rates for grafts are the highest compared with other types of organ transplants.[1] To date, more than 250,000 kidney transplants have been performed in the United States. Despite advancements, complications still arise and the possibility of kidney graft failure remains a concern. Failure may be due to chronic rejection by the patient, graft dysfunction, infection, cancer, liver disease, and/or drug-induced liver toxicity. Therapeutic agents called immunosuppressants suppress the body's immune response in order to reduce the potential of an organ rejection. Two new agents have recently been approved: Gecept and Gelimus (not actual drug names). Gecept, in contrast to Gelimus, has significantly reduced side effects of diarrhea, nausea, constipation, and vomiting. Due to the significant differences in side effects that Gecept circumvents, a comprehensive analysis was conducted to assess costs and outcomes of three different but common maintenance immunosuppression therapies used for post–kidney transplant patients: Gecept, Gelimus, and mycophenolate mofetil (MMF) with reduced-dose cyclosporine (CsA).

METHODS: This was a prospective cohort study that assessed the outcomes of three different treatment regimens post kidney transplants that were successfully completed at two large medical centers. Patients were assessed for up to 365 days after transplantation. To be eligible to participate, individuals must have received Gecept, Gelimus, or MMF with CsA as maintenance immunosuppressive treatment after kidney transplant. In addition, patients who had already undergone one kidney transplant were not included in this study. Based on these parameters, 22 patients qualified for the study, and none were lost during the follow-up period. Health-related quality of life was measured using the Kidney Transplant Questionnaire (KTQ) and number of days free from complications per year (referring to medication adverse effects only). Utility scores were collected from patients who underwent kidney transplants using the standard gamble method, and charges were estimated using the United Network for Organ Sharing (UNOS) data, which extracted its cost data from Millman, Inc., a marketing services company.[2]

RESULTS: Table 6.2 indicates the costs and outcomes collected on the study patients. Table 6.3 shows calculations for both average and incremental ratios. Both Gecept and Gelimus were dominant over MMF with CsA treatment. This is probably due to a number of factors: both of these newer medications are known to have less detrimental side effects than CsA due to their different side effect profiles. In addition, it typically costs more to provide for a combination treatment (MMF with cyclosporine) than a single agent. There are examples when a single agent may cost significantly more than a combination, but this is not the case for this situation. In addition, the incremental ratios for both effectiveness and QALYs indicate that Gecept has better outcomes than Gelimus (more DFMCs and higher QALYs) but at a higher price. Even the higher estimate from the sensitivity analysis, $5,487 per additional QALY, is well below common thresholds for value. See Table 6.4.

TABLE 6.2. **DATA - IMMUNOSUPPRESSION STUDY**			
Data	Gecept	Gelimus	MMF with CsA
Medication costs for 1 year, Mean (SD)	$18,200 ($2,500)	$17,300 ($2,400)	$22,900 ($3,000)
DFMC, Mean (Range)	220 (201–257)	140 (135–176)	110 (101–129)
Utility Score (kidney transplant recipients)	0.72	0.44	0.37

SD = standard deviation; DFMC = days free of medication complications per year; MMF with CsA = mycophenolate mofetil with reduced-dose cyclosporine.

TABLE 6.3. CALCULATIONS – IMMUNOSUPPRESSION STUDY

	Gecept	Gelimus	MMF with CsA
Cost-Effectiveness			
Cost per DFMC	$83	$124	$208
Incremental cost per DFMC: (Δ costs/Δ days)	Gecept is dominant over MMF with CsA	Gelimus is dominant over MMF with CsA	
	Gecept vs. Gelimus: $11 per additional DFMC		
Cost-Utility			
QALY	0.72	0.44	0.37
Average cost per QALY	$25,278	$39,318	$61,892
Incremental cost per QALY: Δ costs/Δ QALYs	Gecept is dominant over MMF with CsA	Gelimus is dominant over MMF with CsA	
	Gecept vs. Gelimus: $3,214 per additional QALY		

MMF with CsA = mycophenolate mofetil with reduced-dose cyclosporine; DFMC = days free of medication complications per year; QALY = quality-adjusted life-years.

TABLE 6.4. SENSITIVITY ANALYSES – IMMUNOSUPPRESSION STUDY

Sensitivity Analysis	Gecept (QALY –10%)	Gelimus (QALY +10%)
Adjusted QALYs	0.648 (0.9 × 0.72)	0.484 (1.1 × 0.44)
Incremental cost per QALY (Δ costs/Δ QALYs)	Gecept vs. Gelimus ($18,200 – $17,300)/(0.648 – 0.484) = $5,488	

LIMITATIONS: There were some limitations to the study. First, the sample population is small and from only two facilities—it reduces potential extrapolation to other populations. Similarly, the length of study is limited in its duration, as the survival rate 3 years post transplant is as high as 90%, but may vary from center to center according to complications that may arise in the interim. Perhaps a longer study period is necessary to capture more accurate data in complication-free days. In addition, annual costs per drug are estimates, and they may fluctuate depending on individual patient dosing, frequency, current market pricing, and price negotiations by various insurance companies. Finally, though the standard gamble method is the gold standard for determining utility scores, the utility scores of this particular study may still differ from a study using a different methodology.

CONCLUSIONS: In this study the use of Gecept was cost-effective compared to Gelimus, and dominant compared to MMF with CsA.

REFERENCES

1. *2008 Annual Report of the U.S. Organ Procurement and Transplantation Network and the Scientific Registry of Transplant Recipients: Transplant Data 1998–2007.* Rockville, MD: U.S. Department of Health and Human Services, Health Resources and Services Administration, Healthcare Systems Bureau, Division of Transplantation. Accessed September 27, 2012 at http://optn.transplant.hrsa.gov/ar2008/112a_dh.htm.
2. *Costs.* Transplant Living. Published by UNOS. Accessed 25 September 2012 at http://www.transplantliving.org/before-the-transplant/financing-a-transplant/the-costs/.

WORKSHEET FOR CRITIQUE OF CUA COMPOSITE ARTICLE 2

1. Complete Title?

_____

_____

_____

_____

2. Clear Objective?

_____

_____

_____

_____

3. Appropriate Alternatives?

_____

_____

_____

_____

4. Alternatives Described?

_____

_____

_____

_____

5. Perspective Stated?

_____

_____

_____

_____

6. Type of Study?

_____

_____

_____

_____

7. Relevant Costs?

8. Relevant Outcomes?

9. Adjustment or Discounting?

10. Reasonable Assumptions?

11. Sensitivity Analyses?

12. Limitations Addressed?

13. Generalizations Appropriate?

_____

_____

_____

_____

14. Unbiased Conclusions?

_____

_____

_____

_____

CRITIQUE OF CUA COMPOSITE ARTICLE 2

1. **Is the title clear?** The title does state the type of study that is being conducted (CUA), but it does not list the comparators.

2. **Is the objective stated?** Yes. Within the introduction, it is stated that "a comprehensive analysis was conducted to assess costs and outcomes of three different but common maintenance immunosuppression therapies used for post–kidney transplant patients: Gecept, Gelimus, and mycophenolate mofetil with reduced-dose cyclosporine."

3. **Are the comparators/alternatives ideal or appropriate?** The comparators are appropriate, as mycophenolate mofetil with reduced-dose CsA are commonly used immunosuppressant medications used as maintenance therapy for post–kidney transplant patients. In addition, the new medications have been found to differ in mechanism of action from both mycophenolate mofetil and cyclosporine, so differences in complications may be attributed to these differences in mechanisms of action.

4. **Were the comparators/alternatives clearly stated? Can the study be replicated?** Though the medications were clearly stated, the doses, frequencies, and duration of treatment were not stated. In addition, the means of data collection was not clearly outlined, only the length of time in which the data were collected (365 days).

5. **Is the perspective of the study indicated?** The perspective of the study was not indicated. However, one might assume it is the payer—In the US, Medicare pays for the majority of the costs for patients who have kidney transplants.

6. **Is the type of study indicated?** The type of study (CUA) is stated in the title. Furthermore, outcomes were measured in QALYs, indicating again that this is

a CUA study. To compare differences in results, incremental cost-effectiveness ratios were calculated based on the days free of medication complications, so the type of study may be regarded as a CEA as well as a CUA study.

7. **Relevant costs: were all the important and relevant costs included?** Since the perspective of the study is not clearly indicated, it is difficult to determine the appropriateness of the costs of the study. Only costs of the medications were included, others costs (e.g., costs of treating medication-related complications) should have been addressed.

8. **Were the important or relevant outcomes measured?** Outcomes were measured by the number of days free from medication-related complications according to patient testimony, and the utility scores were derived from the standard gamble method. However, the outcome "day free from medication-related complications" is not adequately defined or explained. More information on this outcome variable would be useful to the readers. Results from the KTQ were not discussed.

9. **Is adjustment or discounting necessary?** Because the study spanned over the course of 1 year (365 days), adjustment of costs is not necessary, and because results were not extrapolated into the future, neither costs nor outcomes needed to be discounted.

10. **Assumptions stated and reasonable and stated?** It was assumed that utility scores were accurate, as they were derived from patients directly affected by the different medication regimens and thus provide the closest approximation of these utility scores. In addition, medical costs (cost of hospital admission prior and after surgery, procurement of organ, physician costs, costs to treat complications, etc) other than for medications were assumed to be the same between patients.

11. **Sensitivity Analyses: were sensitivity analyses conducted for important estimates or assumptions?** A sensitivity analysis was conducted by adjusting the QALYs of Gecept by −10% and Gelimus by +10%. Gecept was deemed to still be a cost-effective option.

12. **Limitations addressed?** Several limitations were addressed in the limitations section.

13. **Appropriate generalizations: were extrapolations beyond the population studied properly?** Outcomes and costs were collected from a small group of patients from only two health care centers, so caution in extrapolation is warranted.

14. **Were conclusions unbiased?** Conclusions were based on data from a small sample and did not include nondrug costs, but sensitivity analysis on the CUA scores indicated the results to be robust to a range of utility estimates.

QUESTIONS/EXERCISES

Based on the following abstract (condensed summary of a research article), please answer questions 1 through 5:

ABSTRACT

TITLE: Cost-Utility of Asthmazolimide in the Treatment of Severe Persistent Asthma

BACKGOUND: Some patients with severe persistent asthma are not controlled with standard treatment (defined in this study as a combination of long-acting beta-agonists [LABAs] and inhaled corticosteroids [ICS]). Clinical trials have shown improved outcomes for these patients if asthmazolimide (a fictitious drug) is added to their regimen.

OBJECTIVE: The objective of this study was to estimate the cost per QALY of the addition of asthmazolimide to standard treatment for patients enrolled in a randomized controlled trial. The perspective of the study was the third-party payer.

METHODS: Patients with severe persistent asthma in a health plan were prospectively enrolled in the study in 2012 using a pre–post study design. For the first 12 months after enrollment, patients recorded their use of any asthma-related medical services and prescriptions and kept a daily symptom diary. Then patients had asthmazolimide added to their regimen for the next 12-month period and again kept track of their asthma-related medical services and prescriptions and a diary of daily symptoms. Costs of services recorded by the patients were adjusted to 2012 costs to the health plan. QALYs were calculated using utility weights for various asthma-related symptoms that were estimated from previous studies.

RESULTS: A total of 216 patients were enrolled in and completed the study. Asthma-related health plan costs increased after the addition of asthmazolimide (mostly from an increase in prescription costs) by an average of $800 per year. Fewer symptoms and less severe symptoms were reported after the addition of the new drug, resulting in an average increase of 0.1 QALY and an incremental cost per QALY ratio of $8,000.

CONCLUSION: For these 216 patients, the addition of asthmazolimide to the medication regimen resulted in a reduction of symptoms at a reasonable cost to the health plan.

1. Was the title appropriate? Why or why not?

_____

_____

_____

_____

2. Were you able to determine the perspective? If so, what was it?

_____

_____

_____

_____

3. Was either adjustment or discounting appropriate? If so, was it conducted?

_____

_____

_____

_____

4. Were alternatives described in detail?

_____

_____

_____

_____

5. Were generalizations made?

_____

_____

_____

_____

Based on the following informations, please answer questions 6 through 11.

Gastromycin is a potent stimulator of gastric motility. Recent studies have shown the use of IV Gastromycin before endoscopy for gastrointestinal (GI) bleeding ulcers helps clear the stomach of blood. You are asked to compare the use of IV Gastromycin to usual care (no pre-op Gastromycin) before GI endoscopy for bleeding peptic ulcers. The perspective is that of the payer, and the time frame is 1 year.

Assume patients have a 1.0 QALY if not for the need of ulcer surgery

QALYs for the minor surgery and 2-day stay are decreased by 0.10 = 0.90 QALY

QALYs for the major surgery and 3-day stay are decreased by 0.20 = 0.80 QALY

OPTION A—Usual care: Following usual surgery procedures, 70% of the time, the ulcer is located on "first-look"; there is no "second-look" endoscopy needed; minor, tuncomplicated surgery is conducted; and a 2-day hospital stay results—at a cost of $4,000 ($2,000 for surgery; $1,000 per day in hospital times 2 days). The other 30% of the time, a "second-look" endoscopy is needed due to excessive bleeding; the surgery is more complicated, and a 3-day hospital stay results—at a cost of $6,000 ($3,000 for surgery and $1,000 per day in hospital times 3 days).

For each patient, the average cost would be $4,600 [(0.7 × $4,000) + (0.3 × $6,000)]

For each patient, the average QALY would be 0.87 [(0.7 × 0.9 QALY) + (0.3 × 0.8 QALY)]

OPTION B—IV Gastromycin added presurgery: The use of IV Gastromycin adds $500 to the cost of surgery is above the cost of the usual procedures. When using IV Gastromycin, 80% of the time, the ulcer is located on "first-look"; there is no "second-look" endoscopy needed; minor, uncomplicated surgery is conducted; and a 2-day hospital stay results ($4,500). The other 20% of the time, a "second-look" endoscopy is needed due to excessive bleeding, the surgery is more complicated, and a 3-day hospital stay results ($6,500).

For each patient, the average cost would be $4,900 [(0.8 × $4,500) + (0.2 × $6,500)]

For each patient, the average QALY would be 0.88 [(0.8 × 0.9 QALY) + (0.2 × 0.8 QALY)]

6. Calculate the average cost per QALY for each option (no Gastromycin and use of IV Gastromycin).
7. Calculate the incremental cost-utility ratio for IV Gastromycin compared with usual care (no Gastromycin).
8. If OPTION A (no Gastromycin) is the standard treatment, Place an X in the cell that represents the comparison of OPTION B (IV Gastromycin) to the standard (OPTION A).

Cost Outcome	Lower Cost	Same Cost	Higher Cost
Lower outcome			
Same outcome			
Better outcome			

9. If a threshold of $20,000 is used as the value of a QALY, do calculations indicate that IV Gastromycin is a cost-effective option?
10. If a threshold of $50,000 is used as the value of a QALY, do calculations indicate that IV Gastromycin is a cost-effective option?
11. Are the results sensitive to this range of values ($20,000 to $50,000)? Why or why not?

REFERENCES

1. Kaplan RM. Utility assessment for estimating quality-adjusted life years. In Sloan FA (ed). *Valuing Health Care: Costs, Benefits, and Effectiveness of Pharmaceuticals and Other Medical Technologies*. Cambridge: Cambridge University Press, 1995.
2. Murray CJ, Lopez A. Quantifying disability: Data, methods and results. *Bulletin of the World Health Organization* 72(3):481–494, 1994.
3. Sassi F. Calculating QALYs, comparing QALY and DALY calculations. *Health Policy and Planning* 21(5):402–408, 2006.
4. Morrison G. HYE (healthy years equivalent) and TTO (time trade-off): What is the difference? *Journal of Health Economics* 16(5):563–578, 1997.
5. Ried W. QALYs versus HYEs—What's right and what's wrong: A review of the controversy. *Journal of Health Economics* 17(5):607–625, 1998.
6. McGregor M, Caro J. QALYs: Are they helpful to decision makers? *Pharmacoeconomics* 24(10):947–952, 2006.
7. Neumann P, Greenberg D. Is the United States ready for QALYs? *Health Affairs (Project Hope)* 28(5):1366–1371, 2009.
8. Whitehead SJ, Ali S. Health outcomes in economic evaluation: The QALY and utilities. *Br Med Bull* 96(1):5–21, 2010.

9. Drummond MF, Sculpher MJ, Torrance GW, et al. *Methods for the Economic Evaluation of Health Care Programmes* (3rd ed.). Oxford: Oxford University Press, 2005.

10. Dolan P, Gudex C, Kind P, Williams A. Valuing health states: A comparison of methods. *Journal of Health Economics* 15(2):209–231, 1996.

11. Stevens KJ, McCabe CJ, Brazier, J. Mapping between Visual Analogue Scale and Standard Gamble data; results from the UK Health Utilities Index 2 valuation survey. *Health Economics* 15(5):527–533, 2006.

12. Lenert LA. The reliability and internal consistency of an internet capable computer program for measuring health utilities. *Quality of Life Research* 9(7):811–817, 2000.

13. Schackman BR, Teixeira PA, Weitzman G, Mushlin AI, Jacobson I. Quality-of-life tradeoffs for hepatitis C treatment: Do patients and providers agree? *Medical Decision Making: An International Journal of the Society for Medical Decision Making* 28(2):233–242, 2008.

14. Stamuli E. Health outcomes in economic evaluation: Who should value health? *Br Med Bull* 97(1):197–210, 2011.

15. Severens JL, Milne R. Discounting health outcomes in economic evaluation: The ongoing debate. *Value in Health: The Journal of the International Society for Pharmacoeconomics and Outcomes Research* 7(4):397–401, 2004.

16. Brauer C, Rosen A, Greenberg D, Neumann P. Trends in the measurement of health utilities in published cost-utility analyses. *Value in Health: The Journal of the International Society for Pharmacoeconomics and Outcomes Research* 9(4).213–218, 2006.

17. .Neumann P, Fang C, Cohen J. 30 years of pharmaceutical cost-utility analyses: Growth, diversity and methodological improvement. *Pharmacoeconomics* 27(10), 861–872, 2009.

18. Schackman BR, Gold HT, Stone PW, Neumann P. How often do sensitivity analyses for economic parameters change cost-utility analysis conclusions? *Pharmacoeconomics* 22(5): 293–300, 2004.

SUGGESTED READINGS

Brinsmead R, Hill S. Use of pharmacoeconomics in prescribing research. Part 4: Is cost-utility analysis a useful tool? *Journal of Clinical Pharmacy and Therapeutics* 28(4):339–346, 2003

Deverill M, Brazier J, Green C, Booth A. The use of QALY and non-QALY measures of health-related quality of life: Assessing the state of the art. *Pharmacoeconomics* 13(4):411–420, 1998.

Green C, Brazier J, Deverill M. Valuing health-related quality of life. A review of health state valuation techniques. *Pharmacoeconomics* 17(2):151–165, 2000.

Kattan MW. Comparing treatment outcomes using utility assessment for health-related quality of life. *Oncology* 17(12):1687–1701, 2003.

Raisch DW. Understanding quality-adjusted life years and their application to pharmacoeconomic research. *Annals of Pharmacotherapy* 34:906–914, 2000.

Stone PW, Teutsch S, Chapman RH, et al. Cost-utility analyses of clinical preventive services: Published ratios, 1976–1997. *American Journal of Preventive Medicine* 19(1):15–23, 2000.

Moving the QALY Forward: Building a Pragmatic Road. *Value in Health-Special Issue* 12(suppl): S27–S30, 2009.

Torrance G. Measurement of health state utilities for economic appraisal. *Journal of Health Economics* 5(1):1–30, 1986.

Chapter 7

Cost-Benefit Analysis[*]

Objectives

Upon completing this chapter, the reader will be able to:

1. Define and describe cost-benefit analysis (CBA).

2. Address the advantages and disadvantages of CBA.

3. Discuss the methods of measuring productivity and intangible costs, including the human capital (HC) and the willingness-to-pay (WTP) approaches.

4. Compare three types of calculation methods used with CBA: net benefits (or net costs), benefit-to-cost (or cost-to-benefit) ratios, and internal rate of return (IRR).

5. Critique a CBA composite article.

✦ DEFINITION AND HISTORY

As mentioned in Chapter 1, **cost-benefit analysis** (CBA) compares both costs and benefits in monetary units. The theoretical roots of CBA stem from welfare economics. Welfare economics is used to help make decisions regarding public policy by incorporating individual preferences and values to improve social welfare while balancing the effective use of resources.[1] Early social welfare issues in which CBA was used included setting environmental policy. In the 1800s and 1900s, CBA methodology was first used to help set policy for water projects such as irrigation and flood control.[2] CBA was later applied to other public goods such as wildlife, air quality, public parks, and health care. The first use of CBA in health care dates back to the 1960s.[3] In 1961, Weisbrod[4] assessed the costs and benefits of a vaccination

---

[*] This chapter is adapted with the permission of the American College of Clinical Pharmacy from the following *source:* Barner JC, Rascati KL. Cost-benefit analysis. In Grauer DW, Lee J, Odom TD, et al. (eds). *Pharmacoeconomics and Outcomes: Applications for Patient Care* (2nd ed.). Kansas City, MO: American College of Clinical Pharmacy, 2003: 115–132.

program for children in which the benefits of the program were monetized by using wages to value lost productivity and reduced survival. (Note: This is referred to as the **human capital** (HC) approach, which is discussed in more detail later.)

✦ ADVANTAGES AND DISADVANTAGES OF COST-BENEFIT ANALYSIS

An advantage of this type of analysis is that many different outcomes can be compared as long as the outcomes measures are valued in monetary units. The disadvantage is that placing economic values on medical outcomes is not an easy task and there is no universal agreement on one standard method for accomplishing this.

To illustrate the advantage of CBA compared with **cost-effectiveness analysis** (CEA), Table 7.1 shows examples of various programs and interventions and their corresponding cost-effectiveness and cost-benefit ratios. (CBA ratios are expressed as **benefit-to-cost ratios,** where the higher the number, the more cost-beneficial.) Assume you are a decision maker and you must choose one program from Table 7.1 to implement in your organization. Assume that you only had **cost-effectiveness ratios** available to help make the choice. How would you choose? One can quickly see that it would be difficult to compare the programs using only cost-effectiveness ratios because of the varying outcomes (e.g., case prevented, life years saved). On the other hand, the benefit-to-cost ratios can be ranked, and programs with similar, as well as dissimilar, outcomes can be compared. In addition, the decision maker can determine which programs' costs will exceed the benefits and vice versa. If the goal of the decision maker is to maximize the investment, the program with the highest benefit-to-cost ratio (in this case, diabetes medication adherence program) would be chosen. If only the cost-effectiveness ratios were available, it would be more difficult to compare the value of the various interventions.

As the cost of health care continues to increase, many decision makers must make choices regarding which programs will be implemented. Pharmacists are working in many areas of health care providing clinical services and developing specialty clinics in areas such as anticoagulation, diabetes, asthma, osteoporosis,

TABLE 7.1. **COMPARISON OF COST-EFFECTIVENESS RATIOS AND BENEFIT-TO-COST RATIOS**[a]

Program or Intervention	Cost-Effectiveness Ratio	Benefit-to-Cost Ratio
AIDS prevention and awareness program	$230,000/case prevented	8.4:1
Vaccination program for children	$104,000/case prevented	0.3:1
Smoking cessation intervention	$3,700/quit	6.7:1
Diabetes medication adherence program	$67/normoglycemic patient	15.1:1
Breast cancer screening program	$50,000/life year saved	2.4:1

[a]Cost-effectiveness analyses commonly use cost-effectiveness ratios, which are based on the costs of treatment divided by benefits of the treatment. Lower ratios indicate lower costs and are therefore the preferred options. Cost-benefit analyses use benefit-to-cost ratios, which are based on monetary benefits divided by monetary costs. Ratios higher than 1 indicate that the option is cost beneficial. In addition, higher ratios indicate higher benefits for each dollar spent and therefore are preferred over lower ratios. This table indicates an advantage of using benefit-to-cost ratios compared with cost-effectiveness ratios. Because the health outcomes (the denominator) used to calculate cost-effectiveness ratios are measured using different units, it is difficult to compare the programs to determine which one is most cost-effective.

and HIV and AIDS. Although clinical pharmacy programs have shown improvements in clinical outcomes such as glycemic control and bone density, financial pressures are forcing decision makers to consider the following questions: Do the benefits of a program or intervention outweigh the costs? Which program will provide the greatest benefit? CBA is a tool that can be used to address these questions.

The unique aspect of placing a monetary value on the outcome or benefit in CBA also presents a challenge or disadvantage of the method. For example, when comparing the cost-effectiveness ratios for an AIDS prevention and awareness program with the vaccination program for children, it would appear that the vaccination program would be the most cost-effective. But, when examining the benefit-to-cost ratios, the AIDS program is more cost-beneficial. CBA uses methods (which are discussed in more detail later) to value morbidity or mortality lost from a human life. In this example, the benefit (case prevented) was valued higher for AIDS patients than vaccinations for children. The controversy arises regarding the methodology used to place a dollar value on a case prevented or a human life. Thus, the advantage of placing a dollar value on the benefit or outcome is also a disadvantage of the method.

✦ CONDUCTING A CBA

The first step in a CBA is to determine the type of program or intervention to be considered. The second step is to identify alternatives. In many cases, the alternative is to "do nothing." In other cases, the alternative could be to implement a similar program that is smaller or larger in scale or to implement a different program. For example, a clinical pharmacist would like to start an asthma clinic. The alternative could be to compare the costs and benefits of having an asthma clinic with not having an asthma clinic. Another alternative could be to compare implementing an asthma clinic for all persons who had an asthma-related emergency department visit. A third alternative could be to compare implementing an asthma clinic with implementing a diabetes clinic.

To illustrate the components of a CBA, we will use the example of an asthma clinic. The clinic will focus on people with asthma who have had an asthma-related emergency department visit. These people would automatically be referred to a clinical pharmacist, who would provide education on managing asthma. These clinical pharmacy services could include education on triggers, medication adherence, and the use of peak flow meters and inhalers. In this example, the alternative will be no asthma clinic. After the program or intervention and alternatives are identified, the next step is to identify the costs and benefits.

Figure 7.1 shows the basic components of CBA. As shown, there are two categories of costs, **direct medical** and **direct nonmedical,** and three categories of benefits, **direct benefits** (both medical and nonmedical), **indirect benefits** (productivity), and **intangible benefits.** CBA can incorporate as few as one category of benefits or as many as all three of the benefit categories. When only direct medical benefits are measured, some researchers do not consider this to be a "true" CBA. It is sometimes categorized as a cost comparison or **cost analysis.** Some researchers only consider an analysis to be a "true" CBA if, in addition to the direct benefits, a monetary evaluation of the indirect benefits, **other sector** savings, or the actual health benefits (using, for example, **willingness-to-pay** [WTP] measures) are incorporated into the analysis.

Before starting any pharmacoeconomic analysis, it is important to determine the **perspective** of the study. Because of its focus on social welfare and

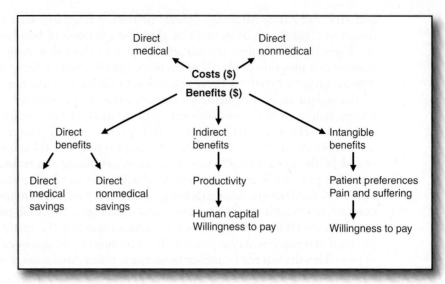

FIGURE 7.1.   Components of cost-benefit analysis (CBA). This schematic represents the types of costs measured when conducting a CBA. Input costs (the numerator) usually consist of direct medical and direct nonmedical costs. The benefits of alternatives can include measures of direct medical and nonmedical costs avoided, indirect costs avoided (measured by human capital [HC] or willingness-to-pay [WTP] methods) and intangible costs avoided (measured by patient preferences or WTP methods). (Adapted with permission from the American College of Clinical Pharmacy. Barner JC, Rascati KL. Cost-benefit analysis. In Grauer DW, Lee J, Odom TD, et al. (eds). *Pharmacoeconomics and Outcomes: Applications for Patient Care* (2nd ed.). Kansas City, MO: American College of Clinical Pharmacy, 2003:115–132.)

policy and the incorporation of indirect (productivity) or intangible benefits, economists recommend that CBAs should be conducted from the **societal perspective.**

✦ DIFFERENCE BETWEEN COSTS AND BENEFITS

In CBA, both costs and benefits are measured in dollar values. This can sometimes cause confusion because benefits are also "cost savings" or "costs avoided." As shown in Figure 7.1, costs and direct benefits are categorized as medical or nonmedical. For example, in the asthma program, a cost to the program could be an increase in medical costs related to visits to the pharmacy. A "cost saving" or benefit as a result of the program could be a reduction in medical costs for asthma-related emergency department visits. It is important to make the distinction between the two and to make sure that costs and benefits are properly placed within the equation.

✦ MEASURING INDIRECT AND INTANGIBLE BENEFITS

Various methods have been developed to estimate the monetary value of health benefits. The two most common methods seen in the pharmacoeconomic literature are the **HC** approach and the **WTP** approach, which are discussed in this chapter. Information on other, less common, methods for estimating the value of health outcomes (e.g., "implied values" and "revealed preferences") are discussed elsewhere.[5]

Human Capital Method

As indicated previously, indirect benefits are increases in productivity or earnings because of a program or intervention. The HC approach is one way to measure indirect benefits. HC estimates wage and productivity losses because of illness, disability, or death. The HC approach assumes that the value of health benefits equals the economic productivity that they permit. There are two basic components to calculating HC: wage rate and missed time (days or years) because of illness. Because the HC approach is based on wages, it is necessary to have some estimate of income. Income estimates can be obtained from several sources, including: the Census Bureau; the Bureau of Labor and Statistics; self-report; or any other data source that provides income estimates based on gender, age, or occupation. Missed time (days or years) because of illness can be obtained by self-report.

Wage Rate Calculations

Depending on the type of study, a yearly wage rate or a daily wage rate can be calculated. A yearly wage rate (income per year) would be calculated for a program or intervention that would reduce long-term disability or death. For example, a pneumococcal vaccination program might result in preventing premature death. Thus, it would be appropriate to use a yearly wage rate and assess the value of the number of years saved because of the intervention. Note that income or wages should include fringe benefits.

A daily wage rate (income per year divided by number of days worked per year) may be calculated for a program or intervention targeted at an acute or chronic illness with short-term disability. A person may not be adversely affected by the disease state on a continual basis, but he or she may have short-term periodic disability. For example, asthma, a chronic disease state, may include episodic asthma attacks. Thus, a person may only experience problems with the disease state on a periodic basis. For this type of disease state, a daily wage rate would be calculated. To calculate a daily wage rate both income and number of days worked per year must be assessed. We may assume that the average person works 240 days a year when accounting for weekends, vacation, and sick leave. A formula to calculate number of days worked per year is:

Number of days in a year (365) − Number of weekend days (104) − Number of vacation days (14) − Number of sick-leave days (7) = 240.

Missed Time (Days or Years) Because of Illness

If a yearly wage rate is calculated, then assessment of the number of years lost because of a disease or illness must be made. If a daily wage rate is calculated, an assessment of the number of missed days because of illness must be calculated. Because many pharmaceutical interventions involve chronic disease states with intermittent episodes, we will use an example calculating the daily wage rate and number of missed days. Missed days because of illness can fall into four groups

TABLE 7.2. **CATEGORIES OF MISSED DAYS**

Categories	Examples
Missed work	Days missed from work (for employed)
Missed housekeeping	Days missed from housekeeping (for unemployed)
Restricted activity days	Percent of time during which work or housekeeping was restricted
	Did not miss an entire day of work or housekeeping but not productive for part of the day
Caregiver time	Parent's time spent as a caregiver to a child who has an illness

(Table 7.2). Notice that for housekeeping and child care, estimates of productivity loss are estimated (imputed) even though no payments are directly associated with these activities.

Using the asthma clinic example, we will calculate an indirect benefit. Assume that the population served by the clinic is made up of adults with an average income (including fringe benefits) of $40,000 and 240 days worked per year. The daily wage rate (average income/number of days worked per year) would be $40,000/240 = $167/day. An average of 20 days a year were missed from work before participating in the asthma clinic, and an average of 7 days a year were missed from work after participating in the asthma clinic. Multiplying the daily wage rate times the number of missed days results in the value of lost productivity. In other words, the value of 20 days lost from work is $3,340, and the value of 7 days lost from work is $1,169. The difference between before and after the program is $2,171, which is the cost savings or the indirect benefit of the program or intervention (see Table 7.3 for the calculation).

Advantages and Disadvantages of the HC Method

Measuring indirect benefits using the HC approach has several advantages. It is fairly straightforward and easy to measure. Income estimates can be obtained or estimated from publicly available sources, and days lost from illness can be readily obtained from the patient or another secondary source.

The HC approach also has several disadvantages. The primary concern with using the HC approach is that it may be biased against specific groups of people, namely unemployed individuals. It assumes that if a person is not working, he or she has little or no economic benefit. Children and unemployed elderly individuals are two groups with which bias can occur.

The HC assumption that the value of health benefits equals the economic productivity they permit may also be biased. The earnings for some individuals

TABLE 7.3. **CALCULATION OF INDIRECT BENEFIT (MISSED WORK)**

Daily Wage Rate	Average Number of Missed Days per Year	Average Value of Lost Productivity ($)
Before: $167	20	3,340
After: $167	7	1,169

Indirect benefit per person = $2,171 (value of increased productivity).

may not equal the value of their output. For example, there is a large difference between the daily wage rate of a professional football player compared with that of an elementary school teacher. Some contend that because the underlying goal of using CBA is to measure the effect of an intervention on society, the HC approach is meant to measure the loss of productivity to society. Thus, wage rates should be based on those of the average population, not the specific patients included in a study. Although using general wage rates would not represent actual productivity losses or benefits to a specific group of patients, it would decrease some of the limitations of inequity already mentioned.

The HC method also does not incorporate values for pain and suffering if these values do not impact productivity. There may be certain disease states or conditions (e.g., menopause, hair loss) that may not impact productivity but do have an impact on a person's **health-related quality of life.** For example, many women experience problems with menopause, including moodiness, hot flashes, and irregular cycles. Although this condition may have a significant impact on quality of life, most women do not miss many days of work because of complications from menopause. Thus, the HC method would not be sensitive enough to capture the benefits of a pharmacist-provided menopause clinic. Although biases exist with this method, it is the most commonly used method to measure indirect benefits.

Willingness-to-Pay Method

The WTP method can value both the indirect and intangible aspects of a disease or condition. The WTP method determines how much people are willing to pay to reduce the chance of an adverse health outcome. The WTP method is grounded in welfare economic theory, and it incorporates patient preferences and intangible benefits such as quality of life differences. **Contingent valuation** (CV), in which the respondent is asked to value a contingent or hypothetical market, is a direct method that is used to elicit the dollar values or the WTP amounts. WTP values can be collected through face-to-face interviews, mail, telephone, or via the Internet. To elicit WTP values, respondents are presented with a hypothetical market describing the benefits of a particular health care intervention (e.g., program, pharmaceutical, medical device). Respondents are then asked to value the health care intervention in a dollar amount, percent of income, or health care premium. Measuring WTP using the CV method should include two general elements, a hypothetical scenario and a bidding vehicle. Cummings et al.[6] and Mitchell and Carson[7] provide additional information on CV.

Hypothetical Scenario

The hypothetical scenario should include a description of the health care program or intervention (e.g., **medication therapy management** program, new drug therapy). The intent of the scenario is to provide the respondent with an accurate description of the good or service that he or she is being asked to value. In addition, the scenario should detail the amount of time the person should expect to spend, as well as the benefit (e.g., percent improvement in the condition) of the intervention. An example of a hypothetical scenario for the asthma clinic might read:

ASTHMA CLINIC SCENARIO

Patients with asthma have improved their condition by learning more about their disease and by taking their medications as directed. Pharmacists can help people with asthma understand their condition and the medications used to treat it. In addition, they can:

- Help you learn how to use a peak flow meter and an inhaler.
- Help you better manage the medications used to treat asthma.
- Help you recognize and handle situations when asthma attacks occur.
- Monitor your asthma by keeping a record on file and following up with you on a regular basis to assess your progress.
- Contact your doctor and report any changes in your health.

An initial visit with your pharmacist would include an educational program on managing your disease state. This type of service is available by appointment only and would last approximately 1 hour. Assume that the program would result in a 50% improvement in your asthma.

Bidding Vehicles

After the program or intervention has been adequately described, respondents are then asked to "bid," or place a value on the program or intervention. Bids can be obtained through a variety of formats, such as open-ended questions, closed-ended questions, a bidding game, or a payment card. Below is a brief description of each of the methods.

Open-Ended Questions Open-ended questions simply ask respondents how much they would be WTP for the program or intervention. This question would immediately follow the hypothetical scenario. Here is an example:

What is the maximum amount that you would be willing to pay for a 1-hour consultation with a pharmacist? _____

The respondent would then write in their maximum WTP amount. This method is used the least because it results in WTP values that vary widely. Many people do not know how to value health care programs because they do not normally pay the full amount out of pocket. The other methods discussed below provide respondents with more guidance in determining their maximum WTP.

Closed-Ended Questions Closed-ended questions are also called "take-it-or-leave-it" or dichotomous choice questions. Respondents are asked whether or not they will pay a specified dollar amount for the program or intervention. Here is an example:

Would you be willing to pay $60 for a 1-hour consultation with a pharmacist?

___Yes___No

This method more closely resembles the marketplace. When consumers shop for products, they must decide based on the price of the product whether to "take-it-or-leave-it." One drawback to this method is that only one question is asked, so only one WTP value can be elicited from a respondent. Thus, a very large sample would be required to determine the overall WTP value.

Bidding Game The bidding game resembles an auction in that several bids are offered to reach a person's maximum WTP. Before soliciting a second response, the bids are adjusted based on the first response. This iteration could go on a number of times, but it is suggested that three times is optimal. Here is an example:

> Would you be willing to pay $60 for a 1-hour consultation with a pharmacist?
>
> ___Yes   If yes, ask: "Would you be willing to pay $80?"
>
> ___No   If no, ask: "Would you be willing to pay $40?"

This method is useful to try to arrive at a person's maximum WTP value. It is time consuming and is best conducted via a face-to-face interview or over the Internet. In addition, the WTP values can be biased depending on how high (or low) the first bid is. This is called "starting point bias."

Payment Card The payment card method provides the respondent with a list of possible WTP amounts (i.e., payment card) to choose from. Here is an example:

> What is the maximum amount that you would be willing to pay for a 1-hour consultation with a pharmacist? Please circle your choice.
>
> | $150 | $90 | $30 |
> |------|-----|-----|
> | $130 | $70 | $10 |
> | $110 | $50 | $0 |

This method is very easy to use and it provides respondents with a range of values to choose from. The advantages of the method can also result in disadvantages. Providing respondents with a range of values can bias their WTP values. The range provided can "suggest" the value of the intervention and can influence what respondents say. Also, "range bias" can influence the WTP amount. For example, if the range of values was from $0 to $75 versus $0 to $150, the respondents' WTP amount can vary depending on which range or starting point was provided.

National Oceanic and Atmospheric Administration Recommendations

The National Oceanic and Atmospheric Administration (NOAA)[8] convened an expert panel to determine guidelines for conducting **CV** studies to determine WTP. Although the organization is primarily concerned with environmental issues, its recommendations apply to the health care sector. NOAA recommends face-to-face interviews and the dichotomous choice (closed-ended) bidding vehicle. Face-to-face interviews are very time consuming and may be cost prohibitive for some researchers. The use of the dichotomous choice format requires a large sample size to accommodate the varying bid levels. Although these are the preferred methods, most studies in the literature have used mail surveys and the payment card format.

Advantages and Disadvantages of the Willingness-to-Pay Method

The main advantage of the WTP approach is that it is a method to place a dollar value on intangible benefits. It is also grounded in welfare economic theory, which embodies patient preferences and choice. However, there are several disadvantages to the WTP methodology. Many critics question the validity of the WTP responses because of the various methods used to elicit dollar values as well as the hypothetical nature of the health care benefit. It is difficult for people to place a dollar value on a health benefit or an increase in health-related quality of life or satisfaction. Because a "hypothetical" or artificial scenario is presented, it is possible that respondents might give a "hypothetical response" or that the respondent may not understand the value of the market (e.g., pharmaceutical care program) being presented. It has been noted that when directly measuring monetary values, there is a difference between a person's WTP for a benefit and his/her willingness to accept (WTA) compensation to forgo the same benefit.[9] The methodological development for collecting **valid** and **reliable** WTP values is ongoing.

Another disadvantage of this method includes the biases involved in measuring WTP. "Compliance bias" occurs when respondents want to "please" the interviewer and may overstate their WTP values. Strategic bias occurs when respondents over- or understate their WTP values to strategically impact the outcome. For example, a respondent may understate a WTP value so that they will not have to pay as much. Other biases with the bidding vehicles (e.g., range bias, starting point bias) were explained previously.

✦ CALCULATING RESULTS OF COSTS AND BENEFITS

After all costs and benefits have been identified and quantified, the results of the analysis must be presented in ways that help decision makers understand the value of the program or intervention. CBA can be presented in the following three formats: **net benefit** calculations, benefit-to-cost ratios, and **internal rate of return** (IRR). When evaluating interventions, it is important to assess the method used. Another issue to consider when choosing a method for displaying the results is the time horizon for the project. If **retrospective data** are collected for more than 1 year or if the project inputs or outcomes are estimated for more than 1 year into the future, it is important to **adjust** or **discount** these costs to one point in time. (See Chapter 2 for examples of adjustment and discounting calculations.)

Net Benefit (or Net Cost) Calculations

The net benefit (or net cost) calculation simply presents the difference between the total costs and benefits. Net benefit = total benefits − total costs; Net cost = total costs − total benefits. Interventions would be considered to be cost-beneficial if:

$$\text{Net Benefit} > 0 \qquad \text{or} \qquad \text{Net Cost} < 0$$

Benefit-to-Cost (or Cost-to-Benefit) Ratio Calculations

CBA results can also be calculated by summing up the total benefits and dividing by the total costs. The ratio may be expressed as a benefit-to-cost ratio or a cost-to-benefit ratio. Depending on how the ratio is calculated, interventions are cost-beneficial if:

$$\text{Benefit-to-cost} > 1 \qquad \text{or} \qquad \text{Cost-to-benefit} < 1$$

Example Using Different Calculation Techniques

Suppose a decision maker had to choose between two proposals for implementation. Also assume that the projects are for 1 year, so discounting is not needed.

Proposal A: Cost = $1,000; Benefit = $2,000
Proposal B: Cost = $5,000; Benefit = $7,500

TABLE 7.4. COMPARISON OF TWO PROPOSALS USING NET AND RATIO CALCULATIONS

	Proposal A	Proposal B
Net benefit	$2,000 – $1,000 = $1,000	$7,500 – $5,000 = $2,500
Net cost	$1,000 – $2,000 = –$1,000	$5,000 – $7,500 = –$2,500
Benefit/cost ratio	$2,000/$1,000 = 2.0	$7,500/$5,000 = 1.5
Cost/benefit ratio	$1,000/$2,000 = 0.5	$5,000/$7,500 = 0.7

Table 7.4 shows the net and ratio calculations for both proposals. Although four calculations are shown in the table, the benefit-to-cost ratio (when compared with the cost-to-benefit ratio) and the net benefit calculation (when compared with the net cost calculation) are used most often because the higher the result, the more cost-beneficial an option becomes.

Using the criteria outlined above for cost-beneficial programs, it is apparent that both programs are cost-beneficial using both the net and ratio methods of calculations. However, when comparing net calculations, proposal B is more cost-beneficial than proposal A (net benefit = $2,500 versus $1,000), but proposal A is more cost-beneficial than proposal B (benefit-to-cost ratio = 2.0 versus 1.5) when using ratio calculations. Thus, the ratio and the net calculation may indicate that different options are the most beneficial.

In this example, in which both proposals are cost-beneficial, the decision maker may consider other issues, such as the amount of money available for investment. Whereas A would require $1,000 input costs, proposal B would require $5,000. Another consideration may involve the return on investment. Proposal A, with a 2:1 benefit-to-cost ratio, has a higher return than proposal B (i.e., 1.5:1 benefit-to-cost ratio). A third consideration is the actual net benefit amount. Proposal B has a higher net benefit than proposal A ($2,500 versus $1,000). The choice between proposal A and B would depend on the goals (both programmatic and financial) of the organization. Caution should be used when interpreting ratio calculations because even when using the same monetary estimates, results can change depending on whether some costs are placed in the numerator as input costs or the denominator as cost savings; this is not a problem when subtracting benefits minus costs in net calculations.

Internal Rate of Return

The internal rate of return (IRR) is the rate of return that equates the **present value** (PV) of benefits to the PV of costs (see Chapter 2 for PV calculations). The goal is to find the rate of return that would make the costs and benefits equal. After the IRR is calculated, it is compared with a specified **hurdle rate.** The decision rule for IRR is to accept all projects with an IRR greater than the hurdle rate. If the IRR is greater than the hurdle rate, then it means that the project can yield a higher rate of return compared with some other investment. For example, the IRR should be higher than the interest rates available for savings accounts or secured bonds.

IRR is difficult to calculate by hand. Computer programs and special functions on calculators are available for determining IRR. Assume that the IRR for the asthma pharmaceutical care program described above is 6.3%. If the market rate of return is 4.5% for other investments, this is the hurdle rate. Because 6.3%

IRR Calculation

$$NPV = 0; \text{ or PV of future cash flows} - \text{Initial Investment} = 0; \text{ or}$$

$$CF1 + CF2 + CF3 + \ldots - \text{Initial Investment} = 0$$

$$(1 + r)1 \; (1 + r)2 \; (1 + r)3$$

Where,

r is the internal rate of return,
CF1 is the period one net cash inflow,
CF2 is the period two net cash inflow,
CF3 is the period three net cash inflow, and so on.

But the problem is we cannot isolate the variable r on one side of the above equation. However, there are alternative procedures which can be followed to find IRR. The simplest of them is described below:

1. Guess the value of r and calculate the NPV of the project at that value.
2. If NPV is close to 0 then IRR is equal to r.
3. If NPV is greater than 0 then increase r and jump to step 5.
4. If NPV is smaller than 0 then decrease r and jump to step 5.
5. Recalculate NPV using the new value of r and go back to step 2.

Find the IRR of an investment having initial cash outflow of $200,000.
   The cash inflows = Year 1 =$60,000; Year 2 = $100,000; and Year 3 =$75,000 respectively.

Solution

Assume that r is 10%.
NPV at 10% discount rate = $193,539 − $200,000 = −$6,461
Since NPV is less than 0 we have to decrease discount rate, thus
NPV at 6% discount rate = $208,575 − $200,000 = +$8,575
But it is greater than 0 we have to increase the discount rate, thus
NPV at 8% discount rate = $200,826 − $200,000 = +$826 = close to 0
IRR ≈ 8%

exceeds 4.5%, the pharmaceutical care program should be chosen because it will yield a greater return, or greater value for every dollar invested. See Exhibit 7.1 for an example of an IRR calculation.

SUMMARY

CBA differs from other pharmacoeconomic methods in that both the costs and benefits are measured in dollars. CBA can be very useful in determining which program or intervention has the greatest benefit. In addition, it is a useful method for comparing multiple programs with varying outcomes. CBA values indirect benefits (productivity) using the HC approach and intangible benefits using the WTP approach. Both methods have several advantages and disadvantages, which can lead to biased or inaccurate estimates of indirect and intangible benefits. Because of the difficulties in measuring and in incorporating indirect and intangible benefits, many of the CBA studies in the literature measure **direct medical costs** and **direct medical benefits only.** As indicated previously, some do not consider this to be a "true" CBA. Example 7.1 summarizes an article that evaluates published CBAs.

A number of studies use **CV** or WTP methods without the incorporation of these results into a CBA. For example, the HC method may be used to estimate **indirect costs** in **cost-of-illness** studies (Example 7.2). Three types of calculations might be conducted to determine if an intervention is cost-beneficial: net calculations, ratio calculations, and IRR calculations. Although CBA has the advantage of monetarily valuing indirect and intangible benefits, this is also a disadvantage because of the difficulty involved in valuing outcomes such as productivity and improvement in health. Exhibit 7.2 provides a summary of the debate of using CBA compared with CEA.

EXAMPLE 7.1 EVALUATIONS OF COST-BENEFIT ANALYSES IN THE LITERATURE

Note: *This is a summary based on the article Zarnke KB, Levine MA, O'Brien BJ. Cost-benefit analyses in the health-care literature: Don't judge a study by its label. Journal of Clinical Epidemiology 50(7):813–822, 1997.*

The objective of this study was to evaluate published health care—related CBAs. The authors searched the literature from 1991 to 1995 to find articles that were labeled as a CBA in the title or the abstract. Ninety-five articles met their inclusion criteria. The most common application of CBA focused on five broad areas (these were not mutually exclusive): prevention strategies (58%), pharmaceuticals (25%), education and counseling (21%), screening strategies (18%), and diagnostic tests (17%). Prevention strategies included various types of vaccination programs for infections such as influenza and hepatitis B. Most of the studies that were categorized as pharmaceutical comparisons were studies that involved the vaccine in the prevention strategies studies. Education and counseling included both asthma and diabetes education programs. Screening strategies focused on cancer screenings, and more recently, screening for HIV and AIDS, particularly in pregnant women.

Of the 95 studies, only 30 (32%) were considered to be "true" CBAs, defined as placing a monetary value on the health outcomes. Most of these (21 articles or 70%) used the HC approach to value benefits, and only four used CV methods such as WTP. The other studies used a variety of methods (e.g., values implied from past decisions and court awards).

EXAMPLE 7.2 HUMAN CAPITAL CALCULATIONS USED WHEN DETERMINING THE BURDEN OF ILLNESS

Note: *This is a summary based on the article Wu EQ, Birnbaum HG, Shi L, Ball DE, et al. The economic burden of schizophrenia in the United States in 2002. Journal of Clinical Psychiatry 66(9):1122–1129, 2005.*

The objective of this study was to estimate annual US costs associated with schizophrenia. A societal perspective was used, and three types of costs were

(continues)

EXAMPLE 7.2   HUMAN CAPITAL CALCULATIONS USED WHEN
DETERMINING THE BURDEN OF ILLNESS (*Continued*)

estimated: (1) "direct medical costs"; (2) **other sector costs** (e.g., law enforcement, homeless shelters); and (3) indirect or productivity costs. Indirect costs were estimated using the HC approach. Market wages were used to calculate the cost of lost productivity from unemployment, reduced workplace productivity, premature mortality from suicide, and family caregiving. Annual costs in 2002 dollars were $22.7 billion in direct medical costs, $7.6 billion for non-health care sector costs, and $32.4 billion in indirect costs, indicating that productivity losses are a major cost component of this illness.

EXHIBIT 7.2

Debate on CBA versus CEA: Summary of article by Johnson [Why not real economics? *Pharmacoeconomics* 30(2):127–131, 2012] and response by Schulpher and Claxton [Real economics needs to reflect real decisions: A response to Johnson. *Pharmacoeconomics* 30(2):133–136, 2012].

Points made by Johnson for the use of CBA:

"Current health technology assessment (HTA) practice obscures efficiency-economic tradeoffs. Health economists' acceptance of CEA instead of CBA is a form of professional misfeasance."

- CBA has been criticized for ethical concerns of putting a value on a human life, but at least it is transparent about the valuation.

- It has been argued that CBA may increase the price of drugs, but if it provides for a more efficient use of resources, that is acceptable.

- CBA has been criticized based on the use of unreliable methods, but these methods have been used for 30 years in environmental and other public good sectors to make decisions.

- One disadvantage of CEA is that comparing the costs of options with the same efficacy still does not determine if any of the options are worth adopting.

Response by Schulpher and Claxton for the use of CEA:

Johnson's paper shows a misunderstanding of ". . . the distinction between CEA and CBA, and fails to identify the real points at issue between the conventional "welfarist" normative principles of economic evaluation and alternative approaches such as social decision making."

- Alternatives to QALY measurements to estimate benefits have been proposed and studied, but these alternatives have rarely been used in applied research, probably due to their practical limitations.

- The threshold of value should represent the health outcomes forgone due to the displacement of existing services to fund any additional cost of new technologies, so comparisons to current options are needed.

- "Welfarist" economics (CBA) is theory-driven. But can researchers really know all of the variables needed and can there really be a broad consensus on monetary values?

- "Social decision making" (CEA) is a more pragmatic view, and more likely to be used by decision makers.

COMPOSITE ARTICLE 1: CBA—VACCINATION

Title: COST-BENEFIT ANALYSIS OF A ROSEOLITIS VACCINATION FOR SENIOR PHARMACY STUDENTS IN THE UNITED STATES

INTRODUCTION: Many studies have highlighted the importance of vaccinating high-risk populations, including health care workers, against various diseases. In the United States, pharmacy students spend their senior year in pharmacy school going to various health care sites (rotations) to obtain experiential training. These students come in contact with many patients and are increasingly being required by their schools to be up-to-date on immunizations and vaccinations for various diseases, such as hepatitis B, influenza, measles, mumps, rubella, and varicella, before starting the first rotation.[1]

A new disease, similar to measles, called "roseolitis" is now being seen in the United States (don't worry; this is made up for the composite article) and is seen in about 1% of the general population per year. People at high risk for other communicable diseases (e.g., influenza, meningococcal disease, hepatitis), such as students living in dormitories, children in day care facilities, military personnel, patients with compromised immune systems, and health care professionals who have direct patient contact, also have a higher risk of contracting roseolitis, but the precise increase in incidence is not yet known for these groups. Symptoms include fever, headache, itching, swelling, and listlessness. The majority of patients (80%) recover fully within 1 week using medication to treat the symptoms (e.g., acetaminophen and antihistamines) and have no lasting effects of the disease. The other 20% develop a serious secondary infection, and about 3% of those with a serious infection die. A vaccine called RVac was developed to reduce the occurrence of roseolitis. (The real article would have clinical references here.)

The objective of this study was to conduct an economic analysis to determine if requiring all US senior pharmacy students to be vaccinated against roseolitis would be cost-beneficial.

METHODS: A CBA was conducted comparing the costs of routine vaccination in 2013 of the senior pharmacy students in the United States with the cost savings (or benefits) of the vaccine from both a payer and a societal perspective. Epidemiologic studies of the new disease have measured the overall incidence per year (1%), the percent of patients with the disease who have severe secondary infections (20%) and the percent with severe infections who die (3%). So far, there is no reason to believe that patients who recover from roselitis have any long-term health problems. It was assumed that pharmacy students would have twice the incidence of the general population.

The development of the vaccine is relatively new, and no information is available on its long-term effectiveness. Because we do not yet know the duration of protection afforded by the vaccine, we assessed all direct medical costs and savings for 1 year (the last year in pharmacy school) using 2013 US$ values.

Productivity costs were estimated using the HC approach. The value of potential future earnings of a pharmacist, $3.2 million, was estimated using PV calculations (3% discount rate) for the year 2013. Direct costs and outcome probabilities were estimated from previously published literature. (Remember this is a "composite" example, not a "real" research article. In a "real" research article, the authors should provide more in-depth detail as to where these estimates came from and how they were estimated.) Sensitivity analyses were conducted for the costs of the vaccine and its administration, the incidence of roseolitis in the senior pharmacy student population, and the effectiveness of the vaccine in preventing roseolitis.

RESULTS: There were approximately 8,000 first professional pharmacy degrees awarded in the United States in 2012, so we will assume this will be the number of seniors in 2013.

Exhibit 7.3 lists base estimates used to determine if it would be cost-beneficial to vaccinate pharmacy students for this disease. Benefit-to-cost ratios are presented (Exhibit 7.4) from the payer perspective (using direct medical costs only) and the societal perspective (including HC values). If only direct medical costs and savings are used to calculate the benefit-to-cost (B/C) ratio using base case assumptions, the ratio is 0.18:1, which means that for every dollar spent on the vaccine, only $0.18 would be saved from a reduction in direct medical treatment costs, indicating that from the payer's perspective, the vaccination is not cost-beneficial. If HC estimates are included in the B/C ratio, the result is now 6.3:1, which means that from a societal perspective, for every dollar spent, more than $6 would be saved, indicating the immunization from this perspective would be cost-beneficial. Exhibit 7.4 also lists the sensitivity analyses calculations using a range of assumptions. Because of the small sample of the population of interest coupled with the low mortality rate from the disease,

some ratios were not calculated. When the difference in the number of deaths was less than one, calculations of productivity cost savings may not be valid. For all sensitivity analyses, the vaccination was not cost-beneficial from a purely payer perspective (range B/C, 0.09 to 0.36) but was cost-beneficial when indirect savings were included (range B/C, 3.6 to 12.6).

CONCLUSIONS: From a societal perspective, the use of the new RVac vaccine to prevent roseolitis in senior US pharmacy students was cost-beneficial, but from a health care payer's perspective, it was not. If a prevention technique is shown to be effective as well as cost saving, it would be readily implemented. However, measures that are not cost-beneficial may also be recommended for implementation based on more complex factors, including relief of pain and suffering and priorities of the public and decision makers. Although all 8,000 senior pharmacy students must be vaccinated to save one life, the value of the one life more than offsets the cost of the 8,000 vaccinations.

EXHIBIT 7.3

Base Case Assumptions

	Without Vaccine	With Vaccine	Difference
Costs			
Cost of vaccine	—	8,000 × $50 = $400,000	$400,000
Administration of vaccine	—	8,000 × $15 = $120,000	$120,000
Total vaccination costs	—		$520,000
Benefits			
Number of cases of roseolitis: 90% effectiveness	8,000 × 0.02 = 160	8,000 × 0.02 × .1 = 16	144 cases avoided
Cost for treatment: $50/doctor visit + $10 medication	160 × $60 = $9,600	16 × $60 = $960	$8,640 saved
Number of severe infections	160 × 0.20 = 32	16 × 0.20 = 3.2	28.8 infections avoided
Cost of infection: $3,000	32 × $3,000 = $96,000	3.2 × $3,000 = $9,600	$86,400 saved
Total direct medical savings $95,040			
Lives saved	32 × 0.03 = 1 life	3.2 × 0.03 = 0.1 life	1 life = $3,200,000
Total direct and indirect savings			$3,295,040

EXHIBIT 7.4

Sensitivity Analyses

	Benefit/Cost Ratio: Payer Perspective	Benefit/Cost Ratio: Societal Perspective
Base case	$95,040 / $520,000 = 0.18	$3,295,040 / $520,000 = 6.3
Cost of vaccine (base = $50)		
$20	0.34	11.8
$100	0.10	3.6
Cost of administration (base = $15)		
$0	0.24	8.2
$30	0.15	5.1
Incidence (base = 2%)		
1%	0.09	a
4%	0.36	12.6
Effectiveness of vaccine (base = 90%)		
50%	0.10	a
100%	0.20	6.4

[a]Sample size too small for meaningful results.

REFERENCE

1. Kirschenbaum HL, Kalis ML. Immunization and other health requirements for students at colleges and schools of pharmacy in the United States and Puerto Rico. *American Journal of Pharmaceutical Education* 65:35–40, 2001.

WORKSHEET FOR CRITIQUE OF CEA COMPOSITE ARTICLE 1

1. Complete Title?

    _____

    _____

    _____

    _____

2. Clear Objective?

    _____

    _____

    _____

    _____

3. Appropriate Alternatives?

_____

_____

_____

_____

4. Alternatives Described?

_____

_____

_____

_____

5. Perspective Stated?

_____

_____

_____

_____

6. Type of Study?

_____

_____

_____

_____

7. Relevant Costs?

_____

_____

_____

_____

8. Relevant Outcomes?

_____

_____

_____

_____

9. Adjustment or Discounting?

_____

_____

_____

_____

10. Reasonable Assumptions?

_____

_____

_____

_____

11. Sensitivity Analyses?

_____

_____

_____

_____

12. Limitations Addressed?

_____

_____

_____

_____

13. Generalizations Appropriate?

_____

_____

_____

_____

14. Unbiased Conclusions?

_____

_____

_____

_____

CRITIQUE OF CBA COMPOSITE ARTICLE 1

1. **Complete Title:** The title did identify the type of study (CBA), what was being assessed (vaccinating for roseolitis), and the population of interest (US senior pharmacy students).

2. **Clear Objective:** The objective of this study was "to conduct an economic analysis to determine if requiring all US senior pharmacy students to be vaccinated against roseolitis was cost-beneficial." This was clear.

3. **Appropriate Alternatives:** This was an example of a "with-or-without" study. The alternatives were to implement routine vaccination for every senior

pharmacy student versus no vaccinations for this group of students. For other vaccination studies, you may see comparisons of vaccinating high-risk populations versus vaccinating everyone or vaccinations at infancy versus vaccinations as an adolescent or adult. Appropriate epidemiologic literature should be cited to validate the choices of alternatives that are most clinically relevant.

4. **Alternatives Described:** The dosing and scheduling of dosing was not described. Readers might assume there was a standard adult dose given to each student. If this new vaccine was given at the same time as other vaccines or immunizations that the students routinely receive, the administration cost might be negligible. The sensitivity analysis using an estimate of $0 for the administration fee shows that this fee makes little difference in the results.

5. **Perspective Stated:** The perspective of the study was explicitly stated as both the payer (which included measuring direct medical costs and savings only) and that of society (which included indirect, or productivity, savings).

6. **Type of Study:** The study was correctly identified as a CBA because outcomes were valued in monetary units as cost savings. Some researchers would not consider the calculations of only direct medical costs and saving as a complete, or true, CBA because intangibles and indirect costs were not included.

7. **Relevant Costs:** It may become more complex to answer this question about CBAs because both inputs and outcomes are measured in dollars. Input costs (left-hand side of pharmacoeconomic equation; Fig. 1.1 in Chapter 1) of the vaccination program included the cost of the vaccine and the cost of administering the vaccine: these are appropriate input costs. Costs to treat any side effects from the vaccine (e.g., redness at site of injection) might have also been included. The authors should have mentioned why these were not included (maybe they were rare or mild). Other costs differences, such as treating secondary infections, were categorized as outcome-related costs savings, or benefits (right-hand side of PE equation), and are addressed by the next question.

8. **Relevant Outcomes:** Outcomes of the vaccine were measured by subtracting the estimated number of health consequences expected with the vaccine from the expected number without the vaccine. The direct medical costs of treating the disease ($60) and treating the secondary infection ($3,000) were multiplied by the number of events avoided as a result of the vaccine. Indirect, or productivity, savings were estimated using the HC approach ($3.2 million per life saved). Intangible costs of pain and suffering and lost productivity for the recovery period were not measured. The time period for data estimation was appropriate.

9. **Adjustment or Discounting:** All direct medical costs were valued in 2013 US dollars. Discounting was used when estimating the value of a pharmacy student's life by determining the net PV of future earnings by the student (indirect benefit).

10. **Reasonable Assumptions:** Because much of the data were not available, many assumptions were made to estimate the B/C ratios. The incidence in this population was assumed to be double the rate of the general population. Based on other similar diseases, this seems reasonable. All costs and consequences of those that survived the disease were assumed to occur in a 1-year time period. It is probable that protection against the new disease from the vaccine lasted for more than 1 year, so savings from future benefits may have been underestimated.

11. **Sensitivity Analyses:** Sensitivity analyses were conducted for the cost of the vaccine and its administration, the efficacy rate of the vaccine, and the incidence of the disease in the senior pharmacy student population. Sensitivity analyses were not conducted on the percentage that had a secondary infection as a result of the disease, the percent of deaths due to the secondary infection, or the value of a life. From the societal perspective, the biggest factor in the calculations was the value attributed to saving a life. If even one life was saved, the benefits were valued at more than six times the cost. On the other hand, for a wide range of assumptions, vaccination was not cost-beneficial from a payer's perspective.

12. **Limitations Addressed:** The authors did not directly address any limitations. Because much of the information used in the equations was not available for the new vaccine, this should have been stated in the limitations. The small sample size was another limitation. When sensitivity analyses were conducted on this small sample, some calculations were not realistic. Intangible costs, such as pain and suffering, were not included in this analysis. If the authors had used a WTP technique, the students may have been willing to pay the whole amount of the vaccine to reduce the probability of becoming sick. If this was the case, the benefit-to-cost ratio may have been higher than one without including the HC valuations.

13. **Generalizations Appropriate:** The authors did not try to extrapolate beyond the population of interest or the year of the study (senior US pharmacy students in 2013).

14. **Unbiased Conclusions:** The authors maintain that even when direct medical savings are less than direct medical costs, payers still consider the intervention and weigh other factors into their decision. If the readers accept that one life would be saved per year as a result of the vaccination of about 8,000 students per year, the societal benefits would far exceed the costs of the program.

COMPOSITE ARTICLE 2: CBA–ALZHEIMER'S DISEASE

Title: WILLINGNESS TO PAY FOR DELAY IN PROGRESSION OF ALZHEIMER'S DISEASE BY UNPAID CAREGIVERS

BACKGROUND: Alzheimer's disease (AD) is a chronic neurodegenerative disorder involving progressive loss of memory and other cognitive functions, personality and behavioral changes, and ability to carry out usual activities. Over time AD leads to a loss of independence and institutionalization is often required. The cost of AD in terms of the burden on family and caregivers is high. Over 5 million Americans have Alzheimer's disease, treatment costs were estimated at $200 Billion in the US in 2012, and unpaid care by relatives and other caregivers amounts to another $210 billion (http://www.alz.org/alzheimers_disease_facts_and_figures.asp [accessed December 30, 2012]).

OBJECTIVE: This study aimed to measure the cost-benefit of a potential new medication that slows the progression of AD, from the perspective of a nonpaid caregiver.

METHODS: In 2012, a sample of 100 staff members and 100 professors at a local university were recruited to answer a hypothetical question about a new (theoretical) AD medication. The scenario (Exhibit 7.5) included a slowing of AD progression with minor, tolerable, adverse events from the medication. They were asked what they would be WTP for year's supply of this medication (assuming it was not covered by medical insurance).

EXHIBIT 7.5

Assume You Are a Caregiver to an Elderly Relative

Starting point

The patient has a diagnosis of mild Alzheimer's disease plus behavioral and psychological symptoms of dementia. He has problems in the following areas: decreased knowledge of current and recent events (e.g., not realizing a major election is taking place); some deficit in memory of his personal history (e.g., forgetting the name of a previous employer); difficulty concentrating; decreased ability to travel, handle finances, etc. He shows no problems in the following areas: orientation to time and place, recognition of familiar persons and faces, and ability to travel to familiar locations. He now requires help with complex occupational and social tasks (e.g., handling finances, planning dinner parties) but can still survive in the community. When family asks him, he denies that anything is wrong. He also shows a flat mood and withdrawal from challenging situations. He is generally happy and interested in life.

Likely outcome after 1 year with no treatment

After 1 year, the patient has the following symptoms: The Alzheimer's disease has progressed and he can no longer survive without some assistance. He is now unable to recall some major relevant aspects of his current life including his address and telephone number, names of his grandchildren and the name of the university he graduated from. He always knows his own name and is usually able to remember the names of his wife and children. He still retains knowledge of many major facts regarding himself and others. He shows some disorientation to time (e.g., date, day of the week, season) and to place. He has difficulty counting back from 40 by fours or from 20 by twos. He now requires assistance with choosing the proper clothing to wear but does not require assistance with toileting or eating. In addition, he shows delusion behavior (once or twice daily he accuses his spouse of being an impostor or thinks that people are stealing things from him), pacing (he frequently walks around the house without purpose), anxiety (several times a day he is afraid to be left alone) and inappropriate physical aggression once or twice a week. He is frequently up all night and must be supervised carefully.

Likely outcome after 1 year with treatment

The patient is currently receiving treatment for these symptoms. His drug therapy involves taking one tablet once per day. He saw the prescribing physician every 2 weeks for a month and then monthly for 3 months, and now he sees him/her only every 3 months. After taking this medication daily for 1 year, he continues to show problems in the same areas, *but the problems have not progressed*. He showed an initial improvement and now, 1 year later, is back where he started.

Adverse effects

In addition, the medication makes him feel queasy, unsteady on his feet and dizzy. These symptoms make him uncomfortable but he has been tolerating them.

Putting yourself in the place of the patient's caregiver, what is the total amount you would be willing to pay for this treatment for 1 year, taking into consideration these adverse effects, to avoid his progressing to the more severe stage?

Adapted from: Wu G, Lanctôt KL, Herrmann N, Moosa S, Oh P. The cost-benefit of cholinesterase inhibitors in mild to moderate dementia: A willingness-to-pay approach. *CNS Drugs* 17(14);1045–1057, 2003.

RESULTS: The mean yearly WTP for this scenario was $5,000 (95% CI 3,000 to 10,000) for staff and $9,000 (95% CI 4,000 to $20,000) for professors. If the cost for a new medication that met this profile was less than $5,000 per year, the majority of caregivers would find it of value.

LIMITATIONS: The sample of respondents was recruited from one location, and may not be representative of the general population. In addition, current caregivers might give different WTP estimates based on their experiences in coping with an AD patient.

CONCLUSIONS: Unpaid caregivers would be willing to pay a significant amount out of pocket to delay the progression of AD.

WORKSHEET FOR CRITIQUE OF CBA COMPOSITE ARTICLE 2

1. Complete Title?

_____

_____

_____

_____

2. Clear Objective?

_____

_____

_____

_____

3. Appropriate Alternatives?

_____

_____

_____

_____

4. Alternatives Described?

_____

_____

_____

_____

5. Perspective Stated?

_____

_____

_____

_____

6. Type of Study?

_____

_____

_____

7. Relevant Costs?

_____

_____

_____

_____

8. Relevant Outcomes?

_____

_____

_____

_____

9. Adjustment or Discounting?

_____

_____

_____

_____

10. Reasonable Assumptions?

_____

_____

_____

_____

11. Sensitivity Analyses?

_____

_____

_____

_____

12. Limitations Addressed?

_____

_____

_____

_____

13. Generalizations Appropriate?

_____

_____

_____

_____

14. Unbiased Conclusions?

_____

_____

_____

_____

CRITIQUE OF CBA COMPOSITE ARTICLE 2

1. **Complete Title:** Did not use the term cost-benefit analysis, but instead WTP. Did not specify a treatment (since it was hypothetical). It did specify that the responses were elicited from unpaid caregivers.

2. **Clear Objective:** "This study aimed to measure the cost-benefit of a potential new medication that slows the progression of AD, from the perspective of a nonpaid caregiver. This was clear.

3. **Appropriate Alternatives:** This was an example of a "with-or-without" study. The scenario described the progression if the AD patient was not treated versus if they were treated with the new medication.

4. **Alternatives Described:** Since the medication is theoretical, it was only described as a once a day dose taken orally.

5. **Perspective Stated:** The perspective of the study was stated as the unpaid caregiver for a patient with AD. In the scenario presented, both costs and benefits of delayed progression would impact the caregiver.

6. **Type of Study:** The study could be categorized as a CBA because outcomes were valued in dollars using a willingness-to-pay technique.

7. **Relevant Costs:** The only input costs considered were the costs of the new theoretical medication. Increased visits to get the medication, and changes in utilization of other services were not addressed.

8. **Relevant Outcomes:** Willingness-to-pay estimates are developed to monetize a variety of benefits—including intangible costs/benefits (e.g., increase in adverse events and decrease in stress and worry of caring for a patient with AD). To what extent the average respondent is able to incorporate all of these outcomes into their estimate is a matter of study and debate.

9. **Adjustment or Discounting:** Since respondents were asked to estimate their WTP for only 1 year, neither adjustment nor discounting was needed.

10. **Reasonable Assumptions:** The main assumptions included (1) the scenario described the most salient aspects of the treatment (2) such a treatment could be developed, and (3) respondents accurately estimated the value of this treatment.

11. **Sensitivity Analyses:** WTP differed by job category of respondent. Professors indicated a higher WTP value than university staff. It has been noted that higher income of respondents may correlate with a higher WTP estimate. It would have been useful to recruit respondents with experience caring for a patient with AD in order to compare their responses to those without this experience.

12. **Limitations Addressed:** As stated, the convenience sample chosen limits generalization, and lack of respondents with experience may reduce validity of estimates.

13. **Generalizations Appropriate:** As stated in the limitations, because respondents were recruited from only one location, generalization may not be appropriate.

14. **Unbiased Conclusions:** It depends on the strength of the WTP methodology as to whether these conclusions are valid. More information on how the scenario was developed, and more testing in different populations would strengthen the findings.

QUESTIONS/EXERCISES

St. Elsewhere Hospital is considering two alternatives and analyzing their consequences over a 3-year period on the hospital budget.

Alternative A = Hire a pharmacist
Alternative B = Buy an automated drug delivery system machine
Alternative A's costs are $80,000 salary plus 20% for fringe benefits per year for the next 3 years.
Alternative A's savings are $120,000 per year for the next 3 years.
Alternative B's costs for the automated system are $200,000 for the first year, $30,000 for the second year, and $30,000 for the third year.
Alternative B's savings are $100,000 per year for each of the 3 years.
Assuming a 5% discount rate, calculate:

1. The net benefit of hiring a pharmacist

_____

_____

_____

_____

2. The net benefit of the automated system

_____

_____

_____

_____

3. The benefit-to-cost ratio for hiring a pharmacist

_____

_____

_____

_____

4. The benefit-to-cost ratio for the automated system

_____

_____

_____

_____

Which option, alternative A or alternative B, would be chosen based on the following:

5. The net benefit calculations? Why?

_____

_____

_____

_____

6. The benefit-to-cost ratios? Why?

_____

_____

_____

_____

REFERENCES

1. Feldman A. *Welfare Economics and Social Choice Theory*. New York: Springer, 1980.
2. Hanley N, Spash CL. *Cost-Benefit Analysis and the Environment*. Cheltenham, UK: Edward Elgar, 1993.
3. Blumenschein K, Johannesson M. Economic evaluation in healthcare. A brief history and future directions. *Pharmacoeconomics* 10(2):114–122, 1996.
4. Weisbrod B. *Economics of Public Health: Measuring the Impact of Diseases*. Philadelphia, PA: University of Pennsylvania Press, 1961.

5. Hirth R, Chernew M, Miller E, Fendrick A, Weissert W. Willingness to pay for a quality-adjusted life year: in search of a standard. *Medical Decision Making: An International Journal of the Society for Medical Decision Making* 20(3):332–342, July 2000.

6. Cummings RG, Brookshire DS, Schulze WD. *Valuing Environmental Goods: An Assessment of the Contingent Valuation Method.* Totowa, NJ: Rowman and Allanheld, 1986.

7. Mitchell RC, Carson RT. *Using Surveys to Value Public Goods: The Contingent Valuation Method.* Washington, DC: Resources for the Future, 1989.

8. National Oceanic and Atmospheric Administration. Report of the NOAA panel on contingent valuation. *Federal Register* 58:4602–4614, 1993.

9. O'Brien BJ, Gertsen K, Willan AR, et al. Is there a kink in consumers' threshold value for cost-effectiveness in health care? *Health Economics* 11:175–80, 2002.

SUGGESTED READINGS

Buxton M, Hanney S, Jones T. Estimating the economic value to societies of the impact of health research: A critical review. *Bulletin of the World Health Organization* 82(10):733–739, 2004.

Lofland JH, Locklear JC, Frick KD. Different approaches to valuing the lost productivity of patients with migraine. *Pharmacoeconomics* 19(9):917–925, 2001.

McIntosh E, Donaldson C, Ryan M. Recent advances in the methods of cost-benefit analysis in healthcare. Matching the art to the science. *Pharmacoeconomics* 15(4):357–367, 1999.

Olsen JA, Smith RD. Theory versus practice: A review of the 'willingness-to-pay' in health and healthcare. *Health Economics* 10(1):39–52, 2001.

Robinson R. Cost-benefit analysis. *British Medical Journal* 307:924–926, 1993.

Tranmer JE, Guerriere DN, Ungar WJ, Coyte PC. Valuing patient and caregiver time: A review of the literature. *Pharmacoeconomics* 23(5):449–459, 2005.

Chapter 8

Health-Related Quality of Life: Health Status Measures*

Objectives

Upon completing this chapter, the reader will be able to:

1. Define the term health-related quality of life (HRQoL).

2. Explain the importance of measuring HRQoL.

3. Compare and contrast the use of HRQoL (i.e., nonutility) measures with the use of direct elicitation utility measures (e.g., standard gamble, time tradeoff) and indirect elicitation preference-based classification systems (e.g., SF-6D, EQ-5D).

4. Compare and contrast generic measures with disease-specific measures.

5. Understand the methods for assessing the psychometric properties of HRQoL instruments, such as reliability, validity and responsiveness.

6. Give examples of common HRQoL measures and discuss their use in pharmacoeconomic research.

7. Give examples of common preference-based classification systems, and discuss their use in pharmacoeconomic research.

8. Discuss the interest by the Food and Drug Administration (FDA) in patient-reported outcomes (PROs) and their relationship to HRQoL measures.

---

*This chapter was originally adapted with permission from Vincze G, Rascati K, Vincze Z. Health-related quality of life. In Vincze Z (ed). *Introduction of Pharmacoeconomics*. Budapest, Hungary: Medicina Publishing House, 2001.

✦ DEFINITIONS

It may be helpful to distinguish between the terms **quality of life** (QoL) and **health-related quality of life (HRQoL)**. The first term, QoL, is a broad concept with many aspects that measures people's overall perception of their life. QoL includes both health-related and non–health-related aspects of their lives (e.g., economical, political, cultural). HRQoL is the part of a person's overall QoL that "represents the functional effect of an illness and its consequent therapy upon a patient, as perceived by the patient."[1] In health-related research and articles, the term QoL is often used interchangeably with the term HRQoL, and both might be used to indicate the narrower definition pertaining to a person's health.

Importance

The use of HRQoL measures has been increasing since the mid-1980s. Traditionally, health has been considered from a biomedical point of view. From this viewpoint, emphasis is placed on activities associated with repairing injury and reducing the impact or length of illness. Although this approach is essential, it does not encompass all of the aspects that are important to health. A broad definition of health proposed by the World Health Organization more than 50 years ago is: "Health is a state of complete physical, mental and social well-being and not merely the absence of disease or infirmity."[2] Many health care providers and health services researchers have adopted this expanded view of health and now include measures of the overall impact of diseases and their treatments. In addition to physical functioning, the overall concept of HRQoL includes other aspects of health, called **domains,** such as psychological and social functioning, that are important to the patient. HRQoL instruments can be used to detect otherwise undiagnosed or undetected diseases such as depression.

✦ HRQoL MEASURES VERSUS UTILITY MEASURES

Table 8.1 summarizes three overarching methods used to measure health states: utility measures, HRQoL measures, and preference-based classification systems.

Utility Measures

In Chapter 6, methods such as the **standard gamble** (SG) and **time tradeoff** (TTO) were described. These methods are used to estimate the **utility** or values that individuals assign to different health states. In both cases, scenarios specific to the study are developed, and face-to-face interviews are conducted to observe when the individual is indifferent between a gamble (e.g., live with disease A until death or receive an intervention which can cure or kill you immediately with probability p) or a tradeoff (live with disease A until death or live a few years less but in a better health state), and as such, these are termed **preference-based** or choice-based measures. These methods are used to estimate a number between 0 and 1 (the utility value) that is multiplied by the length of time in each health state to represent the combined impact of morbidity and mortality outcomes in a linear fashion—usually by calculating **quality-adjusted life years** (QALYs). Respondents (e.g., the general population, patients with a specific disease, providers) are asked

TABLE 8.1. **COMPARISON OF HEALTH MEASURES**

	Utility Measures	HRQoL Measures	Preference-Based Classification Systems
Other designations	Direct elicitation	Nonutility	Indirect elicitation Multi-attribute
More information	Chapter 6	Tables 8.3 and 8.5	Table 8.7
Examples	Describe health states then use one of these to estimate utility value: Standard gamble Time tradeoff Rating scale	Generic Instruments: SF-36 SF-12 Disease-specific instruments: FACT AIMS	Generic classification systems: SF-6D EQ-5D HUI3
Range of scores	0–1.0[d]	Each instrument gives multiple scores per respondent Each instrument has different ranges/scoring	0–1.0[d]
Whose preference?	Societal	Not preference-based-Measure of patient health	Societal[e]

[a]Refer to Chapter 6.
[b]Refer to Tables 8.3 and 8.5.
[c]Refer to Table 8.7.
[d]If worse than death can be <0.
[e]Algorithm based on population preferences used to weight summary scores of health states to obtain utility value.

to imagine possible health states and record their scores to reflect their preferences for these various scenarios. These estimates are then used as a special type of effectiveness measure in the denominator when calculating average **cost-utility** and marginal cost-utility ratios. Collecting and estimating utility estimates via these methods is time-consuming and resource-intensive.

HRQoL Measures

Another technique used to measure the effects of treatments and diseases from a patient's viewpoint is to use HRQoL measures. These have also been termed **nonutility** or **nonpreference** measures.[3] HRQoL measures are generally used to represent a patient's estimation of his or her own health at a point in time. HRQoL is measured from the patient's viewpoint. Respondents to a **health status** assessment survey might be the patient, the patient's relatives or caregivers, or the patient's health care providers, but these questionnaires should always be answered from the patient's standpoint. Most HRQoL surveys are multidimensional and do not result in one overall score (as with **utility measures**), but instead include many scores for each patient based on different aspects, or domains, of the patient's health (e.g., a separate mental health score and physical health score for each respondent). Examples of these domains are given later in this chapter.

It is more difficult to use results from multidimensional health status measures in pharmacoeconomic ratios because measurement of the outcome (i.e., effectiveness) consists of more than one score to represent different aspects of the disease, and the range of possible scores differ between the variety of health status instruments (surveys) available, complicating interpretation issues.

To provide an assessment of a patient's HRQoL, researchers can either select tools that focus on general health status using **generic measures,** or choose tools that focus on specific aspects of the disease under study using **disease-specific measures**. For a comprehensive picture of a patient's HRQoL, it is often desirable to include a combination of both types of assessment tools, the generic (general) health and the disease-specific instruments. Table 8.2 lists advantages and disadvantages of generic versus **disease-specific health status** measures. A source of information on various measures can be found on the PROQOLID (Patient-Reported Outcome and Quality of Life Instruments Database) Website at http:/www.proqolid.org.

General or Generic Measures

The advantage of **generic health status** instruments is that scores can be compared for many disease states and conditions. On the other hand, general measures may not be sensitive to clinically relevant differences for every disease or condition. Examples of generic health status instruments are found in Table 8.3, and some questions from the Medical Outcomes Study Short-Form 36 (MOS-SF-36)

TABLE 8.2. **GENERIC VERSUS DISEASE-SPECIFIC INSTRUMENTS**

Type	Advantages	Disadvantages
Generic or general	Broadly applicable	May not be responsive to changes in health
	Summarizes range of concepts	May not be relevant for specific populations
	May detect unanticipated effects	Results may be difficult to interpret
Disease-specific	More relevant for specific populations	Cannot compare across populations
	More responsive to changes in health	Less likely to detect unanticipated effects

Source: Adapted from Patrick DL, Erickson P. Health Status and Health Policy: Quality of Life in Health Care Evaluation and Health Resource Allocation. Oxford: Oxford University Press, 1993:114.

TABLE 8.3. **EXAMPLES OF GENERAL HRQoL MEASURES**

General Health Status Instruments

Medical Outcome Study Short-Form Health Surveys (MOS-SF)[4–7] (includes SF-12, SF-36, and SF-36 Version 2)

Quality of Well-Being (QWB) Scale[22]

Sickness Impact Profile (SIP)[23]

Dartmouth COOP[24]

TABLE 8.4. **EXAMPLES OF ITEMS FROM THE SF-36 GENERAL HRQoL INSTRUMENT**
Vitality Domain
Answer choices are (1) all of the time, (2) most of the time, (3) a good bit of the time, (4) some of the time, (5) a little of the time, and (6) none of the time
Questions: *How much of the time during the past 4 weeks:*
Q9a. Did you feel full of pep? [reverse wording – higher score = lower HRQoL]
Q9e. Did you have a lot of energy? [reverse wording – higher score = lower HRQoL]
Q9g. Did you feel worn out?
Q9i. Did you feel tired?
Role—Emotional Domain
Answer choices are (1) yes and (2) no.
Questions: *During the past 4 weeks, have you had any of the following problems with your work or other regular daily activities as a result of any emotional problems (such as feeling depressed or anxious)?*
Q5a. Cut down on the amount of time you spent on work or other activities
Q5b. Accomplished less than you would like
Q5c. Did work or other activities less carefully than usual

SF-36v2(tm) Health Survey 1996, 2000 by QualityMetric Incorporated. All rights reserved. SF-36v2™ is a trademark of QualityMetric Incorporated.

Reprinted with permission from Ware JE, Kosinski M, Dewey JE. How to Score Version 2 of the SF-36® Health Survey. Lincoln, RI: QualityMetric Incorporated, 2000. Available at http://www.sf-36.org.

generic survey are listed in Table 8.4. Because the SF-36 is the most common generic HRQoL instrument used in the United States, more detailed information is provided for this survey.

The Medical Outcomes Short-Form Surveys

The SF-36 (the short form of the Medical Outcomes Survey that consists of 36 items) is a multipurpose survey of general or generic health status. It was constructed to fill the gap between much more lengthy surveys and relatively coarse single-item measures.[4-7] The SF-36 yields a profile of eight concepts as well as summary physical and mental health measures (see the Questions/Exercises section for a list of these domains and population norms). The SF-36 also includes a self-evaluation of change in health during the past year. Both standard (4-week) and acute (1-week) recall versions have been published. The SF-36 has proven useful in comparisons of relative burden of different diseases, and preliminary results suggest that it may also be useful in estimating the relative benefits of different treatments.

A slightly different newer version (version 2) and a shorter version consisting of 12 questions (the SF-12) have also been developed. The goal of creating the SF-12 was to be brief enough for practical use yet encompass the important physical and mental measures of the full SF-36. Online information about the SF-36 and SF-12 can be found at http://www.sf-36.org and http://www.qualitymetric.com. Development of algorithms to estimate a single score, the SF-6D will be discussed later in the chapter.

TABLE 8.5. **EXAMPLES OF DISEASE-SPECIFIC HRQoL MEASURES**
Hypertension
• Physical Symptoms Distress Index (PSDI)[25]
• The Subjective Symptom Assessment Profile[26]
Benign Prostatic Hyperplasia
• American Urological Association Symptom Index (AUASI)[27]
• BPH Impact Index[28]
Asthma and Allergy
• Living with Asthma Questionnaire[29]
• Life Activities Questionnaire for Adult Asthma[30]
Diabetes Mellitus
• Diabetes-Specific QoL Instrument (DQOL)[31]
Cancer
• Functional Assessment of Cancer Therapy (FACT)[32]
• Clinically Developed Psychosocial Assessment (CDPA)[33]
Chronic Rheumatic Disorders
• Arthritis Impact Measure Scale (AIMS)[34]
• Toronto Functional Capacity Questionnaire[35]
AIDS
• Functional Assessment of HIV Infection (FAHI)[36]
• HIV Patient-Reported Status and Experience Scale (HIV-PARSE)[37]
• AIDS Health Assessment Questionnaire (AIDS-HAQ)[38]

Disease-Specific Measures

It is often necessary to focus on the impact that a certain disease or condition has on patients, and general health status tools may be inadequate for providing this information. In this case, condition- or disease-specific measures are often used to collect more narrowly focused patient views on the impact of the disease. Examples of specific areas investigated with disease-specific questionnaires include sexual functioning for erectile dysfunction treatment, nausea and vomiting for cancer treatment, and range of movement for arthritis treatment. Examples of disease-specific health status instruments are found in Table 8.5, and some questions from Juniper's Asthma Quality of Life Questionnaire[8] are listed in Table 8.6.

✦ DOMAINS OF HEALTH STATUS

Four essential dimensions, or domains, should be included in all HRQoL instruments: physical functioning, psychological functioning, social and role functioning, and general health perceptions. Examples of other less common domains included in some instruments are economic or vocational status and religious or spiritual status. For readers to better understand the types of questions and domains included, it is recommended that they complete one of the general HRQoL

TABLE 8.6. **EXAMPLES OF ITEMS FROM THE ASTHMA QUALITY-OF-LIFE QUESTIONNAIRE (AQLQ©)**
Activities Domain
How limited have you been during the past 2 weeks in these activities as a result of your asthma?
Question 1. *Strenuous activities (e.g., hurrying, exercising, running upstairs, sports)*
Question 3. *Social activities (e.g., talking, playing with pets or children, visiting friends or relatives)*
Response choices are (1) totally limited, (2) extremely limited, (3) very limited, (4) moderate limitation, (5) some limitation, (6) a little limitation, and (7) not limited at all
Symptoms Domain
Question 6. *How much discomfort or distress have you felt over the past 2 weeks as a result of chest tightness?*
Response choices are (1) a very great deal, (2) a great deal, (3) a good deal, (4) a moderate amount, (5) some, (6) very little, and (7) none
Question 20. *In general, how much of the time during the past week did you wake up in the morning with asthma symptoms?*
Response choices are (1) all of the time, (2) most of the time, (3) a good bit of the time, (4) some of the time, (5) a little of the time, (6) hardly any of the time, and (7) none of the time

Reprinted with permission from Elizabeth Juniper. Juniper EF, Guyatt GH, Ferrie PJ, Griffith LE, et al. Measuring quality of life in asthma. *American Review of Respiratory Diseases* 147(4):832–838, 1993. The questionnaire and more information are available from http://www.qoltech.co.uk/Asthma1.htm

surveys such as the SF-36 or SF-12, which are available online. (See the Questions/Exercises section at the end of this chapter.)

Physical Functioning

Physical functioning questions capture information on the observable limitations or disability experienced by the patient over a defined period of time. Physical functioning covers a broad range of topics, including activities of daily living (e.g., can patients dress themselves?), energy level, confinement because of health problems, and bodily pain.

Psychological (Mental) Functioning

Psychological functioning refers to psychological distress that can be the consequence of a disease or a side effect of a treatment. Anxiety, depression, nervousness, moodiness, life satisfaction, and cognitive functioning are all measures of mental health or psychological functioning.

Social or Role Functioning

Social functioning is defined as the ability to develop, maintain, and nurture social relationships. Social functioning addresses both the participation in social interactions and the satisfaction derived from these interactions. Role functioning questions apply to the patient's duties and responsibilities that are limited by health. The effect of a person's health on his or her ability to work, perform household duties, or complete schoolwork is covered by this concept. Both role functioning and social functioning can be affected by physical or psychological limitations.

General Health Perception

General health perception questions elicit patients' overall beliefs and evaluations about their health. Questions are included that relate to both patients' perceptions about their current health status and their expectations for their future health.

◆ ASSESSING HRQoL INSTRUMENTS

Similar to utility measures, assessments using HRQoL measures may be viewed cautiously by prescribers or decision makers who have been trained to collect and interpret "hard, objective" data, such as blood pressure measurements, radiography results, and blood concentrations of biologic markers. Patient-based assessments of pain, depression, or anxiety are examples of important outcomes that are more subjective in nature. Therefore, it is important to assess the psychometric properties of these HRQoL instruments, including consistency (i.e., **reliability**), precision (i.e., **validity**), and their ability to measure meaningful clinical changes (i.e., **responsiveness**).

Reliability

Reliability refers to the consistency of an instrument. For example, does the instrument produce the same score on multiple administrations? The three common types of reliability measures are test–retest reliability, internal consistency, and interrater reliability.

Test–retest reliability assesses the similarity of health status scores over time when no changes in health have occurred. In other words, if the same person completes an HRQoL instrument and then retakes the same survey at a later time, if the person's health status has not changed, his or her scores from both times should be similar (i.e., consistent).

Internal consistency reliability is a measure of the correlation (agreement) between responses to questions within the same domains. For example, consider Q9g and Q9i in Table 8.4. If these two items are measuring the same aspect (i.e., domain) of health—in this case, "vitality"—these questions should elicit similar answers from the respondent. If the respondent replied that he or she "is worn out" none of the time (score = 6), it is logical that this person would likely answer that he or she "feels tired" none of the time (score = 6).

Interrater reliability calculates the agreement between two respondents when assessing the health status of the same patient. For example, if a young boy has attention deficit hyperactive disorder (ADHD), both his mother and his teacher might be asked to complete the same health status instrument to assess the impact of ADHD on this boy's HRQoL. A comparison of the scores from these two respondents indicates the level of interrater consistency or agreement. For most HRQoL studies, only the patient completes the questionnaire, so interrater reliability is not commonly seen in this type of research.

Note that an instrument can be tested and found to be **reliable** (i.e., it elicits similar scores on readministration) yet imprecise (not **valid**). In other words, scores

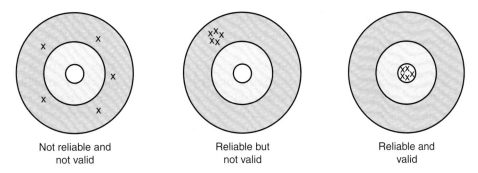

| Not reliable and | Reliable but | Reliable and |
| not valid | not valid | valid |

FIGURE 8.1.   This figure uses three targets to indicate how accurate the scores (*bullets*) are to the real measure of the domain or construct (*bulls-eye* or *center of target*). The left target illustrates scores that are neither reliable (consistent) nor valid (precise). The middle target illustrates the concept of scores that are reliable but not valid. The bullets tend to hit the same area every time, but they are not near the center of the target. The right target illustrates scores that are both reliable and valid—the score is consistently near the center of the target.

calculated using an HRQoL instrument might be reliably (consistently) wrong. If a physician's office had a scale to measure patients' weights, and this scale indicated a weight for each patient that was exactly 25 lb lower than each person's actual weight, this scale would be considered to be reliable (consistent from visit to visit) but not valid (wrong estimation of patients' true weights). Figure 8.1 illustrates the difference between the terms reliability and validity.

Validity

Validity studies are necessary to evaluate whether the scores elicited from the instruments truly represent the underlying constructs (aspects) of HRQoL. In other words, the purpose of validity assessment is to determine whether the instrument is actually measuring what it is supposed to be measuring. Validity refers to the extent to which differences in patients' scores reflect the differences among individuals that the test developer sought to measure. Keep in mind that for an instrument to be valid, it must first be reliable (consistent) (see Fig. 8.1). If researchers do not get reliable (similar) results upon readministration, they cannot assess whether these results actually measure the underlying concept. The validity of an instrument is much more difficult to assess than its reliability. Three common types of validity assessments are content validity, criterion validity, and construct validity.

Content validity pertains to whether the HRQoL instrument offers an adequate representation of the relevant variables of interest. Content validation requires the existence of a standard against which one can compare the concepts. Standards can be based on well-accepted theoretical definitions, on existing accepted standards, or from interviews of those who have experiences with the types of problems under study (e.g., patients with the disease or condition, caregivers, heath care providers). Sometimes content validity is referred to as "face" validity. Upon surface inspection, does the content of the items seem complete and relevant to what is meant to be measured?

Criterion validity demonstrates that HRQoL scores are systematically related to one or more external outcome criteria. This is sometimes called "predictive" validity in that instrument scores correlate with, or predict, health outcomes. Examples of the relationships of HRQoL scores with external evidence (criteria) include high

HRQoL scores (indicating good health) and low use of medical services; and low HRQoL scores (indicating poor health) predicting higher rates of mortality in the following year.

Construct validity is a more abstract and complex concept. A theoretical or conceptual framework should underpin the development of any HRQoL instrument. The ideas (i.e., constructs) under investigation are often an interlocking set of propositions, assumptions, and variables. When construct validation is used, both the HRQoL instrument and the underlying theory must be evaluated. Convergent, discriminant, and known-groups validity may be used to assess construct validity. Convergent validity tests determine if the use of different measures of the same construct provides similar results. For example, the scores of the mental health domain (component) of a common **generic** HRQoL instrument should correlate with those of a **disease-specific** instrument developed to assess mental health. When more than one method of data collection (e.g., face-to-face interview, phone interview, e-mail survey) has been used to measure the same construct, they can be compared with measure convergent validity.

Discriminant validity examines whether these different measures and their underlying construct can be differentiated from other constructs. For example, researchers do not expect a measure of physical functioning to be highly related to mental functioning.

Known-groups validity assesses the differences between two patient groups known or theorized to differ in some way. For example, if a survey was developed to measure anxiety related to childbirth, researchers might expect a higher level (score) of anxiety for first-time mothers than in women who already gave birth to other children.

When enough evidence has been accumulated to show that an instrument reflects the health concept intended to be measured and that it does not measure other unintended concepts, researchers say that a HRQoL instrument has been "validated." However, the process of validation continues as long as new information is produced about the interpretation and meaning of scores.

Responsiveness

The responsiveness of an HRQoL instrument refers to its ability to detect changes in health status. This includes the instrument's ability to not only show numerical differences in scores between patients in dissimilar health states but to also detect changes in a patient's health over time when his or her health status changes. Intertwined with the assessment of responsiveness is the question of what change in score constitutes a clinical difference, sometimes referred to as the **minimally important difference** (MID). Research on the MID for some HRQoL instruments has been published. For example, when scoring items from an asthma questionnaire that uses 7-point response options, a mean change of 0.5 has been shown to represent a minimal clinical difference, 1.0 represents a moderate change, and 1.5 represents a large change in HRQoL.[9]

Other Assessment Issues

HRQoL instruments must contain a sufficient number of questions to adequately measure the domains of interest, but they must also be short enough to be practical (e.g., not be a burden to the respondents). Researchers must find a balance between obtaining the needed information and minimizing respondent burden. Other issues to be considered when choosing, developing, and assessing HRQoL instruments include the applicability of the domains measured to the research question(s), the ease of its use, and the resources needed to obtain responses.

✦ PHARMACOECONOMICS AND HRQoL MEASURES

As mentioned earlier in this chapter, **HRQoL measures** usually result in multiple scores per respondent that correspond to different domains, or dimensions, of a person's health. It is possible that treatment A may be more effective on some dimensions of health, but treatment B may be more effective on others. In addition, the range of possible scores varies by HRQoL instrument, and these scores may not be mathematically linear. These features make it difficult to use HRQoL scores when calculating pharmacoeconomic ratios, which mathematically compute the change in costs divided by the change in outcomes. There are a few scenarios using HRQoL scores that would indicate cost-effectiveness. If the costs of a treatment are the same or lower than the alternative treatment *and* show superior improvement on at least one dimension *and* are no worse on any other dimensions, researchers can claim cost-effectiveness. For other scenarios, cost-consequence tables might be presented instead. For each treatment option, costs are listed in one column, and consequences (measured as scores or score differences from baseline) for each domain are listed in another column, but no ratios are calculated.

✦ PREFERENCE-BASED CLASSIFICATION SYSTEMS

Preference-based classification systems consist of a hybrid of the utility and HRQoL methods for assessing health. As mentioned earlier, direct elicitation of utility or preference-based values (e.g., using the SG or TTO technique) can be time- and resource-intensive, while **HRQoL instruments** (e.g., the SF-36) do not allow for the calculation of one summary utility score that can be used to calculate pharmacoeconomic ratios. As an alternative option, indirect preference-based classification systems, based on a multi-attribute approach, have been developed in order to provide utility value estimates (ranging from 0 to 1.0) based on mathematical algorithms using predeveloped (i.e., less resource-intensive) instruments. Scores are based on self-assessed health status (as with HRQoL measures) but valued using community or general population weights. In the Questions/Exercises section of this chapter, you are asked to indicate your current health state based on five dimensions, and then look up the value of this health state using a table of US population norms. Table 8.7 compares characteristics of the three most commonly used preference-based classification systems: the EuroQol 5D (EQ-5D), the Short-Form 6D (SF6D), and the Health Utilities Index 3 (HUI3).

The EuroQol 5D (EQ-5D) includes five domains/dimensions: mobility, self-care, usual activity, pain/discomfort, and anxiety/depression, each with three levels of functioning (1 = no problems, 2 = moderate problems, 3 = extreme problems), producing a total of 243 possible health states (245 when the states "unconscious" and "immediate death" are added for completeness).[10] Specific questions and scoring are included in the Questions/exercises portion of this chapter. Because only three levels are used for each of the five domains, critics have pointed out that a high percent of respondents choose "11111" (no problems on any of the five

TABLE 8.7. **PREFERENCE-BASED CLASSIFICATION SYSTEMS**

Classification System	SF-6D (from SF-36)	EQ-5D	HUI3
Dimensions (number of levels)[a]			
	Physical (6)	Mobility (3)	Ambulation (6)
	Mental health (5)	Anxiety/depression (3)	Emotion (5)
	Bodily pain (6)	Pain/discomfort (3)	Pain (5)
	Social functioning (5)	Usual activities (3)	Cognition (6)
	Role limitations (4)	Self-care (3)	Dexterity (6)
	Vitality (5)		Hearing (6)
			Speech (5)
			Vision (6)
Number of possible health states	18,000	243	972,000
Elicitation technique	Standard gamble	Time tradeoff/rating scale	Standard gamble
Country where developed	United States	United Kingdom	Canada
Possible range of scores	0.296 to 1.0	−0.11 to 1.0	−0.36 to 1.0
Ceiling effect (percent with score of 1.0)[b] (%)	4.3	36.2	11.4
Average time to administer[b]	7.9 minutes	1.9 minutes	3.4 minutes
Minimal important difference (MID)[c]	0.027	0.040 US / 0.082 UK	0.032
Mean (SD) scores—selected studies[d]			
General US population	NA	0.87 (0.13)	0.81 (0.38)
General UK population	0.80 (0.15)	0.84 (0.23)	NA
General Canadian population	NA	0.83 (NR)	0.85 (NR)
Hearing impaired	0.77 (0.08)	0.79 (0.23)	0.56 (0.15)
Spine disorders	0.57 (0.12)	0.39 (0.33)	0.45 (0.27)
Macular degeneration	0.66 (0.14)	0.72 (0.22)	0.34 (0.28)
Rheumatoid arthritis	0.63 (0.24)	0.66 (0.13)	0.53 (0.29)

[a]Luo N, Wang P, Fu AZ, Johnson JA, Coons S. Preference-based SF-6D scores derived from the SF-36 and SF-12 have different discriminative power in a population health survey. Medical Care 50(7):627–632, 2012.
[b]Fryback D, Dunham N, Palta M, Hanmer J, Buechner J, Cherepanov D, Kind P. US norms for six generic health-related quality-of-life indexes from the National Health Measurement study. Medical Care 45(12):1162–1170, 2007.
[c]Luo N, Johnson J, Coons S. Using instrument-defined health state transitions to estimate minimally important differences for four preference-based health-related quality-of-life instruments. Medical Care 48(4):365–371, 2010.
[d]McDonough CM, Tosteson A. Measuring preferences for cost-utility analysis: How choice of method may influence decision-making. Pharmacoeconomics 25(2):93–106, 2007.
NA = Not available; NR = Not reported ; SF = Short-Form; EQ = Euroquol; HUI = Health Utilities Index.

domains) to describe their current health state, and thus receive a utility score of 1.0. This issue is referred to as a "ceiling effect," which decreases differentiation between respondents in good (but not perfect) health. As a result, the EQ-5D index scores for healthier patients are, on average, higher compared with other methods of estimating utility values (e.g., compared with the SF-6D scores). Testing is currently being conducting on a newer version, the EQ-5D-5L, using five levels of functioning (1 = no problems, 2 = slight problems, 3 = moderate problems,

4 = severe problems, 5 = extreme problems) in order to improve the sensitivity of the instrument to differences in health states.[11]

The Short-Form 6D (SF-6D) is an indirect utility measure developed by Brazier and colleagues using responses from the SF-36 and SF-12 HRQoL measures.[12,13] The current version includes dimensions of physical functioning, role limitations, social functioning, pain, mental health, and vitality, each with four to six levels of functioning and altogether producing a total of 18,000 possible health states. Although the ceiling effect is less of an issue for the SF-6D than the EQ-5D (i.e., higher scores for healthy respondents from EQ-5D than SF-6D) it has been noted that scores obtained for less healthy respondents are, on average, higher when calculated using the SF-6D compared with the EQ-5D.

The Health Utilities Index (HUI) was developed in Canada. The most recent version, the HUI3 includes eight attributes: vision, hearing, speech, ambulation, dexterity, emotion, cognition, and pain, with five or six functioning levels per attribute. The ceiling effect is less of an issue for the HUI3 than the EQ-5D, but more of an issue than for the SF-6D. For respondents with at least one medical condition, the HUI3 scoring values are, in general, lower than the scoring values for the EQ-5D.[14]

Recent research has focused on disease-specific or condition-specific preference-based measures (CSPBMs) in order to provide utility estimates that may be more relevant in some conditions than generic preference-based methods.[15,16]

The appeal in using utility weights, and thus QALYs, as a measure of effectiveness in economic evaluations is in the comparability across different conditions/diseases. It has been shown that different algorithms used by researchers to produce a single utility score provide estimates that are not always comparable, and the difference in methods may lead to different economic conclusions, so caution is warranted.[17,18]

✦ PATIENT-REPORTED OUTCOMES

In 2009, the FDA provided guidance that described current thinking on how the FDA evaluates PROs instruments used in clinical trials to measure treatment benefit. This document defines a PRO as "the measurement of any aspect of a patient's health status that comes directly from the patient."[19] The document gives specific examples of concepts related to treatment benefit that might be measured by PRO instruments from individual symptoms (e.g., pain, seizure frequency) to the overall impact of a condition (e.g., depression, asthma) to feelings about the condition (e.g., worrying about getting worse, feeling different from others). Another US governmental agency, the National Institutes of Health (NIH), developed the Patient-Reported Outcomes Measurement Information System (PROMIS) as a way to provide assessment of and access to PRO measures that can be used by clinicians and researchers (http://www.nihpromis.org). PROs are not routinely collected in routine practice due, in part, to time and logistic concerns, but improved technology may make PRO collection more practical in the future.[20,21]

Some HRQoL instruments can be used to measure PROs, but the terms *PRO* and *HRQoL* are not interchangeable. Some PRO measures are more narrowly focused than HRQoL instruments and may be developed to elicit responses for only one domain or dimension of the treatment benefit, and some HRQoL instruments may be too broad or insensitive to adequately measure the treatment benefit of clinical interest.

SUMMARY

HRQoL instruments attempt to scientifically quantify individuals' perceptions of the consequences of diseases and their treatment. These are nonutility, **nonpreference-based measures,** which reduces their use in economic ratio calculations, but instead provide domain-specific information on health status. HRQoL instruments can measure generic or overall health perceptions or be more narrowly focused on outcomes specific to a disease state or condition. Many researchers use a combination of these two approaches. HRQoL questionnaires should measure at least four dimensions, or domains, of a person's health: physical functioning, psychological functioning, social or role functioning, and general health perceptions. Instruments should be assessed to determine their reliability (consistency), validity (precision), and responsiveness to clinical differences or changes.

Research continues on using **indirect elicitation, preference-based classification systems** to transform multidimensional scores from HRQoL instruments into a single summary utility score so that cost-utility ratios can be calculated. The development of FDA guidelines and NIH assessment initiatives for PROs collected during clinical trials point to the importance of continued research in measuring all aspects of health.

COMPOSITE ARTICLE 1: HRQoL–RHEUMATOID ARTHRITIS

Note: A special supplement appeared in the American Journal of Health-Systems Pharmacy on September 15, 2006. The supplement contains five articles on current treatments for rheumatoid arthritis (RA). In addition, a summary of cost analyses of medications used to treat RA is available: See Bansback NJ, Regier DA, Ara R, et al. An overview of economic evaluations for drugs used in rheumatoid arthritis. Drugs 65(4):473–496, 2006.

Title: COST-EFFECTIVENESS OF INFLAMAWAY VERSUS JOINTREDUCE IN THE TREATMENT OF RHEUMATOID ARTHRITIS

BACKGROUND: Rheumatoid arthritis (RA) is an autoimmune disease that causes chronic inflammation of the joints. The goal of treatment is to reduce joint inflammation and pain, maximize joint function, and prevent joint destruction and deformity. First-line medications, such as nonsteroidal anti-inflammatory (NSAID) medications and injectable corticosteroids, are used to reduce pain and inflammation of the joints. Second-line medications, also known as disease-modifying antirheumatic drugs (DMARDs), may take weeks or months to show effectiveness. DMARDs (including medications such as methotrexate and sulfasalazine) promote disease remission and prevent progressive joint destruction. Two new medications, InflamAway and JointReduce, are now available that help block a protein in the joints that causes inflammation, thereby reducing the inflammatory response.

OBJECTIVE: The objective of this study is to compare the cost-effectiveness of these two new products (InflamAway and JointReduce) from a societal perspective.

METHODS: A total of 400 patients with symptomatic RA were randomized to receive either InflamAway or JointReduce for this 6-month study. Clinical measures include the American College of Rheumatology (ACR)'s scales (http://www.rheumatology.org), the ACR-20, ACR-50 and ACR-70, which correspond to a 20%, 50%, and 70% reduction in symptoms, respectively. Patients were instructed to keep a diary of time missed from work because of RA symptoms, as well as any medical services, medications, and out-of-pocket costs used to treat RA. Patients completed the Arthritis Impact Measurement Scale, Version 2 (AIMS2) at both baseline and 6 months. The AIMS2 is a 78-item questionnaire that has been shown to be reliable, valid, and responsive to changes in health status.

Answers to some of these items can be summarized into a three-component model (physical, affect, and symptom). Example questions from each component are listed in Exhibit 8.1. The complete instrument and scoring guide can be accessed at no charge from PROQOLID (http: /www.proqolid.org). Each domain is scored from 0 (worse health) to 10 (best health), and an improvement of more than 1.0 in each domain indicates a clinical change.

EXHIBIT 8.1

Examples of Items from the Arthritis Impact Measurement Scale, Version 2 (AIMS2)

Physical Component

Hand and finger function domain

During the past month…

1. Could you easily write with a pen or a pencil?

2. Could you easily button a shirt or a blouse?

3. Could you easily turn a key in a lock?

4. Could you easily tie a knot or a bow?

5. Could you easily open a new jar of food?

Answer choices are: (1) all days, (2) most days, (3) some days, (4) few days, and (5) no days

Affect Component

Level of tension domain

During the past month…

1. How often have you felt tense or high strung?

2. How often have you been bothered by nervousness or your nerves?

3. How often were you able to relax without difficulty?

4. How often have you felt relaxed and free of tension?

5. How often have you felt calm and peaceful?

Answer choices are (1) always, (2) very often, (3) sometimes, (4) almost never, and (5) never

Symptom Component

Arthritis Pain Domain

During the past month…

1. How would you describe the arthritis pain you usually had?

Answer choices are (1) severe, (2) moderate, (3) mild, (4) very mild, and (5) none

2. How often did you have severe pain from your arthritis?

3. How often did you have pain in two or more joints at the same time?

4. How often did your morning stiffness last more than 1 hour from the time you woke up?

5. How often did your pain make it difficult for you to sleep?

Answer choices are (1) all days, (2) most days, (3) some days, (4) few days, and (5) no days

The AIMS2 is available at www.qolid.org. Reprinted with permission.

RESULTS: *Outcomes:* The ACR scores at 6 months were not significantly different between Inflam-Away and JointReduce (Exhibit 8.2). Although AIMS2 scores showed clinical improvement for both medications compared with baseline, there were no meaningful differences in the improvements seen with InflamAway compared with the improvement for the JointReduce group (Exhibit 8.3).

Costs: A list of costs for both medications is shown in Exhibit 8.4. The study medication cost for JointReduce was $4,000 more

---

EXHIBIT 8.2

American College of Rheumatology Results[a]

Study Medication	Percent (n) ACR-20 at 6 months	Percent (n) ACR-50 at 6 Months	Percent (n) ACR-70 at 6 Months
InflamAway (n = 200)	70% (n = 140)	55% (n =110)	26% (n =52)
JointReduce (n = 200)	72% (n = 144)	53% (n =106)	25% (n =50)

[a]ACR-20 = at least 20% reduction in symptoms from baseline.

ACR-50 = at least 50% reduction in symptoms from baseline.

ACR-70 = at least 70% reduction in symptoms from baseline.

No statistical differences were found when comparing ARC scores between study medication groups.

EXHIBIT 8.3

Results of Arthritis Impact Measure Scale, Version 2 (AIMS2) Health Status Comparisons

AIMS2 Three-ComponentModel[a]	Average Score at Baseline	Average Score at 6 Months (Difference from Baseline) InflamAway	Average Score at 6 Months (Difference from Baseline) JointReduce	Difference Between JointReduce (n = 200) and InflamAway (n = 200)
Physical component				
Mobility	2.4	3.5 (+1.1)	3.6 (+1.2)	+0.1
Walking and bending	6.2	7.3 (+1.1)	7.2 (+1.0)	−0.1
Hand and finger function	4.1	6.2 (+2.1)	6.1 (+2.0)	−0.1
Arm function	3.1	4.2 (+1.1)	4.1 (+1.0)	−0.1
Self-care	3.0	5.1 (+2.1)	4.5 (+1.5)	−0.6
Household tasks	3.4	4.9 (+1.5)	4.5 (+1.1)	−0.4
Average physical score	3.7	5.2 (+1.5)	5.0 (+1.3)	−0.2
Affect component				
Level of tension	5.6	6.8 (+1.2)	6.9 (+1.3)	+0.1
Mood	4.4	5.6 (+1.2)	5.5 (+1.1)	−0.1
Average affect score	5.0	6.2 (+1.2)	6.2 (+1.2)	0.0
Symptom component				
Arthritis pain	6.0	7.5 (+1.5)	7.5 (+1.5)	0.0

[a]Scores range from 0 to 10, with higher numbers indicating better health. All scores at 6 months show clinical improvement from baseline for both medications. There are no clinically meaningful differences between InflamAway and JointReduce for any component of the AIMS2.

Rheumatoid Arthritis-Related Costs for 6 months in 2006 US Dollars

Categories of Costs	Average Costs per Patient for InflamAway ($)	Average Costs per Patient for JointReduce ($)	p
Cost of study medication	16,000	20,000	0.01
Cost of other RA-related medications	4,000	4,100	0.50
Cost of RA-related office visits	800	750	0.97
Cost of RA-laboratory tests	700	800	0.10
Cost of RA-related emergency department visits	200	150	0.80
Cost of RA inpatient stays	200	300	0.75
Other out-of-pocket costs for patients	100	100	0.99
Lost time from work (days × $200/d)	5,000	5,200	0.97
Total 6-month RA-related costs per patient	27,000	31,400	0.03

Only study medication costs and total costs are statistically different (bolded; $p < 0.05$) between the two groups.

RA = rheumatoid arthritis.

than the study medication InflamAway. Other costs were similar between the two groups, and there were no other statistically different costs categories. The total amount of 6-month RA-related costs for the JointReduce group are $4,400 more than for the InflamAway group. (This difference was mainly because of the higher cost of JointReduce.)

Cost-effectiveness: Total 6-month RA-related costs were lower in the InflamAway group than in the JointReduce group. Both outcome measures (ACR and AIMS2) showed improvement in the patient's condition at the 6-month follow-up, but there was little difference between the two medications when they were compared head to head. Therefore, InflamAway is dominant to JointReduce because it provides similar effectiveness at a lower cost. Therefore, an ICER does not need to be calculated.

CONCLUSION: The two new medications, InflamAway and JointReduce, are expensive compared with older medications, but they have shown greater efficacy in clinical trials. For these study patients, both medications showed health improvements but were very similar to each other in effectiveness (as measured by both the ACR and AIMS2). Because outcomes are similar, the study question might be addressed as a cost-minimization analysis, asking what the lowest cost for the same effect is. In this case, InflamAway is about $4,000 less than JointReduce and is therefore the more cost-effective option.

WORKSHEET FOR CRITIQUE OF HRQoL ARTICLE 1

1. Complete Title?

_____

_____

_____

_____

2. Clear Objective?

_____

_____

_____

3. Appropriate Alternatives?

_____

_____

_____

_____

4. Alternatives Described?

_____

_____

_____

_____

5. Perspective Stated?

_____

_____

_____

_____

6. Type of Study?

_____

_____

_____

_____

7. Relevant Costs?

_____

_____

_____

_____

8.   Relevant Outcomes?

_____

_____

_____

_____

9.   Adjustment or Discounting?

_____

_____

_____

_____

10. Reasonable Assumptions?

_____

_____

_____

_____

11. Sensitivity Analyses?

_____

_____

_____

_____

12. Limitations Addressed?

_____

_____

_____

_____

13. Generalizations Appropriate?

_____

_____

_____

_____

14. Unbiased Conclusions?

_____

_____

_____

_____

Cost-Effectiveness Grid

Which cell represents the comparison of JointReduce to InflamAway for ACR scores? What about AIMS2 scores?

COST-EFFECTIVENESS	Lower Cost	Same Cost	Higher Cost
Lower effectiveness	A	B	C
Same effectiveness	D	E	F
Higher effectiveness	G	H	I

CRITIQUE OF HRQoL ARTICLE 1

1. **Complete Title:** The title did identify the options being compared, InflamAway and JointReduce, and the title did indicate that the type of study was a cost-effectiveness analysis (CEA).

2. **Clear Objective:** The objective was to determine the cost-effectiveness of InflamAway versus JointReduce.

3. **Appropriate Alternatives:** The authors indicated that these were two new medications with the same new mechanism of action. Readers would need to look at references given in "real" articles to determine if these alternatives were clinically relevant.

4. **Alternatives Described:** More information should have been given concerning dosing (method of administration, how often administered, dose of each administration) for both medications.

5. **Perspective Stated:** The perspective of the study was explicitly stated as societal.

6. **Type of Study:** The study was correctly identified as a CEA because the outcomes were measured using both ACR scores and AIMS2 scores (=clinical units). Because the magnitude of clinical improvement for the two drugs was so similar, some authors might call this a cost-minimization analysis.

7. **Relevant Costs:** Based on the societal perspective, direct medical, direct nonmedical (out-of-pocket costs for expenses such as household help), and productivity costs were included. Although much of the utilization data came from the patients' diaries, the authors could have explained how they assigned costs to this utilization data.

8. **Relevant Outcomes:** ACR scores are frequently used in clinical trials to measure changes in RA, but the authors did not describe this method for assessing clinical outcomes (although they gave a web site). The AIMS2 is a common instrument for measuring health status changes in RA. Other survey instruments used in RA are the Disease Activity Score and the Health Assessment Questionnaire. The authors should have indicated why ACR and AIMS2 measurements were chosen to measure changes in RA-related health.

9. **Adjustment or Discounting:** The authors used 2006 costs, so adjustment was not needed. The study only followed patients for 6 months, so discounting was not needed.

10. **Reasonable Assumptions:** An implicit assumption was that the outcomes measured were reliable and valid in this population of patients. Reliability and validity checks should have been conducted and reported. For example, an alpha coefficient (reliability) could have been calculated for the items that comprised the physical component of the Arthritis Impact Measure Scale (AIMS), or the results could have been compared with more objective laboratory measures (e.g., erythrocyte sedimentation rate) in order to measure criterion validity.

11. **Sensitivity Analyses:** No sensitivity analyses were conducted.

12. **Limitations Addressed:** The authors did not address any limitations. More information is needed on the two medications studied. For example, are there differences in side effect profiles? What do the safety profiles look like? Recently, one of the NSAIDs used in patients with RA was withdrawn from the market because of an increased incidence of heart problems. Also, the study did not say if long-term testing had been conducted on these medications. Is 6 months long enough to see the full effect of the products?

13. **Generalizations Appropriate:** The authors did not report the demographics or disease severity of the patients enrolled in the study, so it is difficult to know if these patients represent the "average" RA patient.

14. **Unbiased Conclusions:** These two medications appear to have similar efficacy, but the cost of one study medication is considerably lower than the other. The authors did not give a full description of the study medications or the study population, did not state any limitations, and did not conduct sensitivity analyses. As mentioned, no information on side effects was mentioned, and if these medications have different side effect profiles, this needs to be considered before choosing one option over the other.

Cost-Effectiveness Grid

COST-EFFECTIVENESS	Lower Cost	Same Cost	Higher Cost
Lower effectiveness	A	B	C
Same effectiveness	D	E	F JointReduce compared with InflamAway - ACR JointReduce compared with InflamAway - AIMS2
Higher effectiveness	G	H	I

COMPOSITE ARTICLE 2: HRQoL—CHRONIC LOW BACK PAIN

Note: Some reviews of research relating to the treatment of chronic low back pain and HRQol measures are:
Indrakanti S, Weber M., Takemoto S, Hu S, Polly D, Berven S. Value-based care in the management of spinal disorders: A systematic review of cost-utility analysis. Clinical Orthopaedics and Related Research *470(4):1106–1123, 2012.*
Dharmshaktu P, Tayal V, Kalra B. Efficacy of antidepressants as analgesics: A review. Journal of Clinical Pharmacology *52(1): 6–17, 2012.*
Søgaard R, Christensen F, Videbaek T, Bünger C, Christiansen T. Interchangeability of the EQ-5D and the SF-6D in long-lasting low back pain. Value in Health: The Journal of the International Society for Pharmacoeconomics and Outcomes Research *12(4):606–612, 2009.*

Title: COST-UTILITY OF THE ADDITION OF A BACKTRAMINE TO STANDARD TREATMENT FOR CHRONIC LOW BACK PAIN

Over 28% of the US population (http://www.cdc.gov/nchs/hus/contents2011.htm#052) suffers with low back pain each year, and most people will experience back pain at some time during their lifetime. Acute or short-term low back pain generally lasts from a few days to a few weeks, and is usually the result of trauma to the lower back or a disorder such as arthritis. Symptoms may range from muscle ache to shooting or stabbing pain, limited flexibility and range of motion, or an inability to stand straight. If symptoms last for more than 3 months, the condition is referred to as chronic low back pain (CLBP).

The first line of treatment for CLBP consists of using over-the-counter or prescription pain relievers to reduce discomfort with the possible addition of anti-inflammatory or muscle relaxant medications. When the pain becomes a chronic issue, an antidepressant medication might be added to a patient's regimen, but findings relating to the efficacy of this addition have been mixed.

OBJECTIVE: The objective of this study was to investigate the cost-effectiveness and cost-utility of standard analgesic/anti-inflammatory treatment for chronic back pain compared with standard treatment with the addition of a new serotonin-norepinephrine reuptake inhibitor (SNRI), called Backtramine (not a real medication).

METHODS: All patients enrolled in the study had been on a standard combination of analgesic/anti-inflammatory medications for a minimum of 3 months. The intervention consisted of the addition of a daily placebo or the addition of a daily 60 mg capsule of Backtramine. At baseline and 12-month follow-up, patients were asked to describe their average pain intensity using a numeric analogue scale (range 1 to 10; higher number = more pain intensity) in order to estimate the number of days in pain during the previous year, and to estimate the number of days missed from work due to back pain during the last year. Both the EuroQol 5D (EQ-5D) and the Short Form 6D (SF-6D) were administered at baseline and 12 months. The differences in outcomes were compared with the additional cost of a year's supply of Backtramine. Sensitivity analyses were conducted on both cost and outcomes variables.

RESULTS: Patients from 10 central Texas pain clinics were recruited for this study during 2012. A total of 350 patients on standard care plus placebo and 352 patients on standard care plus Backtramine (combination therapy) were enrolled and completed the study. Exhibit 8.5 illustrates baseline values for both cohorts. Differences between cohorts at baseline were minimal. Utility scores for both cohorts were appreciably lower than the general population. A reduction of pain and a reduction of missed work days were seen for the combination therapy compared with the standard treatment/placebo for some health outcomes, while there was no significant difference for others (Exhibits 8.6–8.8). Specifically, a significant

EXHIBIT 8.5

Characteristics of the Study Population—Baseline

	Standard Care Plus Placebo (n = 350)	Standard Care Plus Backtramine (n = 352)	General Adult Population
Age, mean (SD)	54 (10)	54 (10)	NA
Females, n (%)	125 (50)	126 (50)	NA
Baseline SF-36 Domains (0–100) Mean (SD)[a]			
Physical functioning	65 (25)	64 (25)	88 (20)
Role physical	42 (43)	42 (43)	83 (31)
Bodily pain	51 (21)	50 (28)	79 (23)
General health	57 (25)	56 (26)	76 (20)
Vitality	54 (26)	53 (26)	70 (20)
Social functioning	77 (27)	76 (27)	91 (17)
Role emotional	64 (44)	64 (43)	86 (28)
Mental health	74 (21)	74 (22)	82 (16)
Standardized scales of SF-36 (standardized around 50%), Mean (SD)[a]			
Physical component summary (PCS)	40 (11)	43 (10)	50 (9)
Mental component summary (MCS)	49 (12)	49 (11)	50 (8)
SF-6D (0-1), Mean (SD)[a]	0.60 (0.12)	0.59 (0.12)	0.78 (0.02)
EQ-5D (0-1), Mean (SD)[a]	0.65 (0.20)	0.64 (0.21)	0.85 (0.02)
Pain intensity (1–10) Mean (SD)[b]	6 (2)	6 (2)	NA
Days of pain in the previous year, Mean (SD)	101 (132)	103 (123)	NA
Days of sick leave, Mean (SD)	12 (18)	12 (19)	NA

[a]Higher Scores = better health (less disability).

[b]Higher Scores = worse health (more disability).

NA = Not applicable.

EXHIBIT 8.6

Distribution of Short Form 6D responses across levels of single dimensions (%)

Standard Baseline % at each level

Level[a]	Physical Functioning	Role Limitation	Social Functioning	Pain	Mental Health	Vitality
1	8	30	46	10	31	6
2	17	27	21	14	33	34
3	38	6	22	31	19	25
4–6	38	38	12	46	17	36

Backtrami Baseline

Level	Physical Functioning	Role Limitation	Social Functioning	Pain	Mental Health	Vitality
1	8	30	46	10	30	7
2	18	26	21	15	33	33
3	37	7	21	32	18	25
4–6	37	37	13	43	19	35

Standard 12 Months % at each level

Level[a]	Physical Functioning	Role Limitation	Social Functioning	Pain	Mental Health	Vitality
1	9	29	46	11	30	7
2	16	27	22	12	35	33
3	37	7	22	30	20	26
4–6	38	37	10	47	15	34

Backtramine 12 Months

Level[a]	Physical Functioning	Role Limitation	Social Functioning	Pain	Mental Health	Vitality
1	12	33	48	13	10	10
2	28	33	22	15	35	35
3	35	5	21	34	20	25
4–6	33	29	9	38	15	30

[a] Level 1 = best health; Level 4–6 = worst health

EXHIBIT 8.7

Distribution of EQ5D responses across levels of single dimensions (%)

Standard Baseline % at each level

Level[a]	Mobility	Self-Care	Usual Activities	Pain/Discomfort	Anxiety/Depression
1	55	74	30	16	66
2	45	25	54	65	30
3	1	1	16	19	4

Backtarine Baseline

Level	Mobility	Self-Care	Usual Activities	Pain/Discomfort	Anxiety/Depression
1	55	74	31	16	67
2	44	24	55	66	30
3	2	2	14	18	3

Standard 12 Months % at each level

Level[a]	Mobility	Self-Care	Usual Activities	Pain/Discomfort	Anxiety/Depression
1	55	75	31	15	66
2	44	24	54	65	30
3	1	1	15	20	4

Backtarine 12 Months

Level	Mobility	Self-Care	Usual Activities	Pain/Discomfort	Anxiety/Depression
1	56	76	32	20	68
2	43	24	56	70	32
3	1	0	12	10	0

[a]Level 1 = no problems, Level 2 = moderate problems, Level 3 = extreme problems.

EXHIBIT 8.8

Change in Outcomes

	Standard Care Plus Placebo (n = 350)	Standard Care Plus Backtramine (n = 352)	Difference (95% Confidence Interval)
SF-6D (0–1), Mean (SD)[a]			
Baseline	0.60	0.59	
Follow-up	0.59	0.64	
Difference	−0.01	0.05	0.06 (0.04 to 0.08)
EQ-5D (0–1), Mean (SD)[a]			
Baseline	0.65	0.64	
Follow-up	0.63	0.65	
Difference	−0.02	0.01	0.03 (−0.04 to 0.04) NS
Pain intensity (1–10) Mean (SD)[b]			
Baseline	6.5	6.4	
Follow-up	6.2	5.1	
Difference	0.3	1.3	1.0 (0.5 to 2.3)
Days of pain in the previous year, Mean (SD)[b]			
Baseline	101	103	
Follow-up	104	83	
Difference	3	−20	−23 (−30 to −10)
Days of sick leave, Mean (SD)[a]			
Baseline	12	12	
Follow-up	13	5	
Difference	1	−7	−8 (−10 to −2)

[a]Higher Scores = better health (less disability).

[b]Higher Scores = worse health (more disability).

NS = not significantly different.

increase in average overall utility scores was seen with the SF-6D, indicating an improved QoL, but the improvement was not significantly different when comparing the change in EQ-5D scores. The additional cost per additional QALY produced by the addition of Backtramine would be acceptable at the common threshold of $50,000 per QALY using the SF-6D measure but not using the EQ-5D measure (Exhibit 8.9). Sensitivity analyses indicate that results are sensitive to a number of variables.

CONCLUSIONS: Although the EQ-5D and the SF-6D have both been used and validated as generic outcome assessments in chronic low back pain, it appears they are not interchangeable. Other clinical measures are important when assessing patient outcomes and may be more sensitive to clinical changes in patients with long-term back pain. Sensitivity analysis indicated that a change in assumptions affects the conclusions of this study.

EXHIBIT 8.9

Incremental Ratios and Sensitivity Analyses

	Values ($)	Incremental Ratio ($)
Baseline Calculations		
Incremental cost bactramine	2,800/year	
Incremental outcomes		
SF-6D	2,800/ 0.06 QALY	46,667/QALY
EQ-5D	2,800/ 0.03 QALY	93,333/QALY
Pain-free days	2,800/23 days	122/pain-free day
Workdays	2,800/8 days	350/workday
Sensitivity Analyses—Costs		
Incremental cost bactramine	3,500/year	
Incremental outcomes		
SF-6D	3,500/ 0.06 QALY	58,333/QALY
EQ-5D	3,500/ 0.03 QALY	116,667/QALY
Pain-free days	3,500/23 days	152/pain-free day
Workdays	3,500/8 days	438/workday
Sensitivity Analyses—Outcomes		
Incremental cost bactramine	2,800/year	
Incremental outcomes		
SF-6D	2,800/ 0.05 QALY	56,000/QALY
EQ-5D	2,800/ 0.025 QALY	112,000/QALY
Pain-free days	2,800/20 days	140/pain-free day
Workdays	2,800/5 days	560/workday

WORKSHEET FOR CRITIQUE OF HRQoL ARTICLE 2

1. Complete Title?

_____

_____

_____

_____

2. Clear Objective?

_____

_____

_____

_____

3. Appropriate Alternatives?

_____

_____

_____

4. Alternatives Described?

_____

_____

_____

_____

5. Perspective Stated?

_____

_____

_____

_____

6. Type of Study?

_____

_____

_____

_____

7. Relevant Costs?

_____

_____

_____

_____

8. Relevant Outcomes?

_____

_____

_____

_____

9. Adjustment or Discounting?

_____

_____

_____

_____

10. Reasonable Assumptions?

_____

_____

_____

_____

11. Sensitivity Analyses?

_____

_____

_____

_____

12. Limitations Addressed?

_____

_____

_____

_____

13. Generalizations Appropriate?

_____

_____

_____

_____

14. Unbiased Conclusions?

_____

_____

_____

_____

CRITIQUE OF HRQoL ARTICLE 2

1. **Complete Title:** The title did identify the options and type of study.

2. **Clear Objective:** The objective of this study was to investigate the cost-effectiveness and cost-utility of standard analgesic/anti-inflammatory treatment for chronic back pain compared with standard treatment with the addition of a new serotonin–norepinephrine reuptake inhibitor (SNRI), called Backtramine. This was clear.

3. **Appropriate Alternatives:** The authors indicated why an antidepressant may be added to the regimen and indicated that results from previous studies were mixed.

4. **Alternatives Described:** The SNRI dose (60 mg) and dosing (once-a-day) were stipulated. Not much detail was given about the "standard therapy."

5. **Perspective Stated:** The perspective of the study was not stated. Since the only costs that were measured were costs of medications, it is assumed that the perspective is that of the payer (patient and/or medication insurance).

6. **Type of Study:** The study was correctly identified as a CEA and CUA because the outcomes were measured using both patient-reported clinical units (pain intensity; days in pain; days missed from work) and utilities (EQ-5D and SF-6D scores).

7. **Relevant Costs:** Very narrow measurement of costs. A reduction in pain might also decrease the use of other medical services and increase a patient's productivity—both of which could have been valued in monetary terms. Estimating a specific dollar value for the intangible benefits of pain reduction and improved functioning would be more difficult.

8. **Relevant Outcomes:** There are other clinical measures of pain that are commonly used (e.g., Roland Disability Scale) that were not addressed, and measuring pain at only two points (baseline and 1-year post-index) misses variations that happen during the year. In addition, patients may have trouble recalling days of work missed, or valuing an average level of pain for such a long period. No information was available on adverse events in the two cohorts. For example, common effects of SNRIs are dry mouth, dizziness, and changes in appetite and sleep patterns.

9. **Adjustment or Discounting:** The authors used 2012 costs, so adjustment was not needed. The study only followed patients for 12 months, so discounting was not needed.

10. **Reasonable Assumptions:** An implicit assumption was that the outcomes measured were reliable and valid in this population of patients. Outcomes measures were not as complete or assessed often enough (see #8). It was assumed that the cost of bactramine would be the only medical cost that would be different between the two cohorts (see #7).

11. **Sensitivity Analyses:** Sensitivity analyses were conducted for medication costs and utility estimates. Both were sensitive to the ranges used.

12. **Limitations Addressed:** The authors did not address any limitations. Limitations with the measurement of costs and outcomes have been addressed (see #7 and #8).

13. **Generalizations Appropriate:** Although patients were recruited from 10 clinics, they were all from one geographical area. Comparisons to patients in other US regions could help determine the degree of similarities or differences with other populations.

14. **Unbiased Conclusions:** As with previous studies, results were mixed depending on assumptions. A narrow view of costs was used. The authors should have addressed some of the limitations and given more detail about standard therapy.

QUESTIONS/EXERCISES

Part 1

Go to the following Website to take the SF-36 QoL Survey: http://www.sf-36.org/demos/SF-36.html

The Website will calculate your scores. The codes on the scores are as follows:

BP = bodily pain; GH = general health; MH = mental health; PF = physical functioning; RE = role–emotional; RP = role–physical; SF = social functioning; and VT = vitality.

The first set of scores is your score on a scale of 0 (worst) to 100 (best) QoL. The next two sets of scores are "norm based," which means that compared with the average person taking the survey, you are above average if your score is above 50% or below average if you scored less than 50%.

The average or "norms" (scale ranges from 0 to 100) for the United States were reported by Ware et al.[6] as BP = 71.3, GH = 70.8, MH = 75.0, PF = 83.3, RE = 87.4, RP = 82.5, SF = 84.3, and VT = 58.3.

SF-36v2™ Health Survey 1996, 2000 by QualityMetric Incorporated—All rights reserved. SF-36v2™ is a trademark of QualityMetric Incorporated. (Available at http://www.sf-36.org. Reprinted with permission from Ware JE, Kosinski M, Dewey JE. *How to Score Version 2 of the SF-36® Health Survey*. Lincoln, RI: Quality-Metric Incorporated, 2000.)

Part 2

Take the following EQ-5D Quality-of-Life instrument (reprinted with permission from http://www.euroqol.org):

By placing a checkmark for one box for each numbered item below, please indicate which statements best describe your own health state today.

1. Mobility

   ❏ I have no problems in walking about.
   ❏ I have some problems in walking about.
   ❏ I am confined to bed.

2. Self-care

   ❏ I have no problems with self-care.
   ❏ I have some problems washing or dressing myself.
   ❏ I am unable to wash or dress myself.

3. Usual activities (e.g., work, study, housework, family or leisure activities)

   ❏ I have no problems with performing my usual activities.

   ❏ I have some problems with performing my usual activities.

   ❏ I am unable to perform my usual activities.

4. Pain or discomfort

   ❏ I have no pain or discomfort.
   ❏ I have moderate pain or discomfort.
   ❏ I have extreme pain or discomfort.

5. Anxiety or depression

   ❏ I am not anxious or depressed.
   ❏ I am moderately anxious or depressed.
   ❏ I am extremely anxious or depressed.

For each of the five dimensions, score a 1 if you choose the first (best) response, 2 if you chose the second response, and 3 if you score the third (worst) response. Now look up your score using the information found in the table that follows. For example, if you have no problems with dimensions 1, 2, 3, and 5 (mobility, self-care, usual activities, and anxiety or depression) but have moderate pain, you would look up 11121, and your QoL score would be 0.827 on a scale of 0.000 to 1.000.

US Population-Based Predicted Preference Weights and Standard Errors (SEs) for 243 EQ-5D Health States

State	Value	SE	State	Value	SE	State	Value	SE
11111	1.000	0.000	13211	0.529	0.013	31212	0.415	0.013
11211	0.860	0.008	21322	0.527	0.013	13312	0.414	0.014
21111	0.854	0.008	22312	0.524	0.013	22131	0.410	0.018
11112	0.844	0.008	23111	0.522	0.014	31121	0.409	0.014
21211	0.843	0.009	11123	0.517	0.015	32111	0.407	0.014
11212	0.833	0.010	12113	0.514	0.014	21323	0.401	0.014
11121	0.827	0.008	13112	0.512	0.014	12132	0.400	0.018
21112	0.827	0.009	23211	0.512	0.013	22313	0.399	0.014
12111	0.825	0.008	22321	0.508	0.014	31221	0.398	0.013
11221	0.816	0.009	11223	0.506	0.014	13321	0.397	0.014
12211	0.814	0.008	12213	0.503	0.013	21232	0.397	0.018
21121	0.810	0.008	13212	0.501	0.013	23312	0.397	0.014
22111	0.808	0.009	21123	0.499	0.014	32211	0.396	0.013
11122	0.800	0.009	12322	0.497	0.014	31122	0.382	0.014
12112	0.797	0.008	22113	0.497	0.014	23321	0.380	0.014
21212	0.794	0.011	13121	0.496	0.015	32112	0.379	0.015
12121	0.781	0.007	23112	0.495	0.014	22223	0.378	0.018
21221	0.778	0.010	13221	0.485	0.014	22231	0.378	0.019
22211	0.775	0.010	23121	0.478	0.014	23222	0.376	0.017
11222	0.768	0.011	12123	0.470	0.015	12323	0.372	0.014
12212	0.765	0.009	13122	0.468	0.015	13322	0.370	0.014
21122	0.761	0.009	21223	0.467	0.014	12232	0.368	0.019
22112	0.759	0.010	22213	0.465	0.013	11331	0.365	0.018
12221	0.748	0.009	11131	0.463	0.020	32121	0.363	0.014
22121	0.742	0.008	11231	0.463	0.017	22132	0.361	0.019
12122	0.732	0.008	23212	0.463	0.014	21331	0.358	0.016
21222	0.708	0.013	21131	0.456	0.017	13113	0.355	0.019
22212	0.705	0.012	11313	0.452	0.015	13213	0.354	0.017
22221	0.689	0.012	11132	0.446	0.018	31222	0.350	0.015
12222	0.678	0.012	23221	0.446	0.015	23113	0.348	0.018
22122	0.672	0.012	21231	0.446	0.016	11332	0.348	0.011
11311	0.626	0.013	21313	0.445	0.013	32212	0.347	0.015

State	Value	SE	State	Value	SE	State	Value	SE
21311	0.619	0.011	31111	0.442	0.016	31311	0.344	0.116
11312	0.609	0.011	31211	0.442	0.013	23213	0.337	0.017
22222	0.597	0.019	12223	0.438	0.015	22323	0.333	0.015
11321	0.592	0.013	22322	0.437	0.017	23322	0.331	0.014
21312	0.592	0.011	13222	0.436	0.015	21332	0.331	0.015
12311	0.590	0.012	11232	0.435	0.017	32221	0.330	0.014
21321	0.575	0.012	22123	0.432	0.015	12331	0.329	0.017
22311	0.573	0.012	13311	0.431	0.016	31312	0.327	0.015
11322	0.565	0.012	23122	0.430	0.015	13123	0.321	0.018
12312	0.563	0.012	21132	0.429	0.017	32122	0.314	0.016
11113	0.550	0.015	12131	0.427	0.019	22331	0.312	0.016
11213	0.550	0.012	31112	0.426	0.014	31321	0.311	0.014
12321	0.546	0.013	23311	0.424	0.014	13223	0.310	0.017
21113	0.543	0.013	11323	0.418	0.014	32311	0.308	0.015
21213	0.533	0.011	12231	0.416	0.017	22232	0.308	0.022
13111	0.529	0.016	12313	0.416	0.014	23123	0.304	0.018
12332	0.302	0.016	32213	0.222	0.017	32323	0.120	0.016
11133	0.289	0.022	11333	0.220	0.019	32132	0.118	0.020
11233	0.289	0.019	33212	0.220	0.020	33322	0.118	0.016
13313	0.286	0.018	32322	0.216	0.015	23133	0.117	0.022
31322	0.283	0.014	21333	0.214	0.017	31331	0.112	0.019
21133	0.282	0.020	33121	0.214	0.017	23233	0.106	0.021
32312	0.281	0.015	22233	0.204	0.018	33113	0.102	0.022
23313	0.279	0.017	33221	0.203	0.016	33213	0.102	0.020
23223	0.272	0.017	23232	0.202	0.020	31332	0.096	0.017
21233	0.271	0.018	31313	0.199	0.018	32232	0.086	0.020
31113	0.268	0.019	13331	0.199	0.019	13333	0.084	0.018
13131	0.268	0.022	23331	0.193	0.018	23333	0.077	0.016
31213	0.268	0.017	32123	0.188	0.018	32331	0.077	0.017
13231	0.268	0.019	33122	0.186	0.018	33123	0.069	0.021
32321	0.264	0.014	12333	0.184	0.018	33313	0.063	0.017
22332	0.263	0.017	13332	0.182	0.017	33223	0.058	0.020
23131	0.261	0.020	31131	0.151	0.021	32332	0.049	0.017
32222	0.260	0.018	31231	0.181	0.018	31133	0.037	0.023
12133	0.253	0.021	33311	0.178	0.018	31233	0.036	0.020
13323	0.253	0.017	22333	0.167	0.017	33323	0.030	0.016
13132	0.251	0.020	31323	0.166	0.017	33131	0.016	0.023
23231	0.250	0.019	23332	0.165	0.017	33231	0.015	0.020
33111	0.247	0.019	31132	0.165	0.020	32133	0.001	0.022

(Continued)

State	Value	SE	State	Value	SE	State	Value	SE
33211	0.247	0.017	32313	0.164	0.017	33132	20.001	0.022
12233	0.242	0.019	33312	0.162	0.017	31333	20.003	0.017
13232	0.240	0.019	32223	0.156	0.017	32233	20.110	0.020
22133	0.236	0.020	33222	0.154	0.118	33232	20.012	0.021
23323	0.235	0.017	31232	0.154	0.019	33331	20.024	0.016
31123	0.235	0.018	32131	0.145	0.020	32333	20.038	0.016
23132	0.234	0.020	33321	0.145	0.016	33332	20.040	0.015
32113	0.232	0.018	32231	0.135	0.018	33133	20.100	0.021
33112	0.230	0.019	13133	0.123	0.024	33233	20.100	0.019
31223	0.224	0.017	13233	0.123	0.021	33333	20.109	0.012

SE indicate standard error.

Reprinted with permission from Shaw JW, Johnson JA, Coons SJ. US valuation of the EQ-5D health states: Development and testing of the D1 valuation model. Medical Care 43(3):203–220, 2005.

1. Were you surprised by any of your scores from the SF-36? How about the EQ-5D?

_____

_____

_____

_____

2. Which survey do you think is better at representing your health state? Why?

_____

_____

_____

_____

3. What are one advantage and one disadvantage of using the SF-36 to measure a patient's HRQoL?

_____

_____

_____

_____

4. What are one advantage and one disadvantage of using the EQ-5D to measure a patient's HRQoL?

_____

_____

_____

_____

REFERENCES

1. Schipper H, Clinch JJ, Olweny CLM. Quality of life studies: Definitions and conceptual issues. In Spilker B (ed). *Quality of Life and Pharmacoeconomics in Clinical Trials* (2nd ed.). Philadelphia, PA: Lippincott-Raven, 1996.

2. World Health Organization. *Basic Documents: World Health Organization.* Geneva, Switzerland: World Health Organization, 1948.

3. Deverill M, Brazier J, Green C, Booth A. The use of QALY and non-QALY measures of health-related quality of life: Assessing the state of the art. *Pharmacoeconomics* 13(4): 411–420, 1998.

4. Ware JE, Sherbourne CD. The MOS-36-item short-form health survey (SF-36): Conceptual framework and item selection. *Medical Care* 30(6):473–483, 1992.

5. Ware JE, Kosinski M, Keller SD. A 12-item short-form health survey: Construction of scales and preliminary tests of reliability and validity. *Medical Care* 34(3):220–233, 1996.

6. Ware JE, Kosinski M, Gandek B. *SF-36 Health Survey: Manual and Interpretation Guide.* Lincoln, RI: QualityMetric Incorporated, 2002.

7. Ware JE, Kosinski M, Dewey JE. *How to Score Version 2 of the SF-36 Survey (Standard and Acute Forms).* Lincoln, RI: QualityMetric Incorporated, 2005.

8. Juniper EF, Guyatt GH, Epstein RS, et al. Evaluation of impairment of health related quality of life in asthma: Development of a questionnaire for use in Clinical Trials. *Thorax* 47(2):76–83, 1992.

9. Juniper EF, Guyatt GH, Willan A, Griffith LE Determining a minimal important change in a disease-specific Quality of Life Questionnaire. *Journal of Clinical Epidemiology* 47(1):81–87, 1994.

10. EuroQoL. Available at http://www.euroqol.org.

11. van Hout B, Janssen MF, Feng YS, et al. Interim scoring for the EQ-5D-5L: Mapping the EQ-5D-5L to EQ-5D-3L value sets. *Value in Health: The Journal of the International Society for Pharmacoeconomics and Outcomes Research* 15(5):708–715, 2012.

12. Brazier J, Roberts J, Deverill M. The estimation of a preference-based measure of health from the SF-36. *Journal of Health Economics* 21(2):271–292, 2002.

13. Brazier JE, Roberts, J. The estimation of a preference-based measure of health from the SF-12. *Medical Care* 42(9):851–859, 2004.

14. Luo N, Johnson J, Shaw J, Coons S. Relative efficiency of the EQ-5D, HUI2, and HUI3 index scores in measuring health burden of chronic medical conditions in a population health survey in the United States. *Medical Care* 47(1):53–60, 2009.

15. McTaggart-Cowan HM, Marra CA, Yang Y, et al. The validity of generic and condition-specific preference-based instruments: The ability to discriminate asthma control status. *Quality of Life Research: An International Journal of Quality of Life Aspects of Treatment, Care and Rehabilitation* 17(3):453–462, 2008.

16. Brazier J, Rowen D, Mavranezouli I, et al. Developing and testing methods for deriving preference-based measures of health from condition-specific measures (and other patient-based measures of outcome). *Health Technology Assessment (Winchester, England)* 16(32):1–114, 2012.

17. Pickard AS, Wang Z, Walton SM, Lee TA. Are decisions using cost-utility analyses robust to choice of SF-36/SF-12 preference-based algorithm? *Health and Quality of Life Outcomes* 3:11, 2005.

18. Joore M, Brunenberg D, Nelemans P, et al. The impact of differences in EQ-5D and SF-6D utility scores on the acceptability of cost-utility ratios: Results across five trial-based cost-utility studies. *Value in Health: The Journal of the International Society for Pharmacoeconomics and Outcomes Research* 13(2): 222–229, 2010.

19. U.S. Department of Health and Human Services Food and Drug Administration (FDA). *Guidance for Industry: Patient-Reported Outcome Measures: Use in Medical Product Development to Support Labeling Claims.* Maryland: FDA, 2009. Available at http://www.fda.gov/downloads/Drugs/Guidances/UCM193282.pdf.

20. Lohr K, Zebrack B. Using patient-reported outcomes in clinical practice: Challenges and opportunities. *Quality of Life Research: An International Journal of Quality of Life Aspects of Treatment, Care and Rehabilitation* 18(1):99–107, 2009.

21. Chang C. Patient-reported outcomes measurement and management with innovative methodologies and technologies. *Quality of Life Research: An International Journal of Quality of Life Aspects of Treatment, Care and Rehabilitation* 16(suppl 1):157–166, 2007.

22. Kaplan RM, Anderson JP. A general health policy model: An integrated approach. In Spilker B (ed). *Quality of Life Assessment in Clinical Trials.* New York: Raven Press Ltd, 1990:131–199.

23. Bergner M, Bobbitt RA, Carter WB, et al. The Sickness Impact Profile: Development and final revision of a health status measure. *Medical Care* 19(8):787–805, 1981.

24. Nelson EC, Wasson JH, Johnson DJ, et al. Dartmouth COOP functional health assessment charts: Brief measures for clinical practice. In Spilker B (ed). *Quality of Life and Pharmacoeconomics in Clinical Trials* (2nd ed.). Philadelphia, PA: Lippincott-Raven, 1996:161–168.

25. Anderson RB, Hollenberg NK, Williams GH. Physical Symptoms Distress Index: A sensitive tool to evaluate the impact of pharmacological agents on quality of life. *Archives of Internal Medicine* 159(7):693–700, 1999.

26. Dimenäs E, Dahlöf C, Oloffson B, Wiklund I. An instrument for quantifying subjective symptoms among untreated and treated hypertensives: Development and documentation. *Journal of Clinical Research and Pharmacoepidemiology* 4(3):205–217, 1990.

27. Barry MJ, Fowler FJ, O'Leary MP, et al. The Measurement Committee of the American Urological Association. The American Urological Association symptom index for benign prostatic hyperplasia. *Journal of Urology* 148(5):1549–1557, 1992.

28. Fowler FJ Jr, Barry MJ. Quality of life assessment for evaluating benign prostatic hyperplasia treatments. An example of using a condition-specific index. *European Urology* 24(suppl 1): 24–27, 1993.

29. Hyland ME, Finnis S, Irvine SH. A scale for assessing quality of life in adult asthma sufferers. *Journal of Psychosomatic Research* 35(1):99–110, 1991.

30. Creer TL, Wigal JK, Kotses H, et al. A life activities questionnaire for adult asthma. *Journal of Asthma* 29(6):393–399, 1992.

31. The DCCT Research Group. Reliability and validity of a diabetes quality of life measure (DQOL) for the Diabetes Control and Complication Trial (DCCT). *Diabetes Care* 11(9): 725–732, 1988.

32. Cella DF, Tulsky DS, Gray G, et al. The Functional Assessment of Cancer Therapy Scale: Development and validation of the general measure. *Journal of Clinical Oncology* 11(3): 570–579, 1993.

33. Schain W, Edwards BK, Gorrell CR, et al. Psychological and physical outcomes of primary breast cancer therapy: Mastectomy vs excisional biopsy and irradiation. *Breast Cancer Research and Treatment* 3(4):377–382, 1983.

34. Meenan RF, Gertman PM, Mason JH. Measuring health status in arthritis: The Arthritis Impact Measurement Scales. *Arthritis and Rheumatism* 23(2):146–152, 1980.

35. Helewa A, Goldsmith CH, Smythe HA. Independent measurement of functional capacity in rheumatoid arthritis. *Journal of Rheumatology* 9(5):794–797, 1982.

36. McCain NL, Zeller JM, Cella DF, et al. The influence of stress management training in HIV disease. *Nursing Research* 45(4):246–253, 1996.

37. Berry SH, Bozette SA, Hays RD, et al. *Measuring Patient-Reported Health Status in Advanced HIV Disease: The HIV-PARSE Survey Instrument.* Santa Monica, CA: RAND, 1994.

38. Lubeck DP, Fries JF. Changes in quality of life among persons with HIV infection. *Quality of Life Research* 1(6):359–366, 1992.

SUGGESTED READINGS

Bungay KM, Boyer JG, Steinwald AB, Ware JE Jr. Health-related quality of life: An overview. In Bootman JL, Townsend RJ, McGhan WF (eds). *Principles of Pharmacoeconomics* (3rd ed.). Cincinnati, OH: Harvey Whitney Books Co, 2005.

Coons SJ, Rao S, Keininger DL, et al. A comparative review of generic quality-of-life instruments. *Pharmacoeconomics* 17(1):13–35, 2000.

Fayers PM, Machin D. *Quality of Life: The Assessment, Analysis and Interpretation of Patient-Reported Outcomes* (2nd ed.). West Sussex, England: John Wiley & Sons, 2007.

McDowell I. *Measuring Health: A Guide to Rating Scales and Questionnaires* (3rd ed.). Oxford: Oxford University Press, 2006.

McLeod L, Coon C, Martin S, et al. Interpreting patient-reported outcome results: US FDA guidance and emerging methods. *Expert Review of Pharmacoeconomics & Outcomes Research* 11(2):163–169, 2011.

Speight J, Barendse S. FDA guidance on patient reported outcomes. *BMJ (Clinical Research Ed.)* 340:c2921, 2010.

Spilker B (ed). *Quality of Life and Pharmacoeconomics in Clinical Trials* (2nd ed.). Philadelphia, PA: Lippincott-Raven Publishers, 1996.

Chapter 9

Decision Analysis

Objectives

Upon completing this chapter, the reader will be able to:

1. Give the definition and purpose of decision analysis.

2. List the steps for performing a decision analysis.

3. Draw a decision tree.

4. Calculate average costs and outcomes from a decision tree.

5. Interpret threshold analysis graphs.

✦ WHAT IS DECISION ANALYSIS?

Decision analysis is the application of an analytical method for systematically comparing different decision options. Decision analysis graphically displays choices and facilitates the calculation of values needed to compare these options. It assists with selecting the best or most cost-effective alternative. Decision analysis is a tool that has been used for years in many fields. This method of analysis assists in making decisions when the decision is complex and there is uncertainty about some of the information.[1]

✦ STEPS IN DECISION ANALYSIS

The steps in the decision process are relatively straightforward, especially with the availability of computer programs that greatly simplify the calculations. Articles reporting a decision analysis should include a graphical depiction (decision tree) of the choices and outcomes of interest. For this chapter, the steps in a decision analysis are outlined using an example concerning whether to include a new antibiotic on a hospital **formulary.** For illustrative purposes, the chapter begins with a simple tree that combines the probabilities of two outcomes of interest—the probability of a clinical success and the probability of any adverse events caused by the antibiotic. More complex issues (e.g., the probability of each of the main adverse events) can be incorporated using the same calculation techniques presented in the example.

Step 1: Identify the Specific Decision

The specific decision to be evaluated should be clearly defined by answering the questions: What is the objective of the study? Over what period of time will the analysis be conducted (e.g., the episode of care, a year)? Will the **perspective** be that of the patient, the medical care plan, an institution or organization, or society? For the example problem, the decision is whether to add a new antibiotic to an institutional formulary to treat infections. The perspective is that of the institution, and the time period of interest is the episode of care (about 2 weeks).

Step 2: Specify Alternatives

Ideally, the most effective treatments or alternatives should be compared. In pharmacotherapy evaluations, makers of innovative new products may compare or measure themselves against a standard (i.e., older, more well-established) therapy. This is most often the case with new chemical entities. Decision analysis could compare more than two treatment options (e.g., it could compare the five most common statins) or an intervention versus no intervention (e.g., a diabetes clinic versus no clinic). For the example problem, the use of the new medication (antibiotic A) will be compared with that of the current standard (antibiotic B).

Step 3: Draw the Decision Analysis Structure

Lines are drawn to joint decision points (branches or arms of a decision tree), represented as choice nodes, chance nodes, or terminal (final outcome) nodes. Nodes are places in the decision tree where different options occur; branching becomes possible at this point. There are three types of nodes: (1) in a choice node, a choice is allowed (e.g., treatment A versus treatment B); (2) in a chance node, chance comes into the equation (e.g., the chance or probability of cure or adverse events for different treatment options); and (3) in a terminal node, the final outcome of interest for each option in the decision is represented. The units used to measure final outcomes (e.g., dollars or quality-adjusted life years [QALYs]) must be the same for each option being considered. By convention, software programs use a square box to represent a choice node, a circle to represent a chance node, and a triangle for a terminal branch or final outcome. Figure 9.1 illustrates the decision tree for the antibiotic example.

Step 4: Specify Possible Costs, Outcomes, and Probabilities

For each option, information should be obtained for the probability of occurrence and the consequences of the occurrence. Probabilities are assigned for each branch of the chance nodes, and the sum of the probabilities for each branch must add up to 1.00. Consequences are reported as monetary outcomes, health-related outcomes, or both. Decision analysis articles should provide a listing of the probability, cost, and outcome estimates used in the analysis, including where or how the estimates were obtained (e.g., literature review, clinical trial, expert panel). Table 9.1 lists these data for the antibiotic example.

Step 5: Perform Calculations

At each terminal node, the probability of a patient having that outcome is calculated by multiplying the probability of each arm from the choice node to the

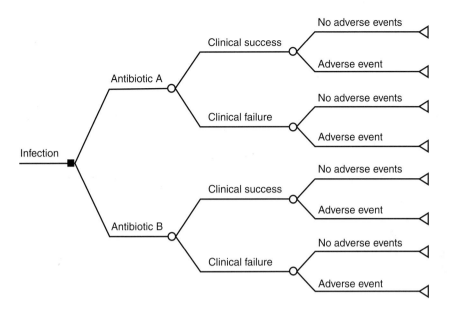

FIGURE 9.1. Decision tree structure for the antibiotic example.

terminal node. The total costs for each terminal node are calculated by adding up the costs over all of the branches from the choice node to the terminal node. The product of the costs multiplied by the probability ($C \times P$) is calculated for each node and then summed for each option.

In our example, each of the two options (antibiotic A versus antibiotic B) has four possible terminal endpoints: success/no adverse events, success/adverse events, failure/no adverse events, and failure/adverse events. Table 9.2 and Figure 9.2 show the calculations used to estimate the average expected cost per treatment. Note that the sum of the probabilities for the four terminal endpoints equals 1.00. For patients taking antibiotic A, the costs can range from $600 (for medication and no adverse events) to $1,600 (for medication and treatment of adverse events), and the average cost is $700 per patient. Similarly, for patients taking antibiotic B, the costs can range from $500 (for medication and no adverse events) to $1,500 (for medication and treatment of adverse events), and the average cost is $650 per patient. These calculations show that antibiotic B is less expensive even when including the costs of treating adverse events. But because antibiotic A is a better clinical option (higher probability of success and lower probability of adverse events), decision makers could use either the **incremental cost-effectiveness ratio** (ICER)

TABLE 9.1. **ESTIMATES FOR THE ANTIBIOTIC EXAMPLE**		
	Antibiotic A	*Antibiotic B*
Probability of clinical success (%)	90	80
Cost of antibiotic per course of therapy ($)	600	500
Probability of adverse events (%)	10	15
Cost of treating adverse events ($)	1,000	1,000

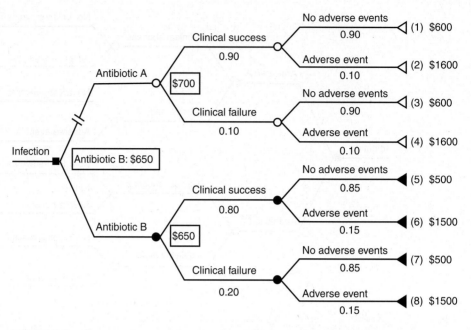

FIGURE 9.2. Average cost per treatment choice for the antibiotic example.

or the **incremental net benefit** (INB) calculations to determine whether to add antibiotic A to the formulary. The calculated ICER would be:

$$\text{ICER} = \frac{\Delta \text{ Costs}}{\Delta \text{ Outcomes}} = \frac{\$700 - \$650}{0.090 - 0.80} = \$500 \text{ more per extra success}$$

If it is decided that each extra successful outcome is worth at least $500 (patient discharged from the hospital faster, prevention of second round of treatment costs with another antibiotic, and so on), then antibiotic A would be added to the

TABLE 9.2. **CALCULATIONS FOR THE ANTIBIOTIC EXAMPLE**			
Outcome	Cost ($)	Probability	Cost × Probability ($)
Antibiotic A			
Success with no adverse events	600	0.9 × 0.9 = 0.81	486
Success with adverse events	600 + 1,000 = 1,600	0.9 × 0.1 = 0.09	144
Failure with no adverse events	600	0.1 × 0.9 = 0.09	54
Failure with adverse events	600 + 1,000 = 1,600	0.1 × 0.1 = 0.01	16
Total for antibiotic A		1.00	700
Antibiotic B			
Success with no adverse events	500	0.8 × 0.85 = 0.68	340
Success with adverse events	500 + 1,000 = 1,500	0.8 × 0.15 = 0.12	180
Failure with no adverse events	500	0.2 × 0.85 = 0.17	85
Failure with adverse events	500 + 1,000 = 1,500	0.2 × 0.15 = 0.03	45
Total for antibiotic B		1.00	650

EXAMPLE 9.1 INCREMENTAL NET BENEFIT
FOR THE ANTIBIOTIC EXAMPLE

As mentioned in Chapter 5, if the incremental cost-effectiveness ratio (ICER) is positive, one medication is both more effective and more costly, and it is up to the readers to determine if the extra cost is worth the extra benefit. Using the incremental net benefit (INB) approach, if it was determined that the value of each additional success with of a cure of infection was between $1,000 and $2,000, the INB calculations for these estimates (i.e., **lambdas**) would be:

$$INB_{\lambda = \$1,000} = (\Delta \text{ Outcome} \times \lambda) - \Delta \text{ Cost} = 0.10 (\$1,000) - \$50 = +\$50$$
$$INB_{\lambda = \$2,000} = (\Delta \text{ Outcome} \times \lambda) - \Delta \text{ Cost} = 0.10 (\$2,000) - \$50 = +\$150$$

This indicates that antibiotic A is cost-effective for this range of values.

---

formulary. See Example 9.1 for incremental net benefit (INB) calculations using a range of $1,000 to $2,000 as the value of successful treatment.

Step 6: Conduct a Sensitivity Analysis

Because some uncertainty surrounds the estimates used to construct these models, a **sensitivity analysis** is conducted. High and low estimates of costs and probabilities are inserted into the decision model to determine the range of answers. These estimates should be sufficiently varied to reflect realistic variations in values. In the base case analysis of our antibiotic example, the total cost of using antibiotic A averaged to $700 versus $650 for antibiotic B (see Table 9.2). By choosing possible high and low ranges for probabilities and costs, numerous one-way sensitivity analyses were conducted. One-way sensitivity analysis calculates the impact of using alternative estimated ranges for one variable at a time while holding the others constant. These calculations are shown in Table 9.3. For example, in the base analysis, the probability of having an adverse event when taking antibiotic A was 10%. When this value was tested for the range of 7% to 15%, the difference in total costs of antibiotic A minus antibiotic B ranges from $20 to $100. For the entire range, the cost of antibiotic A is higher than antibiotic B, so results are **insensitive** to this range of values.

For all other variables listed in Table 9.3, sensitivity was found for the ranges used. For example, in the base analysis, the probability of having an adverse event when taking antibiotic B was 15%. When this value was tested for the range of 10% to 25%, the difference in total costs of antibiotic A minus antibiotic B varied from $100 if the probability was at the lower end of the range (10%) to a cost savings of $50 for the higher end of the range (25%). This means that if the side effects of antibiotic B are as high as 25%, antibiotic A would now be a less costly option because of the extra costs associated with treating more people with adverse events from antibiotic B.

Sometimes a **tornado diagram** is used to compare the impact of various one-way sensitivity analyses.[2] The range that has the biggest impact on the answer is placed at the top of the graph and then the rest appear below in descending rank (hence the funnel or tornado look). A tornado diagram for the variables in Table 9.3 appears in Figure 9.3. The probability of adverse events for antibiotic A (p_AE_A) does not appear in Figure 9.3 because for the entire range (7% to 15%), antibiotic B was less expensive than antibiotic A, so there was no impact on the results.

TABLE 9.3. **SENSITIVITY ANALYSES FOR THE ANTIBIOTIC EXAMPLE**

Variable	Range L=Low Estimate H=High Estimate	Antibiotic A: Overall Costs ($)	Antibiotic B: Overall Costs ($)	Δ Overall Costs: A – B ($)
Base case		700	650	+50
Cost of treating adverse events	L = $500	650	575	+75
	H = $2,500	850	875	−25
Cost per course of therapy for antibiotic A	L = $400	500	650	−150
	H = $800	900	650	+250
Cost per course of therapy for antibiotic B	L = $350	700	500	+200
	H = $750	700	900	−200
Probability of adverse events for antibiotic A	L = 7%	670	650	+20
	H = 15%	750	650	+100
Probability of adverse events for antibiotic B	L = 10%	700	600	+100
	H = 25%	700	750	−50

L = low estimate; H = high estimate.

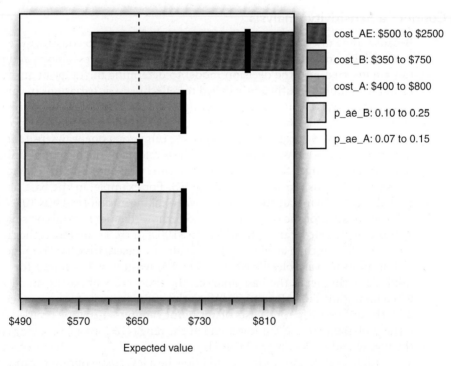

FIGURE 9.3. Tornado diagram for the antibiotic example. This tornado diagram compares the impact of various one-way sensitivity analyses that are shown in Table 9.3 [cost_AE (costs of treating adverse events), cost_B (cost of drug B), cost_A (cost of drug A), prob_ae_A (probability of adverse events for drug A), and p_ae_B (probability of adverse events for drug B)]. The range that has the biggest impact on the answer is placed at the top of the graph (in this example, cost_AE), and then the rest appear below in descending rank (hence the funnel or tornado look). The range of results for the variable p_ae_A does not appear in Figure 9.3 because for the entire range (7% to 15%) antibiotic B was less expensive than antibiotic A, so there was no impact on the choice of antibiotic for this variable.

✦ THRESHOLD ANALYSIS

As seen in Table 9.3, most of the variables used in the antibiotic example were sensitive to the range of estimates used, that is, at one end on the range, antibiotic A was less expensive, but at the other end of the range, antibiotic B was less expensive. **Threshold analysis** helps identify the level within the range at which the decision switches. Figure 9.4 is an example of the threshold analysis looking at the probability of adverse events when using antibiotic B (p_ae_B). At the threshold point of p_ae_B = 20%, the total costs of antibiotic A and antibiotic B are equal (expected value [EV] of $700). If the probability of adverse events for antibiotic B is determined to be higher than this threshold, total costs for antibiotic A are lower than for antibiotic B. On the other hand, if the probability is lower than 20%, antibiotic B would be calculated to be less expensive.

Figure 9.5 shows a threshold analysis for the cost of treating adverse events (cost_AE). When these costs are $2,000, the cost of using antibiotic A and B are equal (EV of $800). If the costs of treating side effects are more than $2,000, then antibiotic A is less expensive than antibiotic B; otherwise, antibiotic B is less expensive.

Two-way sensitivity analyses indicate the impact of varying two estimates at a time and can be depicted using a threshold analyses graph. For the antibiotic example, a depiction of a two-way sensitivity analysis for the probability of adverse events with antibiotic B and the cost of treating adverse events is shown in Figure 9.6. To determine which choice is less costly overall, one would choose a point within each range that is their best estimate and draw intersecting lines from the x and y axis of the graph. For example, if a decision maker estimates that the probability of adverse events for antibiotic B is 17% and the cost of treating adverse

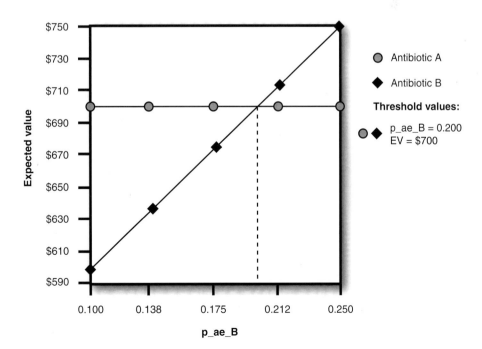

FIGURE 9.4. One-way sensitivity analysis for the probability of adverse events for antibiotic B (p_ae_B).

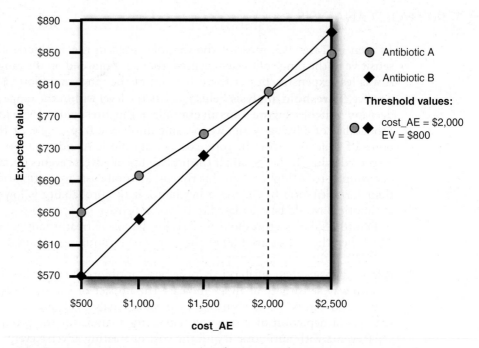

FIGURE 9.5. One-way sensitivity analysis for the cost of treating adverse events of antibiotic treatment (cost_AE).

events is about $1,250, antibiotic B would be the less costly option (see the square in the lightly shaded section of Fig. 9.6). On the other hand, if it is estimated that the probability is 20% and the cost is $1500, then antibiotic A would be less costly (see the circle in the darkly shaded section of Fig. 9.6).

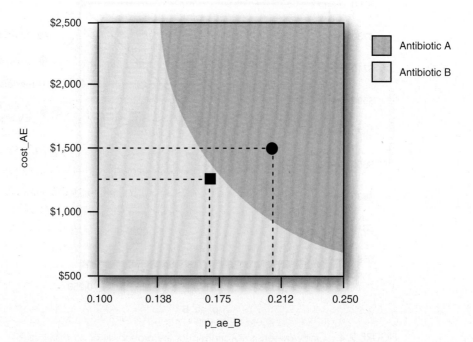

FIGURE 9.6. Two-way sensitivity analysis for the probability of adverse events for antibiotic B (p_ae_B) and the cost of treating adverse events of antibiotic treatment (cost_AE).

SUMMARY

Decision analysis is a technique that can be used to incorporate information and estimates in a systematic way to compare different options. Decision analysis is being used more commonly in pharmacoeconomic evaluations. The use and availability of computer programs to assist with the multiple calculations make it fairly easy for someone to automate their evaluations. Examples of software available for this purpose include Data TreeAge (info@treeage.com), which was used for this book,

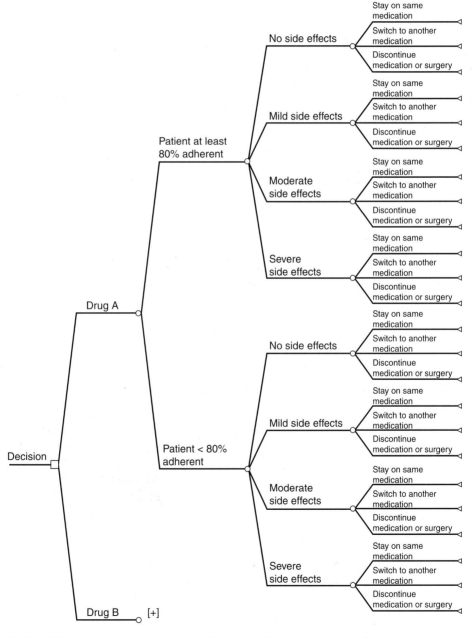

FIGURE 9.7. Decision tree with multiple branches. The plus sign next to the branch for drug B indicates that it uses the same tree structure as the other option (drug A).

and DecisionPro (Vanguard Software Corporation, vginfo@vanguardsw.com). The prices for these software packages range from less than $100 for student versions to almost $1,000 for professional versions. More examples of computer software, vendors, and prices can be found at the Decision Analysis Society's Web site (info// faculty.fuqua.duke.edu/daweb/dasw6.htm). Microsoft Excel can also be used to conduct decision analyses.

It is important to remember that the decision analysis results are only as good as the information used to develop the model. Decision makers should critically evaluate the decision tree structure, the probability and cost estimates, and the **assumptions** used to determine if the results are credible and useful for their purpose. Sensitivity analyses can indicate which uncertain estimates have the largest impact on the results.

While builders of decision trees should try to capture all realistic clinical possibilities and outcomes, the tree may quickly grow in complexity (see Fig. 9.7 for a more complex decision tree). The complexity of model building increases for chronic conditions in which treatment and outcomes are measured over long periods of time. **Markov modeling** (discussed in Chapter 10) serves to break up the analysis into shorter time frames (or cycles) to better represent the nature of the disease or condition.

COMPOSITE ARTICLE 1: DECISION ANALYSIS—MIGRAINE

Title: COST-UTILITY ANALYSIS OF MIGRAINE TREATMENTS FOR PATIENTS IN A MANAGED CARE ORGANIZATION

OBJECTIVE: The purpose of the study is to evaluate two migraine treatments: the orally administered Mi-Tab and the injection Mi-Ject. Both products have been shown by the Food and Drug Administration to be useful in treating migraines. In fact, they contain the same active ingredient. The injection product has a faster onset of action and is slightly more successful in treating migraines, but it also has a higher rate of side effects reported, including redness, inflammation, and itching at the injection site.

METHODS: The perspective of the study is the payer, specifically, the managed care organization (MCO). Both products should be taken at the first sign of a migraine. Information about both products is listed in Exhibit 9.1. The outcome of interest is measured using quality-adjusted life days (QALDs), which incorporates the change in health-related quality of life (HRQoL) for the day of the migraine. If a patient feels a migraine coming and takes the oral product (Mi-Tab), it works, and the patient

has no side effects, then the patient's QALD is measured at 1.0 (no decrease for that day). If the patient is using the injection (Mi-Ject) and has to inject himself or herself, this decreases the patient's QALD by 0.1 because of the inconvenience and pain of an injection. If the patient is nauseated as a result of either product, this decreases the QALD by 0.2. If the patient experiences redness and inflammation at the injection site, this decreases the QALD by 0.2. If the medication does not work and the patient goes to the emergency department (ED) for further treatment or rests in a dark room until the migraine subsides, this decreases the QALD by 0.5. It was assumed that half of the patients would go to the ED if the medication did not work.

RESULTS: A decision tree incorporating the study estimates is found in Exhibit 9.2. The analysis shows that Mi-Tab is less expensive ($110) and has a better outcome (0.93 QALD) on average than the Mi-Ject preparation ($115 for 0.85 QALD); therefore, Mi-Tab is the better

EXHIBIT 9.1

Information about Mi-Tab and Mi-Ject

	Source of Data	Mi-Tab	Mi-Ject
Cost of medication per treatment	Managed care costs	$80	$100
Onset of action	Literature review	30–40 min	5–10 min
Cost of ED visit if medication is unsuccessful	Managed care costs	$500	$500
Probability of success	Literature review	90%	95%
Probability of side effects	Literature review		
Nausea or vomiting		10%	1%
Inflammation at the injection site		N/A	10%
Cost of side effects	Managed care costs		
Nausea or vomiting		$50	$50
Inflammation at the injection site		N/A	$15

ED = emergency department.

EXHIBIT 9.2

Decision Tree for Migraine Composite Article

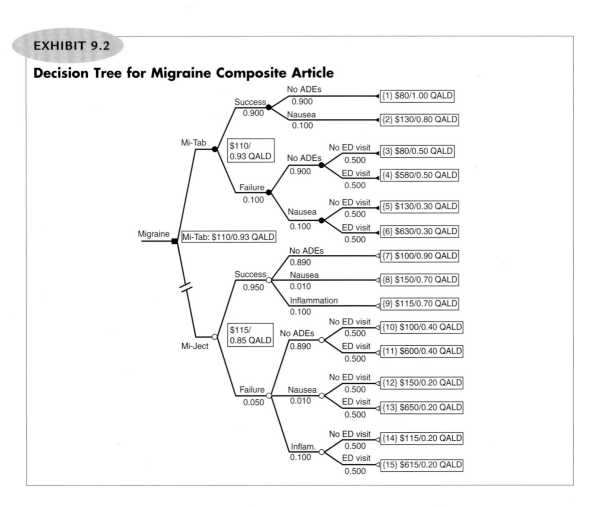

choice. Because success rates were similar and we obtained actual costs for each medication, we varied the probability that the patient would go to the ED if the medication was not successful (range, 40% to 90%), the cost of the ED visit (range, $100 to $1,000), and the probability of inflammation at the injection site (range, 0% to 15%). Threshold analysis results are found in Exhibits 9.3–9.5. For patients with unsuccessful medication treatment, if more than 68% sought treatment from the ED, Mi-Ject would be less expensive, on average, than Mi-Tab (Exhibit 9.3). If the cost of an ED visit was over $680, Mi-Ject would be less expensive (Exhibit 9.4). The cost results were not sensitive to the range of probabilities used for the chance of inflammation at the injection site (Exhibit 9.5).

DISCUSSION AND CONCLUSIONS: Mi-Tab has a small cost advantage over Mi-Ject therapy. In addition, although Mi-Ject had a small advantage in success rate, its QALD value is

decreased because of its form (injections are not pleasant, and patients can have adverse events at the injection site). Therefore, Mi-Tab is a cost-effective choice when treating patients with migraines.

EXHIBIT 9.4

One-way Sensitivity Analysis for the Cost of an Emergency Department (ED) (cost_ED) Visit for a Migraine

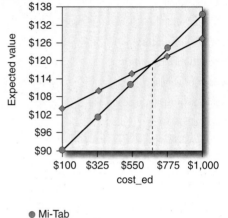

● Mi-Tab
◆ Mi-Ject

Threshold values:

●◆ cost_ed = $680
   EV = $119

EXHIBIT 9.3

One-Way Sensitivity Analysis for the Proportion of Patients who Visit an Emergency Department (ED) if the Medication does not Relieve their Migraine

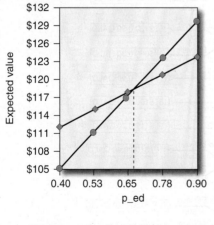

● Mi-Tab
◆ Mi-Ject

Threshold values:

●◆ p_ed = 0.68
   EV = $119

EXHIBIT 9.5

One-Way Sensitivity Analysis for the Probability of Inflammation at the Injection Site for Mi-ject (p_i_ject)

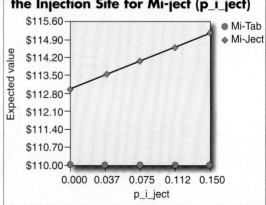

WORKSHEET FOR CRITIQUE OF DECISION ANALYSIS COMPOSITE ARTICLE 1

1. Complete Title?

   _____

   _____

   _____

   _____

2. Clear Objective?

   _____

   _____

   _____

   _____

3. Appropriate Alternatives?

   _____

   _____

   _____

   _____

4. Alternatives Described?

   _____

   _____

   _____

   _____

5. Perspective Stated?

   _____

   _____

   _____

   _____

6. Type of Study?

   _____

   _____

   _____

   _____

7. Relevant Costs?

_____

_____

_____

_____

8. Relevant Outcomes?

_____

_____

_____

_____

9. Adjustment or Discounting?

_____

_____

_____

_____

10. Reasonable Assumptions?

_____

_____

_____

_____

11. Sensitivity Analyses?

_____

_____

_____

_____

12. Limitations Addressed?

_____

_____

_____

_____

13. Generalizations Appropriate?

_____

_____

_____

_____

14. Unbiased Conclusions?

_____

_____

_____

_____

Cost-Effectiveness Grid

Which cell represents the baseline comparison of Mi-Tab to Mi-Ject?

COST-EFFECTIVENESS	Lower Cost	Same Cost	Higher Cost
Lower effectiveness	A	B	C
Same effectiveness	D	E	F
Higher effectiveness	G	H	I

CRITIQUE OF DECISION ANALYSIS COMPOSITE ARTICLE 1

1. **Complete Title:** The title did not identify the two therapeutic options that were being compared. The title did indicate that the type of study was a cost-utility analysis (CUA).

2. **Clear Objective:** The objective was "to perform a cost-utility analysis comparing two migraine treatments, Mi-Tab to Mi-Ject." This was clear.

3. **Appropriate Alternatives:** The authors should explain why these are the appropriate alternatives for the MCO.

4. **Alternatives Described:** The doses of the products should be included in the descriptions, especially if more than one strength of the product is available.

5. **Perspective Stated:** The perspective of the study was explicitly stated as the third-party payer, which would entail measuring direct medical costs only.

6. **Type of Study:** The study was correctly identified as a CUA because the outcomes were measured using QALDs. Some may debate using quality adjustments for a day of therapy versus a year of treatment, but patients have a different number of migraines per year, so results from 1 day of possible impairment was used.

7. **Relevant Costs:** Based on the perspective, only direct medical costs to a third-party provider were assessed. Other costs, such as patient and family costs, direct nonmedical costs (e.g., other sector costs), and productivity (indirect) costs, were not measured. These may be important costs for this condition. Specifically, migraines can lead to a reduction in patients' productivity.

8. **Relevant Outcomes:** It was difficult to calculate outcomes using one measure because although relief from the migraine is the most important outcome, other factors also weigh into the decision (e.g., pain of injection, difference in side effects). QALDs were used as an attempt to compile one outcome measure that could take these into account, but the validity of the decrease in QALDs should be assessed.

9. **Adjustment or Discounting:** Costs and outcomes were assessed at one point in time (for <1 year), so neither discounting nor adjustment was needed.

10. **Reasonable Assumptions:** It was assumed that QALD values were valid and that costs and probabilities were accurate estimates. It was assumed that half of the patients would seek help from an ED if the medication did not help and the other half would rest until the migraine subsided. In reality, when a migraine medication does not work, patients might respond in different ways. Some might try another dose of medication or a different medication, and some might visit a clinic or physician. The authors did not include these options, and there was no information provided on what patients typically do if the medication is unsuccessful.

11. **Sensitivity Analyses:** Sensitivity analyses were conducted for the probability of an ED visit, the cost of an ED visit, and the probability of inflammation at injection site.

12. **Limitations Addressed:** The authors did not directly address any limitations.

13. **Generalizations Appropriate:** Although the authors did not directly address generalizations of the findings, costs were taken from standard US price lists, so generalization to average US third-party payers is reasonable. Because of the transparency of the model, readers could substitute their costs or other probabilities from other trials or the literature and recalculate the answer.

14. **Unbiased Conclusions:** The authors did not overstate the results, although the limitations should have been addressed.

Cost-Effectiveness Grid

COST-EFFECTIVENESS	Lower Cost	Same Cost	Higher Cost
Lower effectiveness	A	B	C
Same effectiveness	D	E	F
Higher effectiveness	G Mi-Tab compared with Mi-Ject	H	I

COMPOSITE ARTICLE 2: DECISION ANALYSIS— ERECTILE DYSFUNCTION

Note: Pooja Desai, a PhD student, helped develop this composite article.

Title: COST-EFFECTIVENESS ANALYSIS OF TWO MEDICATIONS FOR PATIENTS SUFFERING FROM ERECTILE DYSFUNCTION

OBJECTIVE: The aim of this study was to evaluate the cost-effectiveness of a new drug called NomoreED compared with EDGone for the treatment of erectile dysfunction (ED) in male patients over 60 years of age. Both drugs were recently approved by the Food and Drug Administration for the treatment of ED. The perspective of this study is that of the payer (third-party plus patient co-pay).

METHODS: The time frame for the study was 1 month as the patient would discontinue the medication if it did not work in the first month. A decision analysis model was used for this study. Both drugs have the potential to cause serious heart-related adverse effects which are expensive to treat. The information regarding the two medications is provided in Exhibit 9.6. The outcome was measured in quality adjusted life months (QALMs), which incorporates the patient's health-related quality of life due to the presence of ED and the potential adverse effects due to the drugs. The baseline QALM value for male patients over 60 years of age with ED is 0.75. If ED is alleviated the QALM improves to 0.85. The presence of mild side effects (flushing, headache) decreases QALM by 0.05. Serious adverse heart-related events decrease QALMs by 0.40.

RESULTS: The decision tree showing the study estimates for the first month on the medication are found in Exhibit 9.7. The analysis showed that EDGone was less expensive and more effective compared to NomoreED (cost: $271 versus $351; QALMs: 0.811 QALMs versus 0.802 QALMs) and hence would be preferred (see Exhibit 9.8). The drug costs and the cost of treating adverse events were varied over a ±50% range and EDGone was still found to be more cost-effective than NomoreED. The ICERs were not calculated as EDGone is the dominant option.

DISCUSSIONS AND CONCLUSIONS: Treating ED patients with EDGone is less costly than treatment with NomoreED. EDGone also leads to better health outcomes in terms of QALMs. Therefore, treatment with EDGone is the dominant choice when compared to NomoreED.

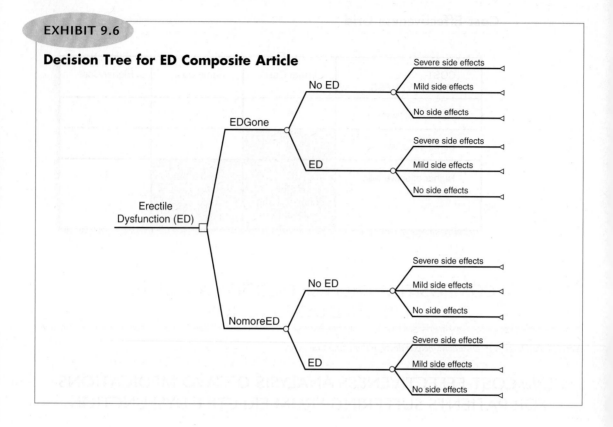

EXHIBIT 9.6

Decision Tree for ED Composite Article

EXHIBIT 9.7

Costs and Probability Estimates for ED Decision Analysis

	EDGone	NomoreED	Source
Cost Estimates			
Cost of medication (6 tablets/month)	$170 ($50 co-pay + $120 third-party)	$150 ($50 co-pay + $100 third-party)	AWP from Red Book
Cost of treating a mild adverse event	$10 (patient costs for OTC medications)	$10 (patient costs for OTC medications)	Expert opinion
Cost of treating a serious adverse event	$10,000 ($1,000 co-pay + $9,000 third-party)	$10,000 ($1,000 co-pay + $9,000 third-party)	Expert opinion
Probability Estimates			
Effectiveness (%)	70%	65%	Literature
Probability of mild adverse events (%)	10%	10%	Literature
Probability of serious adverse events (%)	1%	2%	Literature
Probability of no adverse events (%)	100% − 11% = 89%	100% − 12% = 88%	

EXHIBIT 9.8

Calculations for ED Decision Analysis

Path	Path Probability	Drug Cost	AE Cost	Total Cost	Path Cost	QALY	Path QALM
EDGone							
1	0.007	$170	$10,000	$10,170	$71.19	0.45	0.0032
2	0.070	$170	$10	$180	$12.60	0.80	0.0560
3	0.623	$170		$170	$105.91	0.85	0.5296
4	0.003	$170	$10,000	$10,170	$30.51	0.35	0.0011
5	0.030	$170	$10	$180	$5.40	0.70	0.0210
6	0.267	$170		$170	$45.39	0.75	0.2003
Totals	1.000				$271.00		0.8110
NomoreED							
1	0.013	$150	$10,000	$10,150	$131.95	0.45	0.0059
2	0.065	$150	$10	$160	$10.40	0.80	0.0520
3	0.572	$150		$150	$85.80	0.85	0.4862
4	0.007	$150	$10,000	$10,150	$71.05	0.35	0.0025
5	0.035	$150	$10	$160	$5.60	0.70	0.0245
6	0.308	$150		$150	$46.20	0.75	0.2310
Totals	1.000				$351.00		0.8020

WORKSHEET FOR CRITIQUE OF DECISION ANALYSIS COMPOSITE ARTICLE 2

1. Complete Title?

_____

_____

_____

_____

2. Clear Objective?

_____

_____

_____

_____

3. Appropriate Alternatives?

_____

_____

_____

_____

4. Alternatives Described?

_____

_____

_____

_____

5. Perspective Stated?

_____

_____

_____

_____

6. Type of Study?

_____

_____

_____

_____

7. Relevant Costs?

_____

_____

_____

_____

8. Relevant Outcomes?

_____

_____

_____

_____

9. Adjustment or Discounting?

_____

_____

_____

_____

10. Reasonable Assumptions?

_____

_____

_____

_____

11. Sensitivity Analyses?

_____

_____

_____

_____

12. Limitations Addressed?

_____

_____

_____

_____

13. Generalizations Appropriate?

_____

_____

_____

_____

14. Unbiased Conclusions?

_____

_____

_____

_____

CRITIQUE OF DECISION ANALYSIS COMPOSITE ARTICLE 2

1. **Complete Title:** The title does not give the names of the two therapeutic options that were compared. The title indicates that the study was a cost-effectiveness analysis (CEA). The outcomes were measured in QALM which would make this study a cost-utility analysis (CUA) but a CUA is a subtype of CEA.

2. **Clear Objective:** The objective was clearly stated as "to evaluate the cost-effectiveness of a new drug called NomoreED compared to EDGone for the treatment of erectile dysfunction (ED) in male patients over 60 years of age."

3. **Appropriate Alternatives:** The appropriateness of the two alternatives (ED-Gone and NomoreED) should have been clearly explained by the authors. The authors do mention that both drugs have been approved by the FDA for ED treatment.

4. **Alternatives Described:** The authors mention that six tablets are required per month. However, the strength of the medications should have been clearly described.

5. **Perspective Stated:** The perspective was clearly stated as the payers (third party and patient). Thus, only medical costs, including the patient copays, were included in the analyses.

6. **Type of Study:** The study has been identified as a cost-effectiveness analysis. The outcomes were measured as QALMs and hence it would be better classified as a cost-utility analysis. However the CUA is a type of CEA. There may be debate regarding the quality adjustment of a month instead of a year but the patients likely will discontinue the medication if it is not found to be effective in the first month of use. Thus, QALMs were used as the outcome measure.

7. **Relevant Costs:** Based on the stated perspective, the direct medical costs including the patient copayment were included in the analyses. Other costs, such as lost productivity costs due to heart-related adverse events, were not included.

8. **Relevant outcomes:** The outcome used was QALM. In addition to the proportion of successfully treated patients, it is also important to incorporate the improvement in the health-related quality of life experienced by the patients. Thus, QALM was an appropriate outcomes measure.

9. **Adjustment and Discounting:** The costs were only calculated for a 1-month period and hence no adjustment or discounting was required.

10. **Reasonable Assumptions:** It was assumed that the QALM values were valid and the probabilities obtained from literature were accurate. The analysis was carried out only for a 1-month period. Follow-up for longer periods may be needed.

11. **Sensitivity Analyses:** Sensitivity analyses were conducted by varying the cost of the drugs and the cost of treating the side effects over a ±50% range. Results were not sensitive to these ranges.

12. **Limitations Addressed:** The authors did not directly address any limitations.

13. **Generalizations Appropriate:** The authors used costs from the Red book and the model is quite straightforward. Readers could substitute costs and probabilities relevant to other populations, and recalculate results.

14. **Unbiased Conclusions:** The authors do not overstate their results. Based on these numbers and sensitivity analyses, EDGone is the dominant option over NomoreED for the treatment of ED for this population.

QUESTIONS/EXERCISES

1. The chart represents a sensitivity analysis.
   What is the threshold value for this chart, and what does this mean?

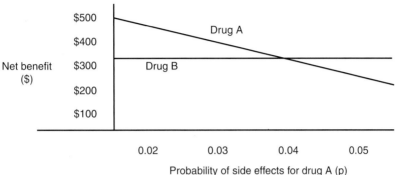

2. Decision tree exercise:
   You are interested in comparing the costs and outcomes over a 1-year time-period of preventative strategies for postmenopausal women with osteoporosis. You plan to compare three options: (1) Oral Cal-More, 10 mg/day; (2) Nasal Cal-More, 200 IU/day; and (3); Long-acting Cal-More, 70 mg, once a week. (Note: These are not real product names.) The main outcome measured is incidence of bone fracture and the effect on QALYs. Each year, about 5% of the patients taking once-a-day oral Cal-More have a fracture (95% do not), about 10% of those taking nasal Cal-More experience a fracture (90% do not), and 5% of those taking long-acting Cal-More experience a fracture (95% do not). The cost of treating a fracture is $3,000, and a fracture decreases a person's QALY by 0.5 QALYs. Once-a-day oral Cal-More causes gastrointestinal (GI) complications in 5% of the patients. Nasal Cal-More causes nasal irritation or bleeding in 10% of the cases. Once-a-week oral Cal-More causes GI complications in 2% of the patients. The average cost of treating GI complications is $200, and QALYs are decreased by 0.2. The average cost of treating nasal problems is $100, and QALYs are decreased by 0.1.

   The costs per year of the three medications are:
   Once-a-day oral Cal-More = $600
   Once-a-day nasal Cal-More = $800
   Once-a-week oral Cal-More = $1,000

   a. Draw the decision tree.
   b. Calculate the average cost for each treatment.
   c. Calculate the average QALY for each treatment.
   d. Calculate the average cost per QALY for each treatment.
   e. Calculate the marginal cost per QALY between options 1 (oral once a day) and 2 (nasal once a day).
   f. Calculate the marginal cost per QALY between options 1 (oral once-a-day) and 3 (oral once a week).

g. If option 1 is considered the standard treatment, place a 2 in the cell that represents the comparison of option 2 (nasal once a day) with the standard (oral once a day) Then place a 3 in the box that compares option 3 (oral once a week) to the standard (oral once a day).

Outcome (QALY)	Cost ($)		
	Lower Cost	Same Cost	Higher Cost
Lower outcome			
Same outcome			
Better outcome			

REFERENCES

1. Rascati KL. Decision analysis techniques: Practical aspects of using personal computers for decision analytic modeling. *Drug Benefit Trends* 33–36, July 1998.
2. Berger ML, Bingefors K, Hedblom EC, et al. *Health Care Cost, Quality, and Outcomes: ISPOR Book of Terms.* Lawrenceville, NJ: International Society for Pharmacoeconomics and Outcomes Research, 2003:226–228.

SUGGESTED READINGS

Alemi F, Gustafson DH. *Decision Analysis for Healthcare Managers* (3rd ed.). Chicago, IL: Health Administration Press, 2006.

Barr JT, Schumacher GE. Using decision analysis to conduct pharmacoeconomic studies. In Spilker B (ed). *Quality of Life and Pharmacoeconomics in Clinical Trials* (2nd ed.). Philadelphia, PA: Lippincott-Raven Press, 1996.

Brennan A, Akehurst R. Modelling in health economic evaluations. What is its place? What is its value? *Pharmacoeconomics* 17(5):445–459, 2000.

Detsky AS, Naglie G, Krahn MD, et al. Primer on medical decision analysis: Part 1—Getting started. *Medical Decision Making* 17(2):123–125, 1997.

Detsky AS, Naglie G, Krahn MD, et al. Primer on medical decision analysis: Part 2—Building a tree. *Medical Decision Making* 17(2):126–135, 1997.

Drummond MF, Sculpher MJ, Torrance GW, et al. Economic evaluation using decision analytic modelling. In *Methods for the Economic Evaluation of Health Care Programmes* (3rd ed.). Oxford: Oxford University Press, 2005.

Jain R, Grabner M, Onukwugha, E. Sensitivity analysis in cost-effectiveness studies: From guidelines to practice. *Pharmacoeconomics* 29(4):297–314, 2011.

Naglie G, Krahn MD, Naimark D, et al. Primer on medical decision analysis: Part 3—Estimating probabilities and utilities. *Medical Decision Making* 17(2):136–141, 1997.

Krahn MD, Naglie G, Naimark D, et al. Primer on medical decision analysis: Part 4—Analyzing the model and interpreting the results. *Medical Decision Making* 17(2):142–151, 1997.

Sculpher M, Fenwick E, Claxton K. Assessing quality in decision analytic cost-effectiveness models. A suggested framework and example of application. *Pharmacoeconomics* 17(5):461–477, 2000.

Chapter 10

Markov Modeling

Objectives

Upon completing this chapter, the reader will be able to:

1. Explain when Markov modeling may be useful.

2. List the steps in Markov modeling.

3. Interpret a pictorial representation of a Markov model.

4. Explain the advantages and disadvantages of Markov modeling.

✦ OVERVIEW

In Chapter 9, relatively simple models and short-term health consequences were presented. For many diseases and conditions, more complex outcomes and longer follow-up periods need to be modeled. For these analyses, patients may move back and forth, or **transition,** between **health states** over periods of time.[1-4] For example, a patient who has a blood clot (embolism) may be given a blood thinner (anticoagulant) to reduce the risk of further embolisms. Three possible health states are the patient dies from the embolism, the patient has blood-related problems from the medications (e.g., internal bleeding), or the patient lives with no complications or side effects. Outcomes past this initial health state can be followed further to see whether patients develop future embolisms or future internal bleeding. Each follow-up interval is called a **cycle**, the time period that is determined to be clinically relevant to the specific disease or condition. **Markov analysis** allows for a more accurate presentation of these complex scenarios that occur over a number of cycles, or intervals.

✦ STEPS IN MARKOV MODELING

There are five steps for Markov modeling: (1) choose the health states that represent the possible outcomes from each intervention; (2) determine possible transitions between health states; (3) choose how long each cycle should be and how many cycles will be analyzed; (4) estimate the probabilities associated with moving (i.e., transitioning) in and out of health states; and (5) estimate the costs and outcomes associated with each option.[1] Each step is discussed in this chapter using a general example (Fig. 10.1) and a more specific diabetes mellitus (DM) example (Fig. 10.2). The DM analysis will model the cost-effectiveness of using a specified diet and exercise plan to increase the length of time that prediabetic patients (impaired glucose tolerance [IGT] is plasma glucose >140 to <200 mg/dL 2 hours after glucose challenge) avoid the transition to DM (plasma glucose >200 mg/dL 2 hours after glucose challenge). For the DM example, patients are followed up for

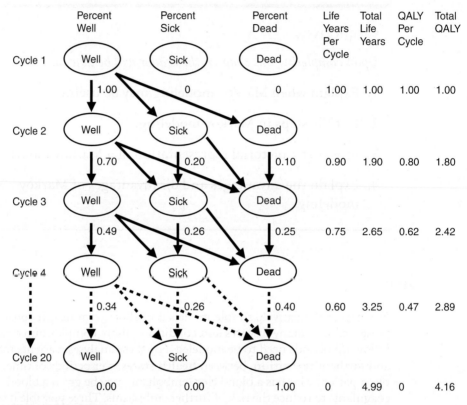

Example Calculations:
Cycle 1 to Cycle 2
 70% of 100% stay well = 70% well
 20% of 100% get sick = 20% sick
 10% of 100% die = 10% dead
Cycle 2 to Cycle 3
 70% of 70% stay well = 49% well
 20% of 70% (14%) get sick plus 60% of 20% stay sick (12%) = 26% sick
 10% of 70% (7%) die plus 40% of 20% (8%) die + 100% of 10% (10%) stay dead = 25% dead
Cycle 3 to Cycle 4
 70% of 49% stay well = 34% well
 20% of 49% (10%) get sick plus 60% of 26% (16%) stay sick = 26% sick
 10% of 49% (5%) die plus 40% of 26% (10%) die + 100% of 25% stay dead (25%) = 40% dead
QALY Calculations
 Cycle 1 = 100% * 1.0 QALY = 1.00 QALY
 Cycle 2 = (70% * 1.0 QALY) + 20% (0.5 QALY) + 10% (0 QALY) = 0.80 QALY
 Cycle 3 = (49% * 1.0 QALY) + 26% (0.5 QALY) + 25% (0 QALY) = 0.62 QALY
 Cycle 4 = (34% * 1.0 QALY) + 26% (0.5 QALY) + 40% (0 QALY) = 0.47 QALY

FIGURE 10.1. Bubble diagram for a general Markov model.

Without Diet and Exercise Program

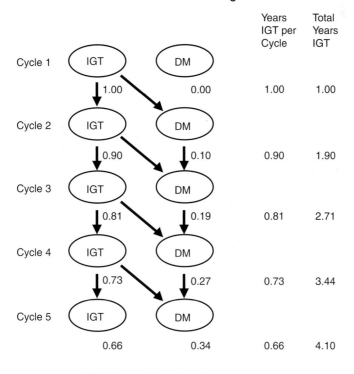

With Diet and Exercise Program

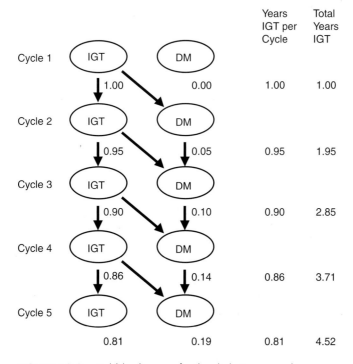

FIGURE 10.2. Bubble diagram for the diabetes example.

IGT = Impared Glucose Tolerance DM = Diabetes Mellitis.

5 years, and it is assumed that none of the patients die during this time frame. The cost of the diet and exercise program is $300 per year. (Estimates and probabilities for this example are used for illustrative purposes only. Published research articles should indicate how these estimates were derived.)

Step 1: Choose Health States

First, a delineation of mutually exclusive health states should be determined by listing different scenarios a patient might reasonably experience. These are referred to as **Markov states.** Patients cannot be in more than one health state during each cycle. A simple general example is "well, sick, or dead." Graphically, by convention, each health state is placed in an oval or circle in a bubble diagram (Fig. 10.1). Time cycles are depicted on the left of the graph. For the DM example, we are concerned with two health states: IGT and DM (Fig. 10.2). A more complex Markov model is illustrated in Example 10.1.

Step 2: Determine Transitions

Next, possible transitions between states are determined based on clinical information. Can patients move (i.e., transition) from one health state to another? For example, if the patient dies, this is called an **absorbing state.** An absorbing state indicates that patients cannot move to another health state in a later cycle. Graphically, arrows are used to indicate which transitions are allowed. In the general example given in Figure 10.1, we assume that everyone starts out in the well state. For cycle 1, each patient can stay well, or can move to the sick or dead states. For the next cycle, patients in the well state can again stay well or move to the sick or dead states. Those in the dead state cannot move back to the other two states. Depending on the disease of interest, patients may or may not be able to move back to the well state after being in the sick state. For example, if a patient gets sick from an infection, it is likely that he or she can recover and become well. If the patient contracts AIDS, he or she may be able to prevent some symptoms or prolong his or her life with medication, but the person would not move back to the well state. For the diabetes example, we will assume that if a patient transitions from the prediabetic state to DM that he or she cannot return to the prediabetic state. Thus, in the diabetes Markov model (Fig. 10.2), DM is an absorbing state.

EXAMPLE 10.1	SUMMARY OF MARKOV MODEL FOR MAINTENANCE TREATMENT FOR GASTROESOPHAGEAL REFLUX DISEASE

Below is a Markov model developed to estimate costs and outcomes associated with 1 year of treatment of gastroesophageal reflux disease (GERD). GERD is characterized by recurrent heartburn and regurgitation (hence the term reflux) and may permanently damage the lining of the esophagus. Both histamine-2 receptor agonists (H2RAs) and proton pump inhibitors (PPIs) are used to treat this disease. In most cases, PPIs are more expensive than H2RAs, so after GERD patients are in remission (no symptoms), lower cost treatments may be used for maintenance therapy.

The authors chose to compare three options for continued therapy: standard-dose H2RAs, low-dose PPIs, and standard-dose PPIs. The nodes with an M inside a circle indicate that a Markov analysis is being used. In this case, the model was run for 12 cycles of monthly treatment.

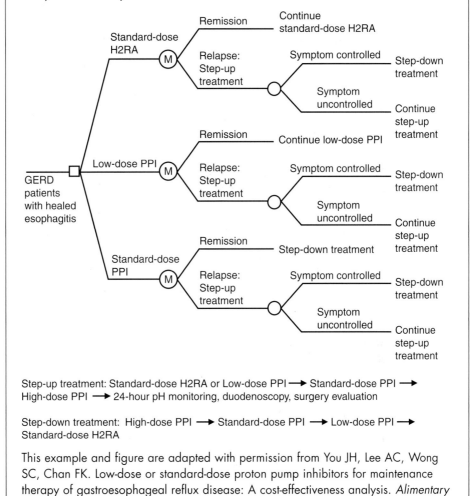

Step-up treatment: Standard-dose H2RA or Low-dose PPI ➝ Standard-dose PPI ➝ High-dose PPI ➝ 24-hour pH monitoring, duodenoscopy, surgery evaluation

Step-down treatment: High-dose PPI ➝ Standard-dose PPI ➝ Low-dose PPI ➝ Standard-dose H2RA

This example and figure are adapted with permission from You JH, Lee AC, Wong SC, Chan FK. Low-dose or standard-dose proton pump inhibitors for maintenance therapy of gastroesophageal reflux disease: A cost-effectiveness analysis. *Alimentary Pharmacology and Therapeutics* 17(6):785–792, 2003. Used with permission of Blackwell Publishing.

Step 3: Choose the Cycle Length and Number of Cycles

The cycle length depends on the disease being modeled. For the example of patients with a blood clot given in the first paragraph of the chapter, a cycle of 1 week might be enough time to determine the number of patients with additional blood clots or bleeding. For chronic diseases, a cycle length of 1 year is commonly used. Again, the number of cycles depends on clinical relevance. Sometimes the model is run for the natural lifetime of the patients or until a certain percent of the cohort is in the absorbing state. For the general example (Fig. 10.1), the model was run until there was no one left in the well or sick health states (20 cycles). For the diabetes example (Fig. 10.2), five 1-year cycles were used to determine the impact of the diet and exercise program on progression to diabetes.

Step 4: Estimate Transition Probabilities

Transition probabilities are used to estimate the percent of patients who are likely to move from one health state to another during each cycle. These probability values usually come from previous research or expert panel estimates. For the general example, the transition probabilities are given in Table 10.1. This matrix of transition probabilities contains zeros when patients are not allowed to move from one state to another. For the diabetes example, estimates were used for those with and without the diet and exercise program. For patients who did not receive the specific diet and exercise program, there was a 10% probability per year (cycle) that they would transition from IGT to DM (90% would stay in the IGT state). For patients who received the program, the probability of DM was reduced to 5% per year (95% would stay in the IGT state). It was assumed that after patients were diagnosed with DM, they could not transition back to IGT. Figure 10.3 shows a different method to depict the general Markov model and includes these probabilities for each arrow that links the health state transitions. Figures 10.4 and 10.5 include the probabilities for the diabetes example.

Step 5: Calculate Costs and Outcomes

Outcomes for each health state should be estimated and given a value. If the outcome of interest is years of life gained or saved and each cycle is for 1 year, then each person who is alive during a cycle gets a value of 1.0 as his or her outcome for that cycle. It is common to adjust each year of life in each cycle for the quality of health that year. In Figure 10.1, for each year in a well state, the value is 1.0, and for each year in the sick state, the value is 0.5, and the value for the dead state is 0. Costs in each health state should be estimated as with simple decision analyses. The total costs and outcomes are then summed for all cycles. Figure 10.2 shows that the 5-year diet and exercise program corresponds with an extra 0.42 years (about 5 months) of being in the IGT state before being diagnosed with DM (4.52 years versus 4.10 years in IGT). The additional costs for patients in the program are $300 per year or $1,500 for 5 years if costs are not discounted. The 5-year cost estimate would be $1,415 if discounted using a 3% **discount rate.** This calculates

TABLE 10.1. TRANSITION PROBABILITIES PER CYCLE FOR GENERAL EXAMPLE

	To Health State			
	Well	Sick	Dead	Total Per Cycle
From Health State				
Well	0.70	0.20	0.10	1.00
Sick	0.00	0.60	0.40	1.00
Dead	0.00	0.00	1.00	1.00

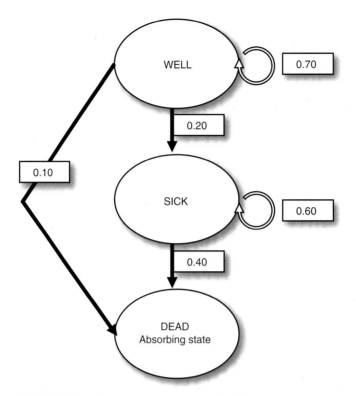

FIGURE 10.3.   Alternate representation of a Markov model for the general example.

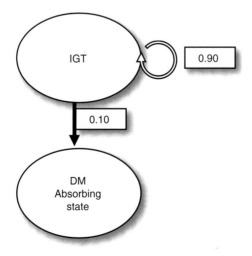

Model and transition probabilities without diet and exercise program

FIGURE 10.4.   Alternate representation of a Markov model for the diabetes example without the diet and exercise program.

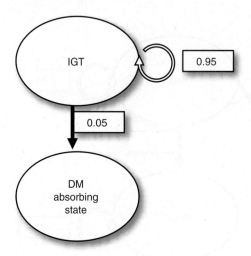

Model and transition probabilities with diet and exercise program

FIGURE 10.5.   Alternate representation of a Markov model for the diabetes example with the diet and exercise program.

to about $3,571 incremental cost for an extra year without DM ($1,500/0.42 years) if costs are not discounted or $3,369 if discounting is conducted ($1,415/0.42 years). As mentioned in Chapter 5 on cost-effectiveness analysis, there is no consensus on whether or not to discount outcomes (in this example, years without DM). Therefore, some researchers may discount outcomes as well as costs in this analysis. The costs of treating patients with DM would be included for both options in a more complete model. Computer software helps with more complex calculations.

✦ DISADVANTAGES OF MARKOV MODELING

By their nature, Markov models can be more complex than simple decision trees and therefore less **transparent** to decision makers. Researchers strive to strike a balance between developing models that are more complex but better able to capture the true nature of the disease state and developing simpler models that are easier to interpret but may not include important clinical factors.

A commonly cited disadvantage of Markov modeling is that it is "memoryless" because the **Markovian assumption** is that the probability of moving from state to state is not based on the previous experiences from former cycles. In practice, a patient's medical history is an important determinant in the probability of his or her future health. More advanced and complex computations, such as using **tunnel states,** allow for integration of health experiences from previous cycles.[4,5] Another disadvantage is that the data needed to estimate probabilities and costs, especially in the long term, are often unavailable. Most clinical studies measure outcomes for a short time, and extrapolation into the future may compound errors in estimations.

✦ ADVANCED ISSUES

An overview of some advanced issues related to Markov modeling is included in this section. Some advanced topics are addressed in more depth elsewhere (see "References" and "Suggested Readings" sections).

Constant Versus Variable Transition Probabilities

For the examples given in this chapter, it was assumed that the probability of transitioning from one Markov state to another was constant over time from cycle to cycle. A **Markov chain** model is used for constant probabilities. However, this may not be consistent with the information that is known about a disease process. For example, the probability of staying asymptomatic may be 90% per year for the first 5 years of a disease and then may decrease to 80% per year for the next 5 years. Also, if the model extends out over a long period, the cohort "ages," and higher mortality rates from aging should be taken into account for future cycles. Time-dependent **Markov process** models can incorporate changes in probabilities for each cycle by incorporating data from a reference table that lists the probabilities for each cycle based on more realistic clinical information.

Calculation Methods

The two basic calculation methods used to determine the results of a Markov analysis are cohort simulation and Monte Carlo simulation.

Cohort Simulation

Cohort simulation uses a hypothetical group (cohort) of patients that usually start out in the same health state. At each cycle, the transition probabilities are applied. (Probabilities may be the same for every cycle if using a Markov chain analysis, or they may vary by cycle if using a Markov process analysis.) The number of patients in each cycle is calculated and summed using matrix algebra. This type of calculation can incorporate discount rates to account for time value associated with costs and outcomes. The composite article for this chapter uses a cohort simulation technique and incorporates discount rates. Cohort simulation models (as well as the **decision analysis** models in Chapter 9) are referred to as **deterministic** analyses. This means that probabilities and costs are set (predetermined) numbers, and variability (i.e., **uncertainty**) in these numbers is not taken into account. Therefore, for a specific model, the analysis always gives the same numerical results.

Monte Carlo Simulation

Monte Carlo simulation is a type of **stochastic** analysis that takes into account uncertainty or variability at the patient level. A random patient is sent through the model, and outcomes and costs are calculated individually for that patient. Then one by one, more random patients are sent through the model. The path through the model that each patient may take is different because of random variation, and results for a specific model can result in different answers each time the simulation is conducted because of the randomness at chance nodes in the model. If a large number of patients (e.g., 100,000) are sent through the model one at a time, the results may be close to the results of the cohort simulation.

First-order Monte Carlo simulation (sometimes called microsimulation or individual simulation) is used to take into account the patient-level variability seen in medical practice. Second-order simulation deals with uncertainty of the statistical parameters (versus uncertainty at the patient level). This may be referred to as probabilistic sensitivity analysis and is beyond the scope of this book. Explanations and examples can be found elsewhere.[6]

Half-Cycle Corrections

The basic Markov models illustrated so far assume that patients stay in one health state for the entire cycle (e.g., 1 year) and transition at the end of each cycle. In reality, patients move between health states in a continuous fashion over each cycle rather than all transitioning at the end of the cycle. In the diabetes example, everyone was given credit for a whole year in the IGT health state for the first cycle before some patients transitioned to DM. In reality, some of these patients would have transitioned to DM before the 1-year mark. Researchers adjust for this potential overestimation of costs and outcomes by using a **half-cycle correction** which moves patients between beginning and ending cycles at the halfway mark. Mathematically, this is accomplished by dividing the costs and outcomes in the first and last cycle by 2.

✦ OTHER ADVANCED TOPICS

Scatterplots and Cost-Effectiveness Acceptability Curves (CEACs)

As shown in Chapter 5, the incremental costs and incremental effects can be represented visually using the four quadrants of the **cost-effectiveness plane.** The horizontal axis divides the plane according to incremental costs (positive above, negative below) and the vertical axis divides the plane according to incremental effects (positive to the right, negative to the left). Previous examples of incremental cost-effectiveness ratios (ICERs) used "point estimates" of both costs and effectiveness measures, without regard to how these points might vary. Using point estimates, there would be one point on the CE plane to illustrate the ICER between two alternatives. Using one point to illustrate each difference in estimates does not take into account any uncertainty in the measurement, or estimates, of costs or effects. Due to imprecise information on the effectiveness of and the resources consumed, both the costs and effects of health interventions are associated with some degree of uncertainty. One method that is typically used to represent the uncertainty in the costs and effects associated with a treatment is a scatter plot of simulated (by bootstrapping or probabilistic modeling) incremental cost and effect pairs on the incremental cost-effectiveness plane. In an example comparing Statin A and Statin B, the point estimate of differences in costs was calculated to be $5,000 higher for Statin A than for Statin B; and the point estimate of differences in effect was calculated to be 0.13 QALY higher for Statin A than for Statin B; which would result in a ICER of $5,000/0.13 = $38,462 per additional QALY. A scatterplot of joint comparisons of potential differences in costs and effects (i.e., plot of cost-effect pairs) for different theoretical patients based on variations (uncertainty) of these variables is illustrated in Figure 10.6. The cost differences range from −$300 (savings of $300 for Statin A) to about $10,000. The effect differences range from

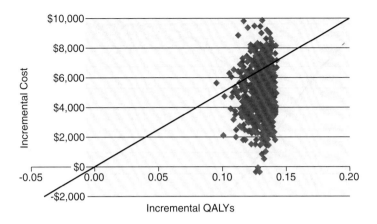

FIGURE 10.6. Scatterplot. Statin A versus Statin B.

0.10 to 0.14 additional QALYs for Statin A compared to Statin B. Over 95% of the points from the cost-effect pairs fall in quadrant I (northeast), indicating that Statin A is more costly and more effective for these points. For the few points that fall in quadrant II (southeast), these paired comparisons show Statin A is less costly and more effective (i.e., dominant). The next question is to determine the probability that the added value is worth the added cost. The angled straight line (ray) in Figure 10.6 indicates where the ICER is $50,000 per QALY (a commonly used threshold or ceiling ratio). To calculate the probability that Statin A is cost-effective compared with Statin B, the proportion of the scatter plot points that fall to the south and east of the ray is determined. In this example the probability (proportion) is 82% that Statin A is cost-effective at the threshold of $50,000. Since the maximum acceptable ceiling ratio, or threshold, is not always stated, (and a standard has not been agreed upon), a sensitivity analysis should be undertaken. This is accomplished by using a cost-effectiveness acceptability curve (CEAC). This curve is constructed by plotting the proportion of the incremental cost-effect pairs that are cost-effective for a range of threshold or ceiling values. Figure 10.7 illustrates the CEAC for the Statin example. As mentioned, at the ceiling of $50,000, 82% of the points are in the cost-effective range. If the maximum threshold was reduced to $35,000/QALY (ray angle moves down and right) the proportion of cost-effect points decreases to 41%, whereas if the ceiling is raised to $65,000/QALY (ray angle increases up and to the left) the proportion increases to 96%. Note that if a QALY is valued at $100,000 the probability of cost-effectiveness of Statin A calculated using joint ratios is 100% (all points would fall below the ray).

SUMMARY

Markov analysis provides a method of adding a time component to decision analyses and is useful when modeling health events that can occur repeatedly over time. It may be a more realistic representation of more complex disease states. Markov modeling can start with clinical (usually short-term) data and incorporate more long-term data from studies of natural disease progression and epidemiology. For a specific research question, the possible health states are defined, the relevant length and number of cycles are determined, transition probabilities between health states are estimated, and both costs and outcomes over a number of cycles

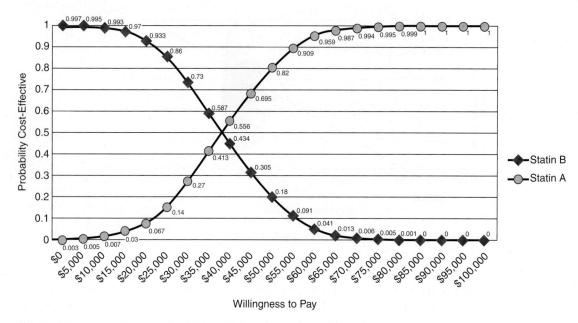

FIGURE 10.7. Cost-effectiveness Acceptability Curve. Statin A versus Statin B.

are calculated and summed. The probabilities of transitioning from one state to another may be held constant over time **(Markov chain analysis)** or may differ depending on the cycle **(Markov process analysis).** A limitation of Markov modeling is the assumption that the probability of moving from state to state is not dependent on previous health states the patient may have experienced, which may not be a realistic depiction for some research questions. More advanced (but more complex) analyses have been used to address this limitation.

COMPOSITE ARTICLE 1: MARKOV MODELING—INITIATION OF HIV THERAPY

Note: Haesuk Park, a PhD student, helped develop this composite article.
More information about this topic can be found in the following references:
Athan E, O'Brien DP, Legood R. Cost-effectiveness of routine and low-cost CD4 T-cell count compared with WHO clinical staging of HIV to guide initiation of antiretroviral therapy in resource-limited settings. AIDS 24:1887–1895, 2010.
Panel on Antiretroviral Guidelines for Adults and Adolescents. Guidelines for the use of antiretroviral agents in HIV-1 infected adults and adolescents. Department of Health and Human Services. Available at http://aidsinfo.nih.gov/contentfiles/lvguidelines/adultandadolescentgl.pdf.
World Health Organization (WHO). HIV/AIDS Programme. WHO case definitions of HIV for surveillance and revised clinical staging and immunological classification of HIV-related disease in adults and children. Available at http://www.who.int/hiv/pub/guidelines/HIVstaging150307.pdf

Title: COST-EFFECTIVENESS OF TWO METHODS TO GUIDE INITIATION OF ANTIRETROVIRAL THERAPY IN SUB-SAHARAN AFRICA

INTRODUCTION: It was estimated that 22.5 million adults and children live with Human immunodeficiency virus (HIV) in sub-Saharan Africa. One indication of the impact of having this virus can be measured by determining the level of CD4 cells in a patient's blood sample.

If CD4 cells become depleted, the patient is left vulnerable to a wide range of infections. In the developed countries, highly active antiretroviral therapy (ART) in the late 1990s brought significant improvement in the quantity and quality of life for patients with HIV. The results of randomized controlled trials and several observational cohort studies demonstrated that ART can reduce transmission of HIV and is a cost-effective intervention. The Department of Health and Human Services Panel recommends ART for patients with CD4 counts ≤500 cells/mm³ ("strong" recommendation for CD4 counts <350 cells/mm³ and "moderate" recommendation for CD4 counts 350 to 500 cells/mm³). In developing countries, the initiation of ART is guided by the patient's CD4 cell count (some treat if ≤200 cells/mm³, others when the count gets ≤350 cells/mm³ or less). Where reliable CD4 cell count testing is not available, the World Health Organization (WHO) has developed clinical staging guidelines for the initiation of ART. Symptomatic stage 3 (advanced immunosuppression) and stage 4 (severe symptoms/AIDS) indicate the need to start ART. The objective of this study was to develop a Markov model of HIV infection and compared the direct health care costs and benefits in life years or quality-adjusted life years (QALYs) gained using two methods to assess the need to start ART: (1) routine CD4 cell count versus (2) WHO clinical staging of HIV. The incremental cost-effectiveness ratios (ICERs) in US dollars per life year (LY) and quality-adjusted life year (QALY) were estimated from the perspective of the public health services in a sub-Saharan African setting.

WHO clinical staging of established HIV infection

HIV-Associated Symptoms	WHO Clinical Stage
Asymptomatic	1
Mild symptoms	2
Advanced symptoms	3
Severe symptoms	4

METHODS: A Markov state transition probability model, following a hypothetical cohort of 10,000 HIV-infected individuals starting with a CD4 cell count more than 350 cells/mm³, was developed comparing the two approaches

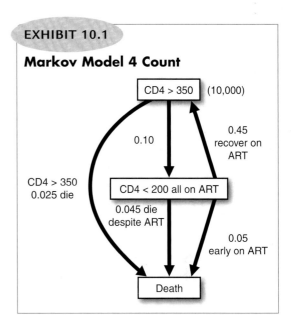

EXHIBIT 10.1

Markov Model 4 Count

to guide initiation of ART (Exhibits 10.1 and 10.2). The Markov model was constructed in Microsoft Excel to estimate the total direct medical costs, patients' life expectancy, and quality of life for the two options. Three health states were used in the model: (1) CD4 cell count of 350/mm³ or more (no treatment), (2) CD4 cell count of 200 or less or WHO stage 3 or 4 (AIDS) (treatment with ART), and (3) death. Patients in the model were reviewed

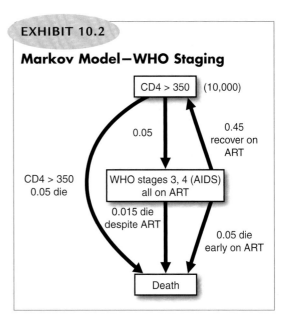

EXHIBIT 10.2

Markov Model—WHO Staging

annually for consideration of ART by either CD4 cell count of 200 mm³ or less or by WHO stage 3 or 4 criteria. It is possible that patients who receive ART could go back to the state of CD4 cell count more than 350 mm³. A portion of patients would progress despite commencement of ART. The transition probabilities were based on published studies and are listed in Exhibit 10.3. The costs of treating HIV patients include the costs of providing ART and other direct health care treatment costs such as treating opportunistic infections, and monitoring and treating adverse effects of therapy. The costs of first-line and second-line ART are derived from published studies in developing countries. All costs used in the model were reported in 2008 US dollars. These estimates appear in Exhibit 10.4. In the base case analysis, future costs and outcomes were discounted at 3% per annum as recommended in a developing country setting. Twenty 1-year cycles were modeled. Sensitivity analyses were conducted for costs, time horizon and the discount rate. The cost-effectiveness threshold used in this analysis is based on an ICER per QALY gained below the per capita gross domestic product (GDP)

EXHIBIT 10.4

Costs, Health Care Utilization, and Utilities

Costs (per year)	
CD4 cell test routine	$15
Drug cost	
ART first-line	$300
ART second-line	$680
Health care cost	
Inpatient	$180
Outpatient	$30
Health care Utilization (per year)	
Inpatient visits	
CD4 cell count > 350	4.0
CD4 cell count ≤ 200	1.0
AIDS	2.0
Outpatient visits	
CD4 cell count > 350	3.0
CD4 cell count ≤ 200	9.0
AIDS	8.0
Utilities	
CD4 cell count > 350	0.890
CD4 cell count < 200	0.830
AIDS	0.730

EXHIBIT 10.3

Transition Probabilities

CD4 Cell Testing to Guide Antiretroviral Therapy

CD4 > 350 → CD4 < 200	10.00%
CD4 > 350 → death	2.50%
CD4 < 200 → CD4 > 350 recover on ART	45.00%
CD4 < 200 → die early on ART	5.00%
CD4 < 200 → die despite ART	4.50%

WHO Staging 3, 4 (AIDS) to Guide Antiretroviral Therapy

CD4 > 350 → WHO stages 3, 4 (AIDS)	5.00%
CD4 > 350 → death	5.00%
WHO stages 3, 4 (AIDS) → CD4 > 350 recover on ART	45.00%
WHO stages 3, 4 (AIDS) → die early on ART	5.00%
WHO stages 3, 4 (AIDS) → die despite ART	1.50%

---

for the Republic of South Africa ($9,800) and Cote d'Ivoire ($1,700). (See Exhibit 10.5 for model and calculations.)

RESULTS: Exhibit 10.6 shows that for baseline calculations, the total costs and effects, in terms of life years (LYs) and QALYs for individuals assessed by WHO staging criteria were $8,710, 10.46 LYs, and 9.17 QALYs, respectively. For those individuals assessed by annual routine CD4 cell count testing, the costs, LYs, and QALYs were $10,013, 11.87 LYs, and 10.46 QALYs, respectively. With these estimates, the ICER of CD4 cell count testing compared with the WHO clinical staging was $923 per life year gained and $1008 per QALY gained. Sensitivity analysis (Exhibit 10.7) shows this result to be robust to the ranges given because the highest

EXHIBIT 10.5

Calculations of the Markov Model
A. Data Markov Analysis: CD4 Cell Count Testing

	Markov State			Outcome		Cost			
Cycle	CD4 > 350	CD4 < 200 all on ART	Death	Life Years	QALYs	CD4 Cell Test Routine ($)	ART Cost ($)	Health Care Cost (Inpatient and Outpatient) ($)	Total Cost (CD4 Cell Test +ART+ Health Care Costs) ($)
0	10,000	0	0	10,000	8,900	150,000	0	8,100,000	8,250,000
1	8,750	1,000	250	9,466	8,367	141,990	475,728	7,317,961	7,935,680
2	8,106	1,330	564	8,895	7,841	133,419	614,290	6,753,287	7,500,996
3	7,691	1,416	893	8,334	7,340	125,016	634,861	6,284,450	7,044,327
4	7,367	1,413	1,220	7,801	6,868	117,020	615,303	5,867,013	6,599,336
5	7,082	1,380	1,538	7,299	6,425	109,491	583,201	5,484,046	6,176,738
6	6,818	1,336	1,846	6,829	6,010	102,431	548,260	5,128,481	5,779,172
7	6,567	1,290	2,143	6,388	5,622	95,821	513,826	4,796,826	5,406,473
8	6,326	1,243	2,430	5,976	5,259	89,635	480,993	4,486,923	5,057,552
9	6,095	1,198	2,706	5,590	4,920	83,848	450,060	4,197,150	4,731,058
10	5,873	1,155	2,973	5,229	4,602	78,435	421,044	3,926,130	4,425,609
11	5,658	1,113	3,229	4,891	4,305	73,370	393,874	3,672,624	4,139,869
12	5,452	1,072	3,476	4,576	4,027	68,633	368,448	3,435,492	3,872,574
13	5,253	1,033	3,715	4,280	3,767	64,202	344,661	3,213,672	3,622,535
14	5,061	995	3,944	4,004	3,524	60,056	322,408	3,006,175	3,388,640
15	4,876	959	4,165	3,745	3,296	56,179	301,591	2,812,076	3,169,846
16	4,698	924	4,378	3,503	3,084	52,551	282,119	2,630,510	2,965,180
17	4,527	890	4,583	3,277	2,884	49,158	263,903	2,460,666	2,773,728
18	4,361	858	4,781	3,066	2,698	45,984	246,864	2,301,789	2,594,637
19	4,202	826	4,971	2,868	2,524	43,015	230,925	2,153,170	2,427,110
20	4,049	796	5,155	2,683	2,361	40,238	216,015	2,014,147	2,270,399
		Per patient		11.870	10.463	178	831	9,004	10,013

B. Data Markov Analysis: WHO Staging

	Markov State			Outcome		Cost			
Cycle	CD4 > 350	WHO Stages 3, 4 (AIDS)	Death	Life Years	QALYs	No Testing ($)	ART Cost ($)	Health Care Cost (Inpatient and Outpatient) ($)	Total Cost (ART+ Health Care Cost) ($)
0	10,000	0	0	10,000	8,900	0	0	8,100,000	8,100,000
1	9,000	500	500	9,223	8,131	0	237,864	7,368,932	7,606,796
2	8,325	695	980	8,502	7,462	0	321,001	6,749,222	7,070,223

(continued)

B. Data Markov Analysis: WHO Staging (Continued)

	Markov State			Outcome		Cost			
Cycle	CD4 > 350	WHO Stages 3, 4 (AIDS)	Death	Life Years	QALYs	No Testing ($)	ART Cost ($)	Health Care Cost (Inpatient and Outpatient) ($)	Total Cost (ART+ Health Care Cost) ($)
3	7,805	757	1,438	7,835	6,863	0	339,364	6,201,304	6,540,668
4	7,365	761	1,874	7,220	6,318	0	331,349	5,706,341	6,037,691
5	6,971	741	2,288	6,653	5,819	0	313,289	5,254,523	5,567,812
6	6,608	712	2,681	6,130	5,360	0	292,079	4,840,038	5,132,117
7	6,267	679	3,054	5,648	4,938	0	270,580	4,458,917	4,729,497
8	5,946	646	3,408	5,204	4,550	0	249,933	4,108,092	4,358,025
9	5,642	614	3,744	4,795	4,192	0	230,551	3,784,993	4,015,544
10	5,354	583	4,063	4,418	3,862	0	212,539	3,487,358	3,699,897
11	5,081	553	4,365	4,070	3,559	0	195,878	3,213,150	3,409,028
12	4,822	525	4,653	3,750	3,279	0	180,498	2,960,512	3,141,010
13	4,576	498	4,925	3,456	3,021	0	166,316	2,727,742	2,894,058
14	4,343	473	5,184	3,184	2,784	0	153,243	2,513,276	2,666,519
15	4,121	449	5,430	2,934	2,565	0	141,197	2,315,673	2,456,869
16	3,911	426	5,663	2,703	2,363	0	130,096	2,133,606	2,263,702
17	3,712	404	5,884	2,490	2,177	0	119,868	1,965,854	2,085,722
18	3,523	384	6,094	2,295	2,006	0	110,443	1,811,292	1,921,735
19	3,343	364	6,293	2,114	1,848	0	101,760	1,668,881	1,770,641
20	3,173	346	6,482	1,948	1,703	0	93,759	1,537,668	1,631,427
			Per patient	10.457	9.170	0	419	8,291	8,710

EXHIBIT 10.6

Base Case Costs, Effects, and Cost-Effectiveness of CD4 Cell Testing Compared with WHO Staging to Guide Initiation of Antiretroviral Therapy for HIV-Infected Individuals Over 20 Years

	Costs ($)	Total Life Years	QALYs	Incremental Cost per Life Year Gained (ICER)	Incremental Cost per QALY Gained (ICER)
WHO staging	8,710	10.457	9.170		
Routine CD4 cell testing	10,013	11.870	10.463	$923	$1,008
Cost-Effect Threshold GDP per Capita 2008					
Republic of South Africa					$9,800
Cote D'Ivoire					$1,700

EXHIBIT 10.7

One-Way Deterministic Sensitivity Analysis

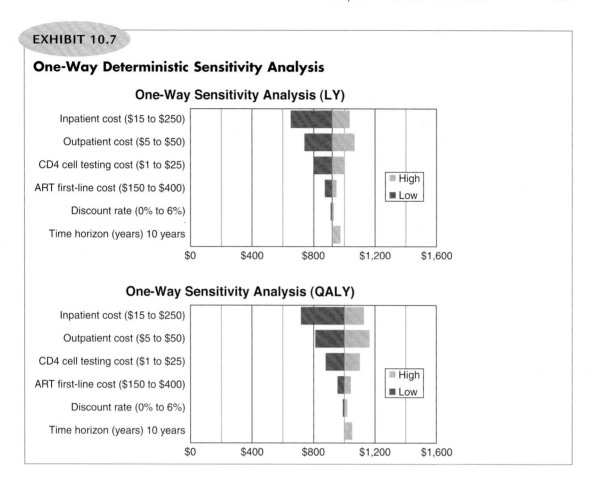

One-Way Sensitivity Analysis (LY)

Inpatient cost ($15 to $250)
Outpatient cost ($5 to $50)
CD4 cell testing cost ($1 to $25)
ART first-line cost ($150 to $400)
Discount rate (0% to 6%)
Time horizon (years) 10 years

High
Low

$0 $400 $800 $1,200 $1,600

One-Way Sensitivity Analysis (QALY)

Inpatient cost ($15 to $250)
Outpatient cost ($5 to $50)
CD4 cell testing cost ($1 to $25)
ART first-line cost ($150 to $400)
Discount rate (0% to 6%)
Time horizon (years) 10 years

High
Low

$0 $400 $800 $1,200 $1,600

incremental cost per QALY gained was $1,165, which is below the threshold value of $1,700.

DISCUSSION AND CONCLUSIONS: Limitations of this study include the assumption of effectiveness of ART. Drug resistance may emerge after 10 years and longer term studies are required. In addition, societal costs were not included. Utilizing routine CD4 cell counts compared to WHO clinical staging in order to guide initiation of ART for patients infected with HIV appears to be a very cost-effective intervention for sub-Saharan Africa. We recommend the implementation of routine CD4 cell testing as an integral part of the scale-up of ART programs in the sub-Saharan African public health services.

WORKSHEET FOR CRITIQUE OF MARKOV COMPOSITE ARTICLE

1. Complete Title?

_____

_____

_____

_____

_____

2. Clear Objective?

_____

_____

_____

_____

_____

3. Appropriate Alternatives?

_____

_____

_____

_____

_____

4. Alternatives Described?

_____

_____

_____

_____

_____

5. Perspective Stated?

_____

_____

_____

_____

_____

6. Type of Study?

_____

_____

_____

_____

_____

7. Relevant Costs?

_____

_____

_____

_____

_____

8. Relevant Outcomes?

_____

_____

_____

_____

_____

9. Adjustment or Discounting?

_____

_____

_____

_____

_____

10. Reasonable Assumptions?

_____

_____

_____

_____

_____

11. Sensitivity Analyses?

_____

_____

_____

_____

_____

12. Limitations Addressed?

_____

_____

_____

_____

_____

13. Generalizations Appropriate?

_____

_____

_____

_____

_____

14. Unbiased Conclusions?

_____

_____

_____

_____

_____

ANSWERS

1. **Complete Title:** Although the title does say the type of study (cost-effectiveness) it does not include what the two options were—CD4 testing versus WHO staging.
2. **Clear Objective:** The objective was clearly stated " ... to develop a Markov model of HIV infection and compared the direct healthcare costs and benefits in life years or quality-adjusted life years (QALYs) gained using two methods to assess the need to start ART."
3. **Appropriate Alternatives:** The authors addressed the two common methods for determining when to start ART and why they were important to compare.
4. **Alternatives Described:** Although the CD4 count assessment was clear with cut-offs, more information could have been given about WHO staging criteria.
5. **Perspective Stated:** The perspective was clearly stated as the "public health services in a sub-Saharan African setting." Thus, only direct medical costs were included.
6. **Type of Study:** The study has been identified as a cost-effectiveness analysis. The outcomes were measured as both life years (LYs) gained—a CEA—and QALYs gained—a CUA. However the CUA is a type of CEA, so the title just including the term CEA is appropriate.
7. **Relevant Costs:** Based on the stated perspective, the direct medical costs of ART and HIV treatment were included.
8. **Relevant Outcomes:** LYs and QALYs are important outcomes in the treatment of HIV since both length and quality of life are affected by the disease and treatment.

9. **Adjustment and Discounting:** All costs were assessed in 2008 US dollars—discounting for the future 20 years was conducted at a rate of 3% (and varied in the sensitivity analysis).

10. **Reasonable Assumptions:** It was assumed that the QALYs values were valid and the probabilities and costs obtained from literature were accurate. It was assumed that the cost-effectiveness threshold would be below the GDP of developing countries.

11. **Sensitivity Analyses:** Sensitivity analyses were conducted by varying the costs, time horizon, and the discount rate. Findings were robust (not sensitive) to these variables/ranges.

12. **Limitations Addressed:** Limitations on long-term effectiveness of ART and that societal costs were not included.

13. **Generalizations Appropriate:** The analysis included input costs and probabilities. A researcher could re-run the analysis with data specific for a different population. The authors did not try to extrapolate beyond sub-Saharan African populations.

14. **Unbiased Conclusions:** The authors do not overstate their results. Based on these numbers and sensitivity analyses, CD4 testing to determine initiation of ART in HIV patients is more effective than using the WHO staging criteria for this population at a reasonable cost.

COMPOSITE ARTICLE 2: MARKOV MODELING— PHOSPHATE BINDERS

Note: Haesuk Park, a PhD student, helped develop this composite article.
More information about this topic can be found in the following references:
Park H, Rascati K, Keith M, Hodgkins P, Smyth M, Goldsmith D, Akehurst R. Cost-effectiveness of lanthanum carbonate versus sevelamer hydrochloride for the treatment of hyperphosphatemia in patients with end-stage renal disease: A US payer perspective. Value in Health: The Journal of the International Society for Pharmacoeconomics and Outcomes Research *2011;14(8), 1002–1009.*
Bernard L, Mendelssohn D, Dunn E, Hutchison C, Grima DT. A modeled economic evaluation of sevelamer for treatment of hyperphosphatemia associated with chronic kidney disease among patients on dialysis in the United Kingdom. Journal of Medical Economics 16(1): 1–9, 2013.

Title: COST-EFFECTIVENESS OF NEW PHOSPHATE BINDER (NEWPB) FOR THE TREATMENT OF HYPERPHOSPHATEMIA IN CHRONIC KIDNEY DISEASE PATIENTS

INTRODUCTION: The clinical and economic burden associated with chronic kidney disease (CKD) is significant. Patients with CKD are at increased risk of premature death and other health issues such as cardiovascular disease and require lifelong care. Hyperphosphatemia (elevated levels of phosphorus in the body) is a common complication of CKD and strongly associated with increased risk of morbidity and mortality in patients with CKD. Phosphate binders (PBs), which lower serum phosphorus level, are a key component in the successful management of hyperphosphatemia. OldPB has been the standard of care for almost 20 years and

is relatively inexpensive but has been associated with an increased risk of cardiovascular events and mortality. NewPB was newly introduced to reduce the long-term safety of OldPB but it is more costly. Recently, a randomized, open-label study evaluated NewPB versus OldPB on mortality and the inception of dialysis. The purpose of this study was to assess the cost-effectiveness of NewPB compared with OldPB in patients with CKD from the US payer perspective.

METHODS: A Markov model was built in Excel 2010 to compare the two PBs (NewPB versus OldPB) in patients with CKD and

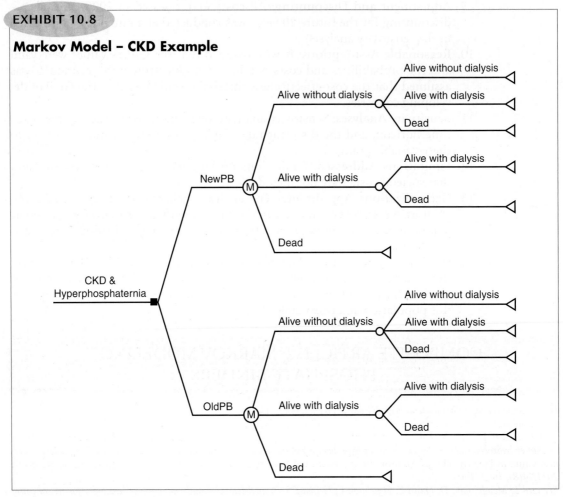

EXHIBIT 10.8

Markov Model – CKD Example

Alive without dialysis
Alive with dialysis
Dead

Alive without dialysis

NewPB — Ⓜ — Alive with dialysis

Alive with dialysis
Dead

Dead

CKD &
Hyperphosphaternia

Alive without dialysis
Alive with dialysis
Dead

Alive without dialysis

OldPB — Ⓜ — Alive with dialysis

Alive with dialysis
Dead

Dead

hyperphosphatemia. Transitions between three relevant clinical states were considered: *alive without dialysis, alive with dialysis* and dead (Exhibit 10.8). In the model, all patients started in alive without dialysis. From this health state, patients could remain in *alive without dialysis* or transit to *alive with dialysis* or progress to dead. Transition probabilities were taken

from a randomized clinical trial (Exhibit 10.9). Outcomes for 10 years were extrapolated using regression analysis beyond the duration of the clinical trial (3 years follow-up) for both

EXHIBIT 10.9

Transition Probabilities – CKD Example

Transition Probability	
Alive without dialysis → Alive with dialysis	
NewPB	10.60%
OldPB	17.40%
Alive without dialysis → dead	10.00%
Alive with dialysis → dead	15.00%

EXHIBIT 10.10

Costs and Utilities – CKD Example

Costs (per Year in 2013 US Dollars)		Probabilistic Sensitivity Assumptions
Drug		
NewPB	$5,000	gamma
OldPB	$2,000	gamma
Dialysis	$20,000	gamma
Utilities		
Alive without dialysis	0.850	beta
Alive with dialysis	0.720	beta

EXHIBIT 10.11

Calculations of the Markov Model
A. Data Markov Analysis: NewPB

	Markov State			Outcome		Cost		
Cycle	Nondialysis	Dialysis	Dead	Life Years	QALYs	Drug Cost	Dialysis Cost	Total Cost (Drug + Dialysis Costs)
0	10,000	0	0	10,000	8,500	$52,000,000	$0	$52,000,000
1	7,936	1,064	1,000	8,571	7,154	$44,571,429	$20,261,131	$64,832,559
2	6,298	1,748	1,953	7,299	5,998	$37,953,230	$31,715,984	$69,669,214
3	4,999	2,156	2,845	6,181	5,011	$32,138,666	$37,249,823	$69,388,489
4	3,967	2,364	3,669	5,209	4,175	$27,086,239	$38,903,419	$65,989,658
5	3,148	2,432	4,420	4,372	3,469	$22,735,115	$38,105,912	$60,841,027
6	2,499	2,402	5,100	3,657	2,875	$19,015,454	$35,845,744	$54,861,198
7	1,983	2,307	5,710	3,049	2,379	$15,855,156	$32,795,733	$48,650,890
8	1,574	2,172	6,254	2,535	1,964	$13,184,091	$29,404,291	$42,588,383
9	1,249	2,014	6,737	2,103	1,619	$10,936,597	$25,961,665	$36,898,261
10	991	1,845	7,164	1,741	1,333	$9,052,796	$22,647,826	$31,700,622
			Per patient	5.472	4.448	$28,453	$31,289	$59,742

B. Data Markov Analysis: OldPB

	Markov State			Outcome		Cost		
Cycle	Nondialysis	Dialysis	Dead	Life Years	QALYs	Drug Cost	Dialysis Cost	Total Cost (Drug + Dialysis Costs)
0	10,000	0	0	10,000	8,500	$20,000,000	$0	$20,000,000
1	7,259	1,741	1,000	8,571	7,070	$17,142,857	$33,154,578	$50,297,435
2	5,270	2,743	1,987	7,268	5,854	$14,535,999	$49,761,499	$64,297,498
3	3,826	3,249	2,925	6,111	4,830	$12,222,468	$56,130,756	$68,353,224
4	2,777	3,427	3,795	5,105	3,972	$10,209,112	$56,395,764	$66,604,875
5	2,016	3,397	4,587	4,241	3,259	$8,482,116	$53,228,764	$61,710,880
6	1,464	3,238	5,298	3,508	2,668	$7,016,915	$48,327,115	$55,344,029
7	1,062	3,007	5,930	2,892	2,181	$5,784,369	$42,742,767	$48,527,136
8	771	2,741	6,488	2,377	1,779	$4,754,494	$37,104,611	$41,859,105
9	560	2,464	6,976	1,949	1,450	$3,898,592	$31,767,790	$35,666,381
10	406	2,192	7,402	1,595	1,181	$3,190,375	$26,913,352	$30,103,727
			Per patient	5.362	4.274	$10,724	$43,553	$54,276

the NewPB and OldPB group. It was assumed that patients continued to receive medication (either NewPB or OldPB) until death. Costs were obtained from a retrospective review of Medicare data, and adjusted to 2013 costs. The quality-of-life estimates were derived from a study reporting utility values for CKD patients with and without dialysis (Exhibit 10.10). Both

EXHIBIT 10.12

Base Case Costs, Effects and Cost-Effectiveness of NewPB Cell versus OldPB for CKD with Hyperphosphatemia Over 10 Years

	Costs ($)	Total Life Years	QALYs	Incremental Cost per Life Year Gained (ICER)	Incremental Cost per QALY Gained (ICER)
NewPB	59,742	5.472	4.448	$49,759	$31,579
OldPB	54,276	5.363	4.274		

costs and outcomes were discounted at 5% per year. Patient outcomes were modeled for 10 years, and incremental cost-effectiveness ratios (ICERs) per life year gained and per QALY gained were calculated for NewPB relative to OldPB (see Exhibit 10.11 for model and calculations).

RESULTS: Exhibit 10.12 shows that the total costs and effects, in terms of life years and QALYs for patients treated with NewPB over 10 years and applying for a discount rate of 5%, were $59,742, 5.472 LYs, and 4.448 QALYs, respectively. For those patients treated with OldPB, the costs, life years and QALYs were $54,276, 5.363 LYs, and 4.274 QALYs,. respectively. With these estimates, the ICER of NewPB compared

with OldPB was $49,759 per life year gained and $31,579 per QALY gained. The results of probabilistic sensitivity analyses are shown in Exhibit 10.13 and 10.14. Exhibit 10.13 presents the scatter-plot diagrams with a maximum willingness-to-pay (WTP) of $50,000/QALY, which is the joint distribution of the mean incremental costs and mean incremental effects. All of the estimates fell in quadrants I and II of the cost-effectiveness plane (although the vast majority fell in quadrant I). These results suggest that when varying costs and utility values within reasonable ranges, NewPB was either more costly and more effective, or in a few cases, less costly and more effective than OldPB. The mean values for each group were used to generate acceptability curves over a range of WTP values (Exhibit 10.14).

EXHIBIT 10.13

Cost-Effectiveness Plane of NewPB versus OldPB for CKD Patients with Hyperphosphatemia with a Maximum Willingness-to-Pay Level of $50,000 per QALYs

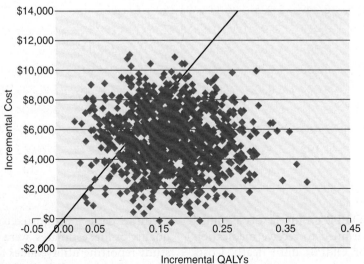

EXHIBIT 10.14

Cost-Effectiveness Acceptability Curves of NewPB versus OldPB for CKD Patients with Hyperphosphatemia

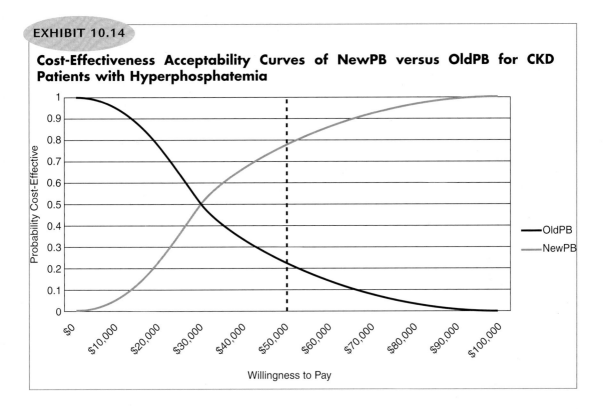

The cost-effectiveness acceptability curve illustrates a 79.5% probability of NewPB being cost-effective at the $50,000 WTP threshold.

DISCUSSION AND CONCLUSIONS: Limitations of this study include the assumption of efficacy data. The efficacy data from the randomized clinical trial was based on a relatively short duration of follow-up. Estimated outcomes for 10 years were modeled based on this short-term data. Hospitalization and cardiovascular event data were not collected in the randomized clinical trial. Overall, this analysis indicates that the long-term benefits of NewPB versus OldPB in terms of overall survival and inception of dialysis in patients with CKD and hyperphosphatemia from the perspective of the US payer. The results of this analysis demonstrate that NewPB represents a cost-effective alternative to OldPB for the treatment of hyperphosphatemia in patients with CKD in the US.

WORKSHEET FOR CRITIQUE OF MARKOV ANALYSIS COMPOSITE ARTICLE 2

1. Complete Title?

_____

_____

_____

_____

_____

2. Clear Objective?

_____
_____
_____
_____
_____

3. Appropriate Alternatives?

_____
_____
_____
_____
_____

4. Alternatives Described?

_____
_____
_____
_____
_____
_____

5. Perspective Stated?

_____
_____
_____
_____
_____

6. Type of Study?

_____
_____
_____
_____
_____

7. Relevant Costs?

_____

_____

_____

_____

_____

8. Relevant Outcomes?

_____

_____

_____

_____

_____

9. Adjustment or Discounting?

_____

_____

_____

_____

_____

10. Reasonable Assumptions?

_____

_____

_____

_____

_____

11. Sensitivity Analyses?

_____

_____

_____

_____

_____

12. Limitations Addressed?

_____

_____

_____

_____

_____

13. Generalizations Appropriate?

_____

_____

_____

_____

14. Unbiased Conclusions?

_____

_____

_____

_____

_____

ANSWERS

1. **Complete Title:** The title does include the type of study (cost-effectiveness) and the population (CKD patients). Although it lists one alternative (NewPB) it does not list the other alternative (OldPB).
2. **Clear Objective:** The objective was clearly stated as " ... to assess the cost-effectiveness of NewPB compared with OldPB in patients with CKD."
3. **Appropriate Alternatives:** Both medications are fictional—authors provide some comparisons of OldPB and NewPB.
4. **Alternatives Described:** No dosing given—may have to go to randomized controlled trial publication to determine dosing.
5. **Perspective Stated:** The perspective was clearly stated as the US payer perspective. Thus, only direct medical costs were included.
6. **Type of Study:** The study has been identified as a cost-effectiveness analysis. The outcomes were measured as both life years (LYs) gained—a CEA—and QALYs gained—a CUA. However the CUA is a type of CEA, so the title just including the term CEA is appropriate.

7. **Relevant Costs:** Based on the stated perspective, the direct medical costs of medication and dialysis treatment were included. Costs of treating side effects of medications should have been addressed.

8. **Relevant Outcomes:** LYs and QALYs are important outcomes in the treatment of CKD patients since both length and quality of life are affected by the disease and treatment.

9. **Adjustment and Discounting:** All costs were adjusted to 2013 US dollars and discounting for the future 10 years was conducted at a rate of 5%.

10. **Reasonable Assumptions:** It was assumed that the QALYs values were valid and the probabilities and costs obtained from literature were accurate. It was assumed that results from short term trials would extrapolate to 10 years. It was assumed that the cost-effectiveness threshold would be below $50,000.

11. **Sensitivity Analyses:** Sensitivity analyses were conducted by varying the costs and utility values using a technique called probability sensitivity analysis—results are illustrated in the scatterplot. The discount rate could also have been varied.

12. **Limitations Addressed:** Limitations on using short term efficacy data are addressed. Other outcomes cost (e.g., costs of side effects of medications), and effect of different rates of discounting were not addressed.

13. **Generalizations Appropriate:** The analysis included input costs and probabilities. A researcher could re-run the analysis with data specific for a different population. The authors did not address generalization—the appropriateness depends on the generalizability of the trial population used for data estimates.

14. **Unbiased Conclusions:** The authors do not overstate their results. Based on these numbers and sensitivity analyses, NewPB is, on average, more expensive that than OldPB, but provides better outcomes (LYs and QALYs) at a reasonable cost.

QUESTIONS/EXERCISES

An online coaching program has been developed for patients with borderline hypertension. A total of 100 patients are randomized to receive the coaching, and 100 patients serve as control subjects. It has been shown that for the first year after beginning the program, 90% with coaching were not considered hypertensive (normal or borderline blood pressure) and 10% were prescribed medication to control their blood pressure. In the control group (no coaching), 80% were not considered hypertensive after 1 year and 20% were prescribed blood pressure medication. Patients in the coaching group continue to receive coaching even if they are prescribed medication. The cost per year per patient for the coaching program is $50. The cost per year per patient for medication is $500. Assuming that these probabilities are constant for the next 4 years and that after patients begin medication, they must continue it for the rest of the study (absorbing state), answer the following questions. (Some cells have been filled in to help you get started.)

FOR 100 PATIENTS IN THE COACHING PROGRAM:

Prevention Coaching Program	Subjects without Hypertension (n)	Subjects with Hypertension (n)	Cost of Coaching Program	Cost of Medication	Total Costs
Cycle 1	100	0	$5,000	$0	$5,000
Cycle 2	90	10	$5,000	$5,000	$10,000
Cycle 3	81	19	$5,000	$9,500	$14,500
Cycle 4					
Cycle 5					
Total					

FOR 100 PATIENTS WITHOUT THE COACHING PROGRAM:

Prevention Coaching Program	Subjects without Hypertension (n)	Subjects with Hypertension (n)	Cost of Coaching Program	Cost of Medication	Total Costs
Cycle 1	100	0	$0	$0	$0
Cycle 2	80	20	$0	$10,000	$10,000
Cycle 3	64	36	$0	$18,000	$18,000
Cycle 4					
Cycle 5					
Total					

1. What are the total costs for the patients in the coaching group if no discounting is conducted? If a 5% discount rate (beginning cycle 2) is used?

2. What are the total costs for the patients in the control group (no coaching) if no discounting is conducted? If a 5% discount rate (beginning cycle 2) is used?

3. If the online counseling costs are considered input costs and benefits are calculated as cost savings due to less medication costs, what is the benefit-to-cost ratio of the program with and without discounting?

_____

_____

_____

_____

_____

4. Would using a half-cycle correction be appropriate in this example? Why or why not?

_____

_____

_____

_____

5. What other costs and outcomes would be included in a more clinically relevant (and more complex) model?

_____

_____

_____

_____

_____

REFERENCES

1. Petitti DB. Complex decision problems. In *Meta-Analysis, Decision Analysis, and Cost-Effectiveness Analysis.* Oxford: Oxford University Press, 1994.
2. Briggs A, Sculpher M, Claxton M. *Decision Modelling for Health Economic Evaluation.* Oxford: Oxford University Press, 2006.
3. Naimark D, Krahn MD, Naglie G, et al. Primer on medical decision analysis: Part 5—Working with Markov processes. *Medical Decision Making* 17(2):152–159, 1997.
4. Sonnenberg FA, Beck JR. Markov models in decision making: A practical guide. *Medical Decision Making* 13(4):322–338, 1993.
5. Hawkins N, Sculpher M, Epstein D. Cost-effectiveness analysis of treatments for chronic disease: Using R to incorporate time dependency of treatment response. *Medical Decision Making* 25(5):511–519, 2005.
6. Berger ML, Bingefors K, Hedblom EC, et al. (eds). *Health Care Cost, Quality, and Outcomes: ISPOR Book of Terms.* Lawrenceville, NJ: International Society for Pharmacoeconomics and Outcomes Research, 2003.
7. Desgagné A, Castilloux A, Angers J, LeLorier J. The use of the bootstrap statistical method for the pharmacoeconomic cost analysis of skewed data. *Pharmacoeconomics* 13(5, pt 1): 487–497, 1998.
8. Fenwick E, Marshall DA, Levy AR, Nichol G. Using and interpreting cost-effectiveness acceptability curves: An example using data from a trial of management strategies for atrial fibrillation. *BMC Health Services Research* 6:52, 2006.

SUGGESTED READINGS

Caro JJ, Briggs AH, Siebert U, et al. Modeling good research practices—Overview: A report of the ISPOR-SMDM modeling good research practices task force-1. *Value Health* 15:796–803, 2012.

Drummond MF, Sculpher MJ, Torrance GW, et al. Economic evaluation using decision analytic modelling. In *Methods for the Economic Evaluation of Health Care Programmes* (3rd ed.). Oxford: Oxford University Press, 2005.

Kuntz KM, Weinstein MC. Modelling in economic evaluations. In Drummond MF, McGuire A (eds). *Economic Evaluation in Health Care*. Oxford: Oxford University Press, 2002.

Petrou S, Gray A. Economic evaluation using decision analytical modelling: Design, conduct, analysis, and reporting. *BMJ (Clinical Research Ed.)* 342:d1766, 2011. doi:10.1136/bmj.d1766

Chapter 11

Retrospective Databases

Objectives

Upon completing this chapter, the reader will be able to:

1. Compare and contrast the use of data from randomized, controlled trials (RCTs) versus observational studies for pharmacoeconomic analyses.

2. Give examples of types of retrospective databases available for pharmacoeconomic research.

3. Explain additional issues to be addressed when critiquing research that uses retrospective databases.

4. Critique a study that uses a retrospective database.

✦ OVERVIEW OF RETROSPECTIVE DATABASES

When clinicians and other decision makers need to determine whether a medication or treatment "works," they look for information that can help answer this question. A hierarchy of research methods is used to collect and analyze this information. For data on what "works," decision makers and clinicians can look to studies that use a variety of research methods, including **randomized, controlled trials** (RCTs), **observational** (retrospective and prospective) **studies,** meta-analyses, and expert opinions or panels. Advantages and disadvantages of meta-analyses and expert opinions or panels can be found elsewhere.[1] This chapter compares and contrasts the advantages and disadvantages of collecting and using data from RCTs (**efficacy** data) with those of observational studies (**effectiveness** data) for pharmacoeconomic research.

✦ RANDOMIZED, CONTROLLED TRIALS

RCTs are required by the Food and Drug Administration (FDA) to approve for sale any prescription drug product in the United States. RCTs are listed at the top of the research methods hierarchy because they provide the strongest evidence that a drug is "efficacious." Efficacy indicates whether the drug "can work" in a controlled study. As the name implies, patients are randomly chosen (i.e., randomized) to get either the medication of interest or another medication or a placebo (an inactive compound). **Randomization** is used to decrease baseline differences between patient groups. If patients are assigned to their group in a random manner, there is a high likelihood that the groups will be similar in age, gender, disease severity, and so on. If researchers find a difference in the clinical outcomes between the two groups, the randomization process increases our confidence that these differences are, in fact, because of the difference in the effects of the medication and not the difference in patient characteristics.

✦ OBSERVATIONAL STUDIES

Observational studies follow what happens to patients who receive medical care in a "real-world" environment. Observational studies measure the "effectiveness" of treatments. Effectiveness indicates whether the treatment "does work" in everyday medical practice. Observational studies can be **prospective** or **retrospective.** Prospective observational studies record treatments and outcomes as they occur. Retrospective observational studies analyze treatments and outcomes that have already occurred. Patients are not randomly assigned to which treatment they receive, and treatment or **selection biases** may occur. For example, patients with a more severe form of a disease or who have been treatment resistant to standard therapy may receive (be "selected" to receive) the newer medication.

✦ ADVANTAGES AND DISADVANTAGES OF RCTs

As mentioned above, one main advantage of RCTs is that the random assignment of patients improves the chances that patient characteristics are similar between study groups at baseline. This, in turn, makes the efficacy differences, if found, more credible. But there are limitations that should be considered when using data from RCTs for pharmacoeconomic studies.

The time frame of RCTs may be too short to determine long-range outcomes, especially for chronic diseases such as diabetes and heart disease. In addition, the sample size may be too small to detect some differences in outcomes such as rates of side effects. Patients who are recruited to participate in RCTs may not be representative of the average patient population because of the study's inclusion and exclusion criteria (i.e., rules of who can or cannot participate in the study). The criteria used to select patients for the study may state that patients cannot have any other diseases (comorbidities) except for the disease of interest in the study or that they cannot be taking any other medications except for the study drugs. In addition, there may be other restrictions such as age or level of literacy. Patients enrolled in an RCT may behave differently or receive different levels of services compared with usual medical care. For example, patients are more likely to take their medications consistently when being monitored in a study (which increases the amount of medication used by study participants). Because of the study protocol (plan), patients may receive more monitoring (e.g., physician visits, laboratory tests) than is customary in routine medical practice.

✦ ADVANTAGES AND DISADVANTAGES OF OBSERVATIONAL STUDIES

Observational studies can overcome some of the restrictions of RCTs, but they have their own limitations (Table 11.1). Observational studies, especially if they are retrospective, are less expensive and less time-consuming than RCTs because researchers do not have to enroll patients into the study. **Retrospective databases** allow researchers to analyze many years' worth of patient information from a large number of records in a short period at a relatively low cost. Observational data can reflect a more realistic picture of treatment patterns for a wider population of patients and factor in patients' true adherence to treatment regimens.

Sensitivity analyses can be easily conducted by simply changing the computer programming code for the baseline analysis. For example, inclusion or exclusion criteria (e.g., age range, diagnoses, adherence to medication) for patient data used in the baseline analyses can be expanded or restricted to determine if results are **robust** (i.e., **insensitive**) for these different criteria ranges.

The major limitations with using observational data are that the information may be incomplete, inaccurate, or biased. Health care databases consist of information provided by patients and health care providers. Most retrospective databases are collected and used primarily for payment (**reimbursement**) of treatment and services rather than to assess patient outcomes. Patient information may be incomplete if a patient switches insurance companies during the study period or becomes ineligible to receive services during part of the study period. Data may also be incomplete if the patient pays out of pocket for some of his or her health care expenses, if the service is not covered by the patient's insurance plan, or if the patient has more than one form of insurance (e.g., both Medicaid and Medicare, insurance from an employer and the spouse's employer).

Data provided on diagnoses may be inaccurate. Reimbursements for medical services, such as a physician visit or a hospitalization, require the provider or a staff

TABLE 11.1. COMPARISON OF RANDOMIZED PROSPECTIVE TRIALS VERSUS RETROSPECTIVE DATABASE STUDIES: SOME POSSIBLE ADVANTAGES AND DISADVANTAGES

Type of Study	Advantages	Disadvantages
Prospective randomized, controlled trial	More scientifically rigorous	Only select patients
	Needed for FDA approval	Short-term follow-up
	Less chance of baseline differences	High cost of recruitment and follow-up
	Can collect clinical and PRO outcome data	Protocol-driven costs unrealistic in standard practice
		Only highly adherent patients
		Small sample size
Retrospective database	Includes broader range of patients	Selection bias
	Lower cost to conduct study	May be only one population
	Larger sample size	May be missing data
	Longer time period	Data may be miscoded
	Easier to recalculate with different criteria (sensitivity analyses)	Clinical or PRO outcome data may be lacking

FDA = Food and Drug Administration; PRO = patient-reported outcome.

member to indicate the diagnosis code (or codes) for the service using International Classification of Disease, Ninth Edition (ICD-9) or Current Procedural Terminology (CPT) codes. Each visit or service may be associated with one or more diagnoses. Miscoding of diagnoses may occur, intentionally or unintentionally. Different payment structures by various insurance systems may lead to undercoding or overcoding of diseases. If a patient is in a capitated insurance system (one that pays the providers the same amount per billing cycle regardless of the patient's level of use or non-use of medical services), there may be a tendency for the providers to record only one diagnosis per visit because adding other diagnoses will not result in a higher reimbursement. Some insurance companies allow a maximum number of diagnoses recorded per claim, so comorbidities may be underdocumented. On the other hand, if the amount of reimbursement is tied to the severity and number of diagnoses, additional or unimportant diagnoses codes may be recorded.

Even if steps are taken to ensure that the information extracted for the study are largely accurate and complete, selection bias is still an issue. There may be differences in the group who had medication A prescribed compared with those who had medication B prescribed. Some differences are easily compared using the databases (e.g., age range, gender), but there may be differences that are not measured (e.g., past rate of adherence to other medications or treatments) or not recorded in the database (e.g., rate of smoking, family history of diseases).

Sometimes a phenomenon known as **channeling bias** occurs, in which patients with certain characteristics are more likely to be channeled to one medication over another. An example of channeling bias may occur if medication A is thought to cause an unwanted side effect such as weight gain more often than medication B. For patients who are already overweight or prone to gain weight, prescribers might opt for medication B in the hope of decreasing the chance of this side effect. When patient groups are different at baseline, the outcomes measured for the study may be partially based on these patient differences. Various statistical calculations (multivariate regression, instrumental variable analysis, and propensity score matching) are available to reduce the impact of these biases.[2]

✦ TYPES OF RETROSPECTIVE DATABASES

Three types of retrospective databases are often used in pharmacoeconomic research: electronic medical records, national health survey data, and health insurance claims records. Insurance claims databases may come from private insurers, such as managed care providers, or from federal or state-funded (public) insurance programs. The estimates of medical service use between these different types of databases may not always be highly correlated,[3] and each have their own unique advantages and disadvantages. Some examples of pharmacoeconomic research using these three categories of databases are found in Table 11.2. Two Websites that list information describing medical databases available for analysis are *Bridge to Data* at www.bridgetodata.org and *Accelerate* at http://accelerate.ucsf.edu/research/celdac.

Electronic Medical Records

Some health care organizations hire transcribers or use electronic methods to transform patient medical records into an electronic form that can be accessed via computers by health providers throughout its system. Electronic medical record (EMR) systems provide detailed information about patient encounters and are a

TABLE 11.2. EXAMPLES OF STUDIES THAT USED RETROSPECTIVE DATABASES

Electronic Medical Records

Wells BJ, Lobel KD, Dickerson LM. Using the electronic medical record to enhance the use of combination drugs. *American Journal of Medical Quality* 18(4):147–149, 2003.

Kim Y, Rascati K, Prasla K, Godley P, Goel N, Dunlop D. Retrospective evaluation of the impact of copayment increases for specialty medications on adherence and persistence in an integrated health maintenance organization system. *Clinical Therapeutics* 33(5):598–607, 2011.

National Databases

Hurst F, Jindal R, Abbott K, et al. Incidence, predictors, costs, and outcome of renal cell carcinoma after kidney transplantation: USRDS experience. *Transplantation* 90(8):898–904, 2010.

Cheng L, Rascati K. Impact of Medicare Part D for Medicare-age adults with arthritis: Prescription use, prescription expenditures, and medical spending from 2005 to 2008. *Arthritis Care & Research* 64(9):1423–1429, 2012.

State Medicaid

Gilligan A, Malone D, Warholak T, Armstrong E. Health disparities in cost of care in patients with Alzheimer's disease: An analysis across 4 state Medicaid populations. *American Journal of Alzheimer's Disease and Other Dementias* 28(1):84–92, 2013.

Rascati K, Akazawa M, Johnsrud M, Stanford R, Blanchette C. Comparison of hospitalizations, emergency department visits, and costs in a historical cohort of Texas Medicaid patients with chronic obstructive pulmonary disease, by initial medication regimen. *Clinical Therapeutics* 29(6):1203–1213, 2007.

Veterans Administration

Chan K, Lai M, Ho S, et al. Cost-effectiveness analysis of direct-acting antiviral therapy for treatment-naïve patients with chronic hepatitis C genotype 1 infection in the Veterans Health Administration [published online ahead of print May 22, 2013]. *Clinical Gastroenterology and Hepatology*.

Ajumobi A, Vuong R, Ahaneku H. Analysis of nonformulary use of PPIs and excess drug cost in a Veterans Affairs population. *Journal of Managed Care Pharmacy* 18(1):63–67, 2012.

rich source of data for pharmacoeconomic research. Although EMR information may be more complete than other database methods (i.e., insurance claims data), it is costly to implement the system and time-consuming to retrieve the information needed for a study.[4]

National Health Surveys

In the United States, various national health surveys, such as the National Ambulatory Care Survey (NAMCS) and the National Hospital Ambulatory Medical Care Survey (NHAMS), are conducted by the Center for Disease Control's National Center for Health Statistics (NCHS) to provide information on patterns of medical utilization.[5,6] The Medical Expenditure Panel Survey (MEPS) is a national health survey cosponsored by NCHS and the Agency for Healthcare Research and Quality (AHRQ) that produces estimates of health care use and health care expenditures for noninstitutionalized civilians living in the United States. MEPS includes three separate but related surveys. First, surveys are completed by a nationally representative sample of the population using the Household Component (HC) Survey. Supplemental information for these respondents is collected from their medical care providers through the Medical Provider Component (MPC) Survey and their insurance providers via the Insurance Component (IC) Survey. The MEPS survey includes questions from the SF-12 and EQ-5D (see Chapter 8) to evaluate a patient's **health status**.[7,8]

Researchers have noted that national health surveys may be missing some variables of interest (e.g., amount of patient copayments or deductibles), that the data collected for some medical services are more accurate than others, and that analysis of the survey data is a challenge because of its statistical complexity.[9,10] On the whole, national health surveys provide high-quality information on health care utilization and health care costs, and they are generally representative of the US population.

✦ INSURANCE AND CLAIMS RECORDS

Insurance records, or **claims data,** are often used for pharmacoeconomic research because the data files usually contain specific information on a large number of patients. Claims for different services and settings (e.g., hospitalizations, outpatient visits, prescriptions) can be merged to better indicate each patient's overall medical utilization. The claims data may be collected by private insurers (e.g., Aetna or Blue Cross) or by public insurers (e.g., Medicaid, Department of Defense, or Veterans Administration). A major advantage of using claims data is that a large amount of patient information is available in an easily retrievable format, and the costs of setting up the data collection system have already been financed by the insurance company that needs the data to pay patient claims. A major disadvantage of using insurance claims data is that they are often missing clinical information (e.g., laboratory results, patient's **health-related quality of life** changes) that may be needed to answer the research question.

✦ CRITIQUING RETROSPECTIVE DATABASE STUDIES

There are additional issues to be considered when reading and critiquing a pharmacoeconomic study that uses information from retrospective databases. Five of these issues are discussed below.

Clear Explanation of the Database

Researchers should address the type of information (e.g., prescription data, medical service data, hospitalization data, laboratory values) that is available in the database or databases they used for their study and for what period of time the data were collected. They should also describe the population that is covered by the database(s). For example, if the database contains information from the Veterans Administration, the majority of recipients would be older men, and the costs for individual prescriptions may be lower than average because of discounts offered to the federal government.

Any relevant **formulary** or payment restrictions specific to the insurance plan should also be discussed. For example, some state Medicaid plans have limits on the maximum number of prescriptions the plan will pay for each month. Other insurance plans may have a strict formulary, which can result in most patients being prescribed the medication that was chosen by the plan as being preferred. If the patient can only receive a nonformulary (or nonpreferred) item by overcoming specific requirements (e.g., getting a physician to fill out paperwork for special authorization or requiring that the patient has "failed" on other medications), this can lead to a difference in the groups that get the formulary versus nonformulary medications, which, in turn, makes comparisons difficult.

Clear Explanation of Patient-Selection Criteria

Just as with RCTs, it is imperative that researchers include the criteria (i.e., rules) used to select patients for the study. If specific diagnoses or the use of specific medications were used as a proxy to infer that patients had a specific condition or disease, these diagnoses or medications should be listed. Exclusion criteria for patients should also be stated. Examples of exclusion variables are the patient's age, comorbid diagnoses, concomitant medications, and noncompliance with treatment.

Eligibility of Patients

Some patients may not be "eligible" to receive insurance benefits during the entire period of study. Patients might switch to another insurance plan or become ineligible for their current plan (e.g., they no longer work full time for their employer or no longer meet the criterion for "need" according to the Medicaid definition). It is important to describe what steps are taken to address this issue. Many researchers list ineligibility at any time during the study period as an exclusion criterion.

Clinical or Outcome Measures

As already mentioned, medical claims databases are primarily used for reimbursement purposes, so they may not contain patient outcome variables such as blood pressure measurements or **patient-reported outcomes** (PROs). Sometimes clinical outcomes are inferred by using information from billed medical services. For example, when comparing the outcomes of various oral antidiabetic medications, markers such as a diagnosis of ketoacidosis or a diabetes-related emergency department visit or hospitalization may serve as an indication that the disease is not well controlled. These markers may not be as accurate as clinical outcomes measures (e.g., fasting blood glucose or hemoglobin A1c levels) and may be skewed by other patient factors. For example, a patient without a primary care physician may be more likely to go to an emergency department for routine care, and a patient who lives alone may spend an extra day in the hospital before being discharged.

Another issue that arises is that of "double-counting" outcomes. The incremental cost-effective ratio (ICER) is calculated by dividing the difference in costs by the difference in outcomes. When comparing the effectiveness of medications, any additional hospitalizations or emergency department visits are a marker of an unwanted outcome (i.e., lower effectiveness), which appears in the denominator of the ICER, while also increasing the costs in the numerator of the equation.

Sensitivity Analyses

Retrospective database studies allow the researcher to be flexible when selecting study design parameters such as the length of the follow-up period, retrospective matching techniques, and patient inclusion and exclusion criteria. Sensitivity analyses of key design choices are relatively easy to execute and should be included. Because it may be difficult to identify whether a medication or service is specifically related to the disease or condition of interest (e.g., was the oral corticosteroid prescribed for asthma or an allergic reaction?), an additional sensitivity analysis is often seen in retrospective database analyses. This additional analysis compares results using **disease-specific** costs and outcomes (e.g., those with a specific ICD-9) with those using total costs and outcomes the patients have incurred for all diseases and conditions for the period of interest.

SUMMARY

Two types of research methods—RCTs and observational studies—are often used to collect the information needed for pharmacoeconomic decisions. RCTs are essential as a first step for determining the efficacy of a new medication or treatment. In other words, they are used to answer the question: "Can the drug work under controlled conditions?" If the answer is no, the medication is not approved by the FDA.

RCTs are said to possess a higher level of **internal validity** than observation studies in that the evidence is strong that any difference in outcomes for the study groups is attributable to the intervention and not other factors. After the medication is available to be prescribed, decision makers are also interested in the effectiveness of the product, asking: "Does the drug work in routine medical practice?" The answer may be different than that found by the RCT because of a broader range of patients taking the medication, a difference in patient behavior (e.g., adherence), and a different level of services received (e.g., less frequent monitoring).

Observational studies are said to have a higher level of **external validity** than RCTs. This means that results are more **generalizable** (more representative) to a broader range of patients. Although there are major differences between these two research methods, both are useful, and comparisons of clinical findings for many disease states and conditions have shown that results from the two methods produce similar answers.[1,11]

The use of retrospective databases to analyze observational health care information is less time-consuming and less expensive than conducting RCTs. Retrospective information can come from three major categories of databases: EMRs, national health surveys, and insurance claims. Each type has advantages and disadvantages. Because of the potential limitations associated with using these databases, some additional issues must be addressed when evaluating studies that use them. Five of these issues were discussed in this chapter. A more extensive checklist and further guidelines are available elsewhere.[12-15]

COMPOSITE ARTICLE 1: RETROSPECTIVE DATABASE—COPD

Title: COST-EFFECTIVENESS OF TWO MEDICATIONS USED FOR CHRONIC OBSTRUCTIVE PULMONARY DISEASE IN A STATE MEDICAID POPULATION

BACKGROUND: Chronic Obstructive Pulmonary Disease (COPD) is a disease characterized by airflow limitation that is not fully reversible, resulting in disabling symptoms such as chronic cough, sputum production, and dyspnea. During 2000, COPD was responsible for 8 million physician office and hospital outpatient visits, 1.5 million emergency department (ED) visits, 726,000 hospitalizations, and 119,000 deaths. COPD is the fourth leading cause of death in the United States, with an age-adjusted death rate of 42.7 per 100,000.

The National Medical Expenditure Panel Survey (MEPS) indicated that inpatient hospitalizations and ED visits accounted for the majority of total expenditures among patients with COPD. Therefore, medication treatments that prevent or reduce the risk of hospitalizations or ED visits would likely have a substantial impact on the overall clinical and economic burden of the disease. Recent RCTs have indicated that the use of Pulmolair may decrease the number of exacerbations of breathing difficulties compared with Bronchocort. (Note: Neither is the name for an actual mediation; assume relevant clinical references to indicate these are appropriate and clinically relevant choices.) The objective of this study was to compare the costs and effects of these two medications on COPD-related exacerbations from a state Medicaid perspective.

METHODS: *Design and Sample:* The study used patient-level administrative medical and pharmacy data captured from the state Medicaid database. This database encompassed inpatient and outpatient medical service claims as well as outpatient prescription claims for patients who were enrolled in the state Medicaid program. The study involved the use of a retrospective design to compare the costs and outcomes among patients who were continuously enrolled for at least 24 months in the state Medicaid program (12 months before their index date and 12 months after their index date).

Patients 40 to 64 years old with a primary or secondary diagnosis of COPD-related (ICD-9-CM codes 491.xx, 492.xx, or 496.xx) medical costs anytime during the observational period and with at least one prescription claim for either Pulmolair or Bronchocort were eligible for inclusion. Patients with a diagnosis for cystic fibrosis (ICD-9-CM, 277.xx) or respiratory

tract cancer (ICD-9-CM, 160.xx-164.xx, 231.xx) were excluded from the analysis. Patient data were included in the study if the patient's first dispense date (index date) for either medication occurred within the index period between April 1, 2005, and March 31, 2006.

The index date was defined as the first pharmacy claim for either Pulmolair or Bronchocort. If a patient had both index medications dispensed within 60 days of their index date, he or she was classified as being on combination therapy and was excluded from further analysis. Total COPD-related costs were calculated by summing the amount that Medicaid paid for COPD-related medications and COPD-related medical services in the year after each patient's index date. Outcomes were measured as the number of breathing exacerbations suspected based on the number of COPD-related hospitalizations, the number of COPD-related ED visits, and the number of prescriptions for an oral "burst" of steroids. The Charlson Index Severity Score was calculated based on preindex ICD-9s classifications and weightings to adjust for comorbidities.

Statistical Analyses: Medical and prescription claims for 1 year after each patient's index date were assessed to determine the total COPD-related costs and the number of COPD-related exacerbations (hospitalization, ED visit, or burst of steroids). Propensity score matching was conducted to adjust for baseline differences. Variables included in the matching were demographics (age, gender, and race) presence of comorbid respiratory diseases (e.g., asthma), presence of comorbidity of other diseases (Charlson score), preindex utilization of other respiratory medications (e.g., theophylline), and the number of COPD-related preindex exacerbations (hospitalizations, ED visits, bursts during the 1-year period before the index date).

RESULTS: *Patient Sample:* A total of 4,332 patients had one index medication (1,322 Pulmolair and 3,010 Bronchocort) and at least one record of a COPD-related medical visit within 1 year before or after their medication index date. Propensity scores helped select the 1,322 Bronchocort patients who best matched the 1,322 Pulmolair patients. Comparison of baseline demographics and preindex comorbidities by index medication category are listed in Exhibit 11.1, and preindex utilization and costs by index medication category can be found in Exhibit 11.2.

Exacerbations: The number and types of COPD-related exacerbations in the 1-year period after the index dates for the propensity-matched cohorts are listed in Exhibit 11.3. Although patients on Pulmolair had a higher average number of oral steroid bursts in the 1 year after the index date (2.81 versus 2.50), they had fewer COPD-related ED visits (1.51 versus 1.90) and fewer COPD-related hospitalizations (0.15 versus 0.30) than patients taking Bronchocort.

Costs: One-year postindex COPD-related prescription costs, COPD-related medical service

EXHIBIT 11.1

Baseline Demographic Information and Preindex Comorbidities for Matched Cohorts

	Pulmolair (n = 1,322)	Bronchocort (n = 1,322)
Gender, n (% female)	991 (75%)	1,018 (77%)
Ethnicity		
White, n (%)	674 (51%)	674 (51%)
Black, n (%)	278 (21%)	317 (24%)
Hispanic, n (%)	278 (21%)	238 (18%)
Other, n (%)	92 (7%)	93 (7%)
Age, mean (SD)	53.20 (6.63)	53.55 (6.72)
Charlson score, mean (SD)	1.99 (1.36)	1.97 (1.33)
Comorbidities		
Acute respiratory, n (%)	1,071 (81%)	1,084 (82%)
Asthma, n (%)	885 (67%)	912 (69%)
Influenza, n (%)	555 (42%)	568 (43%)
Other upper respiratory, n (%)	846 (64%)	860 (65%)

SD = standard deviation.

EXHIBIT 11.2

One-Year Preindex COPD-Related Utilization and Costs for Matched Cohorts

	Pulmolair (n = 1,322)	Bronchocort (n = 1,322)
One-Year Preindex Utilization		
COPD hospital visits, mean (SD)	0.10 (0.24)	0.10 (0.28)
COPD ED visits, mean (SD)	1.51 (2.53)	1.54 (2.51)
Burst of oral steroids, mean (SD)	2.31(2.93)	2.36 (2.06)
SABAs, mean (SD)	1.95 (2.43)	2.04 (2.83)
Theophylline prescriptions, mean (SD)	2.19 (2.00)	2.26 (2.30)
One-Year Preindex Costs		
COPD prescription costs, mean (SD)	$173 (196)	$172 (181)
COPD medical costs, mean (SD)	$785 (2,452)	$776 (2,534)
COPD total costs, mean (SD)	$958 (2,466)	$948 (2,546)

COPD = chronic obstructive pulmonary disease; ED = emergency department; SABA = short-acting beta-agonist; SD = standard deviation.

costs, and total COPD-related costs for the matched cohorts are provided in Exhibit 11.3. Patients with an index prescription for Pulmolair had higher COPD-related prescription costs ($491 versus $374) but lower COPD-related medical costs ($1,067 versus $1,541), resulting in lower total COPD-related costs ($1,558 versus $1,915) compared with patients with an index medication for Bronchocort. Pulmolair was the better option because it was associated with both a lower number of COPD-related exacerbations (i.e., increased effectiveness) and overall lower COPD-related costs. Therefore, the calculation of an incremental cost-effectiveness ratio was not warranted.

LIMITATIONS/CONCLUSION: *Limitations:* As with any retrospective data analysis, there are inherent limitations. It was assumed that

EXHIBIT 11.3

One-Year Postindex COPD-Related Utilization and Costs for Matched Cohorts

	Pulmolair (n = 1,322)	Bronchocort (n = 1,322)
One-Year Postindex Utilization		
COPD hospital visits, mean (SD)	0.15 (0.38)	0.30 (0.48)
COPD ED visits, mean (SD)	1.51 (2.53)	1.90 (2.90)
Burst of oral steroids, mean (SD)	2.81 (2.93)	2.50 (2.06)
Number of COPD Exacerbations, mean (SD)	4.47 (6.50)	4.70 (6.70)
One-Year Postindex Costs		
COPD prescription costs, mean (SD)	$491 (471)	$374 (440)
COPD medical costs, mean (SD)	$1,067 (3,577)	$1,541 (5,906)
COPD total costs, mean (SD)	$1,558 (3,673)	$1,915 (5,930)

COPD = chronic obstructive pulmonary disease; ED = emergency department; SD = standard deviation.

the data were complete when, in reality, patients may have gone outside of the state Medicaid system for health care. Patients age 65 years and older were not included in the analysis because of their high probability of receiving additional care from the federal Medicare system. Data were collected from one state Medicaid system and may not be generalizable to other COPD patients.

Conclusion: In this state Medicaid system, 1-year COPD-related costs and exacerbations were compared for a matched sample of patients starting on either Pulmolair or Bronchocort. Pulmolair was found to be the better option because it was associated with both lower costs and fewer breathing exacerbations. Research in other patient populations is needed.

WORKSHEET FOR CRITIQUE OF RETROSPECTIVE DATABASE COMPOSITE ARTICLE 1

1. Complete Title?

_____

_____

_____

_____

2. Clear Objective?

_____

_____

_____

_____

3. Appropriate Alternatives?

_____
_____
_____
_____

4. Alternatives Described?

_____
_____
_____
_____

5. Perspective Stated?

_____
_____
_____
_____

6. Type of Study?

_____
_____
_____
_____

7. Relevant Costs?

_____
_____
_____
_____

8. Relevant Outcomes?

_____
_____
_____
_____

9. Adjustment or Discounting?

_____

_____

_____

_____

10. Reasonable Assumptions?

_____

_____

_____

_____

11. Sensitivity Analyses?

_____

_____

_____

_____

12. Limitations Addressed?

_____

_____

_____

_____

13. Generalizations Appropriate?

_____

_____

_____

_____

14. Unbiased Conclusions? Include answers to the five additional question used for analyses using retrospective databases.

_____

_____

_____

_____

Cost-Effectiveness Grid

Which cell represents the comparison of Pulmolair with Bronchocort?

COST-EFFECTIVENESS	Lower Cost	Same Cost	Higher Cost
Lower effectiveness	A	B	C
Same effectiveness	D	E	F
Higher effectiveness	G	H	I

CRITIQUE OF RETROSPECTIVE DATABASE COMPOSITE ARTICLE 1

1. **Complete Title:** The title did identify the type of study (cost-effectiveness analysis [CEA]) and that patients were in a state Medicaid program, but it did not specify which medication regimens were included in the analysis.

2. **Clear Objective:** The objective of this study was to conduct a CEA to determine the number of COPD-related exacerbations. This was clear.

3. **Appropriate Alternatives:** Appropriate literature should be cited to validate the choices of alternatives that are most clinically relevant.

4. **Alternatives Described:** The dosing and scheduling of doses were not described. Patients may have been more adherent to one medication than the other. The average doses and adherence for each alternative should be included.

5. **Perspective Stated:** The perspective of the study was explicitly stated as the state Medicaid program.

6. **Type of Study:** Some would identify this as a CEA because outcomes were measured as exacerbations avoided (see double-counting debate in question 8).

7. **Relevant Costs:** Because the perspective was the state Medicaid program, costs paid by this system were the relevant costs to measure. As a sensitivity analysis, it would have been informative for the researchers to also calculate the total costs per patient in addition to the total COPD-related costs per patient because some cost differences might not have been captured by the restriction of specific ICD-9 codings.

8. **Relevant Outcomes:** Outcomes were measured by comparing the "number of exacerbations," defined as a hospitalization, an ED visit, or a burst of oral

steroids. With retrospective databases, outcomes are usually restricted to measures found in pharmacy/medical claims. Laboratory measures (such as forced expiratory volume) and health-related quality of life (HRQoL) measures or patient preference measures are not usually included in these databases. In this example, double counting (the difference in the number of exacerbations in the denominator and the difference of the costs of exacerbations in the numerator) was not an issue because incremental cost-effectiveness ratios were not calculated.

9. **Adjustment or Discounting:** Costs and outcomes for a 1-year period were analyzed, so neither adjustment nor discounting was needed.

10. **Reasonable Assumptions:** When using retrospective databases, many assumptions are usually standard (e.g., that the data are accurate and complete). Patients may get services outside the system, or the coding may be inaccurate. Some plans' claims databases have limits on the services that it will pay for (e.g., most will not pay for smoking cessation products, so this cannot be factored into COPD exacerbations). In this example, COPD is a disease that affects an older population, and data for patients age 65 years and older were not included because of the dual-eligibility situation.

11. **Sensitivity Analyses:** Sensitivity analyses were not conducted. As mentioned in question 7 (relevant costs), a sensitivity analysis should have been performed for the total costs to Medicaid for these patients. Researchers could have also varied the age range (e.g., included those older than age 65 years) or adherence criterion (e.g., eliminated those with poor adherence to Pulmolair or Bronchocort).

12. **Limitations Addressed:** Some limitations, such as age range and low generalizability, were addressed. One limitation that is common in RCTs, that of inadequate sample size, is less of an issue when using large retrospective databases.

13. **Generalizations Appropriate:** The authors did not try to extrapolate beyond the state Medicaid patients between 40 and 65 years old.

14. **Unbiased Conclusions:** The conclusions were based on the results presented and were not overstated. As listed in this chapter, *five additional issues* should be addressed when critiquing studies that use retrospective databases. The first issue involves describing the database. Although this study includes the types of data available from Medicaid and some demographics of the patients who were in the matched cohort, it does not describe the overall state Medicaid population (e.g., number of people covered) nor any restrictions (e.g., maximum number of prescriptions allowed per month or formulary restrictions). The next two issues consider patient criteria and patient eligibility. This study outlined the medications and ICD-9 codes that were used to assess COPD-related outcomes and costs and specified that only patients eligible for the entire study period were included in the analyses. The last two issues, regarding clinical outcome measures and sensitivity analysis, were addressed in the answers to questions 8 and 11.

Cost-Effectiveness Grid

COST-EFFECTIVENESS	Lower Cost	Same Cost	Higher Cost
Lower effectiveness	A	B	C
Same effectiveness	D	E	F
Higher effectiveness	G Pulmolair compared with Bronchocort	H	I

COMPOSITE ARTICLE 2: RETROSPECTIVE DATABASE—BISPHOSPHONATES

Title: PHARMACOECONOMIC ANALYSIS OF BISPHOSPHONATES IN A LARGE MANAGED CARE ORGANIZATION

BACKGROUND: Bisphosphonates are used to decrease the incidence of fractures, but direct head-to-head comparisons of the effectiveness of these medications are lacking.

OBJECTIVE: The objective of the study was to compare costs and fractures rates for 5 years following initiation of two oral bisphosphonates (BP1 and BP2) in a large managed care population.

METHODS: Claims data were obtained from 10 geographically diverse health plans in the United States. Criteria included a diagnosis for osteoporosis, prescriptions for BP1 or BP2 and 5 years of follow-up medical claims. The date of the first pharmacy claim for an osteoporosis medication was used as the index date. Members were followed for 5 years after the index date. Cost inputs included costs for BP1 or BP2 medications using 2013 cost estimates. Outcomes included the percent of patients who had at least one fracture during the 5-year follow-up.

RESULTS: A total of 10,000 members were included ($n = 5,500$ on BP1, $n = 4,500$ on BP2). There were no statistically significant differences between BP1 and BP2 in the percentages of subjects with at least one fracture during the follow-up period (BP1 = 6.1%; BP2 =6.2%). In addition BP1 cost an additional $3,000 over the 5-year time span (BP1 = $12,000; BP2 = $9,000), indicating that BP2 was a more cost-effective option based on fracture rates.

CONCLUSION: This retrospective analysis found a difference in the cost of bisphosphonates, but no significant difference in fracture prevention rates.

WORKSHEET FOR CRITIQUE OF RETROSPECTIVE DATABASE COMPOSITE ARTICLE 2: BISPHOSPHONATES

1. Complete Title?

_____

_____

_____

_____

2. Clear Objective?

_____

_____

_____

_____

3. Appropriate Alternatives?

_____

_____

_____

_____

4. Alternatives Described?

_____

_____

_____

_____

5. Perspective Stated?

_____

_____

_____

_____

6. Type of Study?

_____

_____

_____

_____

7. Relevant Costs?

_____

_____

_____

_____

8. Relevant Outcomes?

_____

_____

_____

_____

9. Adjustment or Discounting?

_____

_____

_____

_____

10. Reasonable Assumptions?

_____

_____

_____

_____

11. Sensitivity Analyses?

_____

_____

_____

_____

12. Limitations Addressed?

_____

_____

_____

_____

13. Generalizations Appropriate?

_____

_____

_____

_____

14. Unbiased Conclusions? Include answers to the five additional questions used for analyses using retrospective databases.

_____

_____

_____

_____

CRITIQUE OF RETROSPECTIVE DATABASE COMPOSITE ARTICLE 2: BISPHOSPHONATES

1. **Complete Title:** The title did not identify the type of analysis or the specific bisphosphonates compared.

2. **Clear Objective:** The objective of the study was clear—to compare costs and fractures rates for 5 years following initiation of two oral bisphosphonates (BP1 and BP2) in a large managed care population.

3. **Appropriate Alternatives:** Appropriate literature should be cited to validate the choices of alternatives that are most clinically relevant. There are more than two bisphosphonates on the market—why did they choose to compare these two?

4. **Alternatives Described:** The dosing and scheduling of doses were not described. Patients may have been more adherent to one medication than the other. The average doses and adherence for each alternative should be included.

5. **Perspective Stated:** The perspective of the study was not stated, but based on the costs measured (medication costs) it was from the perspective of the payer—probably based on reimbursement data in the large managed care database.

6. **Type of Study:** Some would identify this as a CEA because outcomes were measured as fracture rates. It might be argued that this was a cost minimization since the outcomes measured were found to be the same.

7. **Relevant Costs:** Only medication costs were measured—other costs due to side effects or fractures should have been addressed.

8. **Relevant Outcomes:** Outcomes were measured by comparing the percent of patients that had at least one fracture over the 5-year period. Time to first fracture, type of fracture, and total number of fractures would be important to measure. In addition, bone density values before and after starting medication can assess its effectiveness—but these types of values are rarely found in retrospective claims databases.

9. **Adjustment or Discounting:** Five years of retrospective medication costs were estimated using adjustment to 2013 values. No discounting was needed.

10. **Reasonable Assumptions:** When using retrospective databases, many assumptions are usually standard (e.g., that the data are accurate and complete). By only looking at patients that stayed in one health plan for at least 5 years, some of the population with osteoporosis would not be included—the authors should explain how many patients would have been included with less strict eligibility criteria.

11. **Sensitivity Analyses:** Sensitivity analyses were not conducted.

12. **Limitations Addressed:** Limitations were not addressed.

13. **Generalizations Appropriate:** The authors did not address generalizability, but data from 10 geographically diverse managed care populations would probably be fairly generalizable.

14. **Unbiased Conclusions:** The conclusions were based on the results presented and were not overstated, but the analysis was not complete—only medication costs and one outcome were measured. As listed in this chapter, *five additional issues* should be addressed when critiquing studies that use retrospective databases. The first issue involves describing the database. Although this study indicated it was from 10 geographically diverse managed care groups, it did not include other information (e.g., number of people covered, demographic characteristics). The next two issues consider patient criteria and patient eligibility. This study outlined the medications and diagnosis that were used to identify osteoporosis patients. Fracture diagnoses could have been expanded upon, and different types of fractures could have been assessed. The severity associated with a hip fracture is much higher than with a wrist fracture. The last two issues, regarding clinical outcome measures and sensitivity analysis, were addressed in the answers to questions 8 and 11.

QUESTIONS/EXERCISES

Go to an online search Website (such as MEDLINE). Search for articles with the words "retrospective database" in their titles. Choose one of the articles (or if you are using this book as part of a course, your professor may assign an article). After reading the article, answer the following questions:

1. Was there a clear explanation of the database used for the study?
2. Was there a clear explanation of the inclusion and exclusion criteria use to select patients?
3. Was the eligibility period of patients discussed?
4. How were outcomes measured?
5. Were sensitivity analyses conducted?

REFERENCES

1. Concato J, Shah N, Horwitz RI. Randomized controlled trials, observational studies, and the hierarchy of research designs. *New England Journal of Medicine* 342(25):1887–1892, 2000.
2. Golberg-Arnold R, Kotsanos JG, Motheral B, et al. Panel 3: Methodological issues in conducting pharmacoeconomic evaluations: Retrospective and claims database studies. *Value in Health* 2(2):82–87, 1999.
3. Lin SJ, Lambert B, Tan H, Toh S. Frequency estimates from prescription drug datasets. *Pharmacoepidemiology and Drug Safety* 15(7):512–520, 2006.
4. Maclean JR, Fick DM, Hoffman WK, et al. Comparison of two systems for clinical practice profiling in diabetic care: Medical Records versus claims and administrative data. *American Journal of Managed Care* 8(2):175–179, 2002.
5. National Health Care Survey. Available at http://www.cdc.gov/nchs/nhcs.htm; accessed August 2007.
6. National Ambulatory Care Survey. Available at http://www.cdc.gov.nchs/about/major/ahcd/namcsdes.htm; accessed August 2007.
7. Medical Expenditure Panel Survey. Available at http://www.meps.ahrq.gov/mepsweb.htm; accessed August 2007.

8. Cohen SB. Design strategies and innovations in the medical Expenditure Panel Survey (MEPS). *Medical Care* 41(7 suppl):III5–III12, 2003.
9. Liang SY, Phillips KA, Haas JS. Measuring managed care and its environment using national surveys: A review and assessment. *Medical Care Research and Review* 63(6 suppl):9S–36S, 2006.
10. Gilchrist VJ, Stange KC, Flocke SA, et al. A comparison of the National Ambulatory Medical Care Survey (NAMCS) measurement approach with direct observation of outpatient visits. *Medical Care* 42(3):276–280, 2004.
11. Benson K, Hartz AJ. A comparison of observational studies and randomized, controlled trials. *New England Journal of Medicine* 342(25):1878–1886, 2000.
12. Motheral B, Brooks J, Clark MA, et al. A checklist for retrospective database studies: Report of the ISPOR Task Force on Retrospective Databases. *Value in Health* 6(2):90–97, 2003.
13. Berger ML, Mamdani M, Atkins D, Johnson ML. Good research practices for comparative effectiveness research: Defining, reporting and interpreting nonrandomized studies of treatment effects using secondary data sources: The ISPOR good research practices for retrospective database analysis task force report—Part I. *Value in Health* 12:1044–1052, 2009.
14. For Part II of the ISPOR Retrospective Database Analysis Task Force Report: Good research practices for comparative effectiveness research: Approaches to mitigate bias and confounding in the design of non-randomized studies of treatment effects using secondary data sources: The ISPOR good research practices for retrospective database analysis task force—Part II. Available at http://www.ispor.org/TaskForces/RetrospectiveDBPractices2.asp.
15. For Part III of the ISPOR Retrospective Database Analysis Task Force Report: Good research practices for comparative effectiveness research: Analytic methods to improve causal inference from nonrandomized studies of treatment effects using secondary data sources: The ISPOR good research practices for retrospective database analysis task force report—Part III. Available at http://www.ispor.org/TaskForces/RetrospectiveDBPractices3.asp.

SUGGESTED READINGS

Aspinall SL, Good CB, Glassman PA, Valentino MA. The evolving use of cost-effectiveness analysis in formulary management within the Department of Veterans Affairs. *Medical Care* 43(7 suppl):II20–II26, 2005.

Berggren F. Assessing the use of retrospective databases in conducting economic evaluations of drugs: The case of asthma. *Pharmacoeconomics* 22(12):771–791, 2004.

Eisenberg SS. Usefulness of database studies as applied to managed care. *Journal of Managed Care Pharmacy* 11(1 suppl A):S9–S11, 2005.

Else BA, Armstrong EP, Cox ER. Data sources for pharmacoeconomic and health services research. *American Journal of Health-System Pharmacy* 54(22):2601–2608, 1997.

Esposito D, Migliaccio-Walle K, Molsen E. Reliability and Validity of Data Sources for Outcomes Research & Disease and Health Management Programs. *International Society for Pharmacoeconomics and Outcomes Research,* 2013.

Finder S. Providing cost-effective therapy using pharmacoeconomic evaluations: The public sector approach. *Clinical Therapeutics* 19(1):160–166, 1997.

Hillestad R, Bigelow J, Bower A, et al. Can electronic medical record systems transform health care? Potential health benefits, savings, and costs. *Health Affairs* 24(5):1103–1117, 2005.

Hing E, Cherry DK, Woodwell DA. National Ambulatory Medical Care Survey: 2004 summary. *Advance Data* 23(374):1–33, 2006.

Kaboli PJ, McClimon BJ, Hoth AB, Barnett MJ. Assessing the accuracy of computerized medication histories. *American Journal of Managed Care* 10(11, pt 2):872–877, 2004.

Motheral BR, Fairman KA. The use of claims databases for outcomes research: Rationale, challenges, and strategies. *Clinical Therapeutics* 19(2):346–366, 1997.

Retchin SM, Wenzel RP. Electronic medical record systems at academic health centers: Advantages and implementation issues. *Academic Medicine* 74(5):493–498, 1999.

Sax MJ. Essential steps and practical applications for database studies. *Journal of Managed Care Pharmacy* 11(1 suppl A):S5–S8, 2005.

Smith MW, Joseph GJ. Pharmacy data in the VA health care system. *Medical Care Research and Review* 60(3 suppl):92S–123S, 2003.

Chapter 12

Pharmacy Services

Objectives

Upon completing this chapter, the reader will be able to:

1. Discuss the history and development of research on the value of pharmacy services.

2. List issues specifically related to critiquing pharmacy service research.

3. Understand the importance of measuring costs and patient outcomes associated with medication therapy management (MTM) services mandated for high-risk Medicare patients.

4. Critique an example of a pharmacoeconomic study that evaluates pharmacy services.

✦ WHAT ARE PHARMACY SERVICES?

One of the definitions given in Chapter 1 for pharmacoeconomics is that it identifies, measures, and compares the costs and consequences of pharmaceutical *products* and *services*.[1] In most chapters, the research examples have focused on the evaluation of pharmaceutical products. However, this chapter focuses on the pharmacoeconomic research that evaluates pharmaceutical services.

A variety of terms have been associated with pharmaceutical or pharmacy services in the literature, including clinical pharmacy services, cognitive pharmacy services, **pharmaceutical care** services, disease-state management, and **medication therapy management** (MTM). Pharmacy services consist of a variety of functions performed by a pharmacist that may or may not be associated with the dispensing of a particular prescription order. Examples include pharmacokinetic monitoring (e.g., using algorithms to estimate blood concentrations of medications), patient education to improve medication taking behaviors, and drug use monitoring and review to ensure the appropriate use of medication. MTM is a term used by Medicare to include a wide range of services provided to its recipients. MTM is discussed in more detail later in this chapter.

✦ HISTORY OF PHARMACY SERVICES

The need for research that evaluates the effects of pharmacy services was identified as early as 1971 by the Task Force on the Pharmacist's Clinical Role,[2] and research articles that estimate the value of pharmacy services have been published since the late 1970s.[3] Most early studies were used to justify the value of the provision of "clinical pharmacy" services (e.g., pharmacokinetic dosing) in institutional (hospital) settings. In 1990, Hepler and Strand[4] proposed the concept that pharmacists should provide pharmaceutical care, just as physicians provide medical care and nurses provide nursing care. Pharmaceutical care is "the responsible provision of drug therapy for the purpose of achieving definite outcomes that improve a patient's quality of life."[4] Research on the value of providing pharmaceutical care services was extended to outpatient and community pharmacy settings. The federal government has recognized the importance of MTM services and included the provision of these services to high-risk patients as part of the Medicare Part D outpatient prescription drug benefit that took effect in January 2006.[5]

✦ REVIEW OF THE RESEARCH

How is a value placed on pharmacy services? A variety of approaches have been used, including **contingent valuation** (CV), prospective studies, modeling, and a combination of these methods.

CV or **willingness-to-pay** (WTP) methodologies (see Chapter 7) have been used to estimate what patients would pay for pharmacy services. A review of 10 research articles using CV to place a value on pharmacy services was published in 1999.[6] The advantage of using CV or WTP methods is that they combine the range of benefits (e.g., better **health-related quality of life,** less sick time, less use of medical resources) perceived by patients into one monetary amount. The disadvantage found by these authors is that because of the different ways the questions were presented and the inherent biases of CV (e.g., starting point bias), results vary widely and the **validity** of some results is questionable. The authors provided suggestions to researchers on how to improve the quality and usability of future CV studies. One study published after this review incorporated an appropriate methodology to determine the amount patients would be willing to pay to reduce their risk of medication-related problems. The average amount people were willing to pay out of pocket ranged from $4 to $5 per prescription, and the amount they were willing to pay through increased insurance premiums was $29 to $36 per year.[7]

Other researchers have used the approach of measuring how much money would hypothetically be saved in **direct medical costs** when community pharmacists performed interventions (e.g., detecting a drug–drug interaction or a preexisting allergy to the medication) before dispensing medications. Rupp[8] developed a methodology for pharmacists (or pharmacy students) to record pharmacist interventions and assembled a panel to estimate cost savings attributable to these interventions. He found that about 1.9% of all prescriptions filled required an intervention, and the estimated savings for each intervention was $123 in direct medical costs (i.e., physician, emergency department, or hospital services) avoided, resulting in a value of about $2.30 per screened prescription.

Dobie and Rascati[9] used this methodology and the same panel to assess pharmacists' interventions in rural pharmacies. Although they found that interventions were recorded for fewer prescriptions (0.8%), the estimated savings per intervention were higher ($425), or about $3.40 per screened prescription. These studies did not estimate the cost of the pharmacists' time involved with providing these interventions but only estimated the monetary benefits from costs avoided, so no benefit-to-cost ratios were calculated. A more recent study by Lee et al.[10] used a similar method of assessing the potential for harm that would have occurred if pharmacist recommendations were not made and accepted in a Veterans Affairs (VA) medical center (including inpatient, outpatient, and skilled-nursing facilities). On average, each pharmacist recommendation avoided about $700 in overall medical and pharmacy costs.

Three publications have emanated from the American College of Clinical Pharmacy (ACCP) Task Force on Economic Evaluation of Clinical Pharmacy Services. The first summarized the economic literature on pharmacy services before 1988, the second between 1988 and 1995, and the third from 1996 to 2000.[11-13] Each task force publication contains an appendix, in table form, that summarizes the key points for each evaluated article, including; the objective, analytic methods, type of comparison group, input costs included, resource use and economic outcomes, economic results, and reviewers' comments. In the most recent Task Force publication, 59 research articles were summarized. Most studies were conducted in a community hospital ($n = 16$) or a university hospital ($n = 13$), and the most common pharmacy service evaluated was "general pharmacotherapeutic monitoring" ($n = 28$). Most research articles ($n = 50$) found a positive economic impact attributable to the service, and 16 benefit-to-cost (B:C) ratios were listed. The range of B:C ratios was 1.7:1 to 17.0:1, with a median of about 5:1, indicating that for every one dollar spent providing pharmacy services, $5 was saved.[13]

Summaries of Specific Multipharmacy Projects

Economic results of some multisite outpatient pharmacy service studies have been published, with varying results.[14] Three large prospective studies with positive clinical and economic findings will be discussed here in more detail. These studies are the Impact of Managed Pharmaceutical Care on Resource Utilization and Outcomes in Veterans Affairs Medical Centers (IMPROVE) study, the Asheville Project, and the Patient Self-Management Program (PSMP) Program.

The IMPROVE Study

The IMPROVE study was designed to assess general health outcomes of VA patients who received pharmaceutical care in ambulatory clinics.[15] Nine VA sites across the country participated in the study. Patients at a high risk for drug-related problems were randomized to either the pharmaceutical care service in addition to usual care (intervention group; $n = 523$) or usual care alone (control group; $n = 531$) and followed for 1 year. Pharmacists contacted each patient in the pharmaceutical care group an average of about three times during the follow-up year. No significant difference in health-related quality of life (measured using the SF-36; see Chapter 8) was seen between the two groups. An assessment of some disease-specific laboratory values indicated an improvement in glucose and cholesterol levels in the intervention group compared with the control group. Overall medical costs for both groups increased in the follow-up year, but the costs for the pharmaceutical care group increased less than for those who received usual care only ($1,020 versus $1,313, respectively).

The Asheville Project

The Asheville Project was implemented for employees of the City of Asheville, NC, and for employees of the Mission-St. Joseph's (MSJ) Health System, and it targeted two diseases: diabetes and asthma.[16,17] Employees were provided with consultations by pharmacists from 1 of 12 local pharmacies, who performed medication review and monitoring in addition to education and physical assessments. The patients, in return for participating in the project, received a copay waiver for their diabetes or asthma medications and supplies. Patients who received these pharmacy services had improved clinical indicators (better control of their blood glucose or improvement in forced expiratory volume), reduced direct medical costs, and reduced **indirect costs** (as measured by a decrease in sick days).

The Patient Self-Management Program

Because of the success of the Asheville Project, 80 community pharmacy providers with diabetes training were selected from five communities (in four different states) to be included in a pilot project, the PSMP, which encouraged patients with diabetes to actively participate in the management of their disease (e.g., to meet with their pharmacist to set clinical goals for themselves).[18] A total of 256 patients participated in the program and showed clinical improvement in many areas (e.g., improvement in blood glucose levels, improvement in cholesterol levels, and higher influenza vaccination and eye examination rates), and average annual health care costs per patient were $918 less than projected.

✦ ISSUES IN VALUING PHARMACY SERVICES

Wide Variation in Services

When researchers say the purpose of their study is to evaluate the provision of pharmacy services, they can be referring to a wide variety of activities. Some studies may assess a specific service that is directed toward a particular disease or condition (e.g., determining the correct antibiotic to use for infections based on laboratory culture results), a specific service that is directed toward a variety of diseases (e.g., telephone calls to increase patient adherence to their chronic medications), or a group of general services directed toward multiple diseases (e.g., MTM). Because of these variations, it is imperative that researchers explain in detail what pharmacy service activities are being examined and how they are being provided. In fact, the provision of the same set of services may differ from pharmacist to pharmacist or from pharmacy site to pharmacy site which may partially explain why results from service evaluation studies are so wide ranging.

Type of Pharmacoeconomic Study

Because the purpose of most pharmacy service economic evaluations is to determine whether the service is worthwhile financially, cost-benefit analyses (CBAs) are commonly conducted. Input costs include the resources used to provide the service, and benefits are often measured as direct medical costs avoided because of the provision of the service. As mentioned in Chapter 7 on CBA, some health care economists do not consider this method as a true CBA unless health consequences are also valued in dollars, and they refer to this type of study as a cost analysis or cost avoidance study.

Costs Associated with Providing Services

Estimating the cost of providing health care services usually involves the measurement of labor costs of the health care providers. Even if no new personnel are hired to provide the services in question, the time associated with providing the services should be measured and valued because the professionals could instead be performing other productive activities instead of these services (see the discussion of **opportunity costs** in Chapter 2). It is important to include both the estimated salary per hour of the health care professional as well as the cost of fringe benefits to the company or institution for these professionals. If new computer equipment or programming or new space is needed to provide the services, these costs should also be included in estimations. Free online software (the PharmAccount service cost calculator) is available, which provides a step-by-step approach for analyzing of the costs of delivering pharmacy services.[19]

Benefits Associated with Services

It is often difficult to tie patient benefits directly to health care services that are provided. In some cases, it can be determined quickly if the correct drug and dose was chosen (e.g., intravenous antibiotics used in hospitalized patients). For other services, such as general medication monitoring, the association with better health outcomes and lower costs might not be apparent immediately, and may be attributable, in part, to other factors such as improved diet or increased exercise. The use of comparison groups who do not receive the service but are similar at baseline to the patients receiving the service increases the confidence in the findings.

Pharmacy Budget Silo Mentality

Another barrier to economic research pertaining to pharmacy services is referred to as **silo mentality,** that is to consider only one budget or silo (in this case, the pharmacy budget) rather than overall resource use. In many cases, the provision of pharmacy services increases the pharmacy budget because of increases in pharmacy personnel time and possibly additional or more expensive medications that may be recommended by the pharmacist. As we have seen with the IMPROVE study and the Asheville Project, pharmacy services can lead to a decrease in overall health care costs because of a decrease in the use of other nonpharmacy budgetary resources such as emergency department and hospitalization services.

✦ MEDICARE MEDICATION THERAPY MANAGEMENT

A development in the provision of pharmacy services is the recognition by Medicare of the need for MTM. The Medicare Prescription Drug Improvement and Modernization Act (MMA), which was passed in late 2003, in addition to creating a Medicare Part D outpatient prescription drug benefit that began in 2006, called for the implementation of MTM strategies for high-risk patients. Eleven national pharmacy groups met in 2004 to develop a profession-wide consensus on the definition of MTM.[20] MTM includes a broad range of professional activities and may occur in conjunction with or independently from the dispensing of a medication. The five core elements of MTM include[21]:

- Medication therapy review
- A personal medication record
- A medication action plan
- Intervention and referral
- Documentation and follow-up

Some updates (Version 2.0) were developed in 2008.[22] The newer version places an increased emphasis on the patient's role in medication self-management, care transitioning and collaborative health care team partnerships.

Although consensus on the definition of MTM services is emerging, there is no consensus on how to bill for or receive payment for these services. Pharmacies and pharmacists currently negotiate with the various drug plans to determine the fee structures and reimbursement rates, and federal standard-setting organizations (e.g., the Agency for Healthcare Research and Quality) are developing guidelines and quality assurance measures for these services.[5,23]

As early as 2003 (3 years before implementation of the Medicare Part D prescription benefit), researchers tried to predict what effect MTM services would have on costs and patient outcomes. Etemad and Hay[24] used information from past literature to create a **Markov model** (see Chapter 10) to predict the cost per life year saved because of MTM services. Their base case results indicated that although the costs of paying pharmacists for these services were estimated at almost $48 billion per year (all costs in year 2000 dollars) and costs of medications would increase by about $22 billion (about $109 billion increase because of better patient compliance coupled with a $87 billion decrease because of discontinued medications), medical costs (e.g., hospitalizations, emergency department visits) would decrease by $53 billion. The net annual cost projected because of the provision of MTM services was $17 billion ($48 billion + $22 billion − $53 billion), and it was estimated that these services would provide an increase of about 8 million life-years, for a **cost-effectiveness ratio** (CER) of about $2,000 per life year saved. Many **sensitivity analyses** were conducted on model variables. Results ranged from MTM services being **dominant** (i.e., decrease in overall costs while increasing life-years) to a maximum cost of $13,000 per life year saved, which is well below the common $50,000 threshold (see Example 6.1 in Chapter 6).

Touchette et al.[25] surveyed MTM programs to determine what had been implemented in the first 4 months of the program. The researchers received responses from managers of 21 MTM programs used by 70 health insurance plans. These 21 MTM programs covered 12 million of the 21 million Medicare patients enrolled in Part D by April 2006. Many different methods were used to define high-risk Medicare patients in need of MTM services. The majority of MTM programs provided both information mailed to the patient and in-house call centers for patient health management. Only 4 of the 21 programs used contracts with local pharmacies to provide face-to-face MTM services, but they were large programs and covered 7.5 million Medicare beneficiaries (although the authors admit they could not give an estimate of how many of these 7.5 million patients met the criteria for MTM services nor how many received them at the local level).

There is continued debate on the cost-effectiveness of MTM services by setting (call centers, mailings, clinics, community pharmacies). When assessing changes in medication expenditures from a group of health plans, Winston and Lin found that costs savings were higher for patients who received care from community pharmacists than from call centers and mailings. Drug costs decreased most for face-to-face services, decreased somewhat for call center services, and were unchanged for those who received MTM via mailings.[26] Another study surveyed patients about their preferences for receiving MTM services. Respondents were willing to spend about $30 to trade telephone MTM for clinic-based MTM, and they were willing to pay $13 more for MTM service at a community pharmacy compared with clinic-based MTM.[27]

Oladapo et al. conducted a literature search for post-2005 studies on clinical pharmacy services (including MTM services) with results reported in terms of cost-benefit ratios, net benefits/savings, return on investment, cost savings or cost avoided ($n = 21$ studies).[28] While the majority of these studies reported positive economic values with the provision of MTM or clinical pharmacy services, they also had limitations. These include: absence of a control or comparison group; insufficient detail on the services provided; restriction of input costs to only personnel costs and failure to input other costs involved in the provision of the service; failure to evaluate clinical outcomes and convert them to monetary units; focus on direct drug costs only; absence of incremental CBAs and sensitivity analyses; and failure to evaluate indirect costs.

A preliminary study by CMS retrospectively investigated how enrollment in a standalone Prescription Drug Plan (PDP) or Medicare Advantage Prescription Drug Plan (MAPD) MTM program with or without receipt of an annual comprehensive medication review (CMR) influenced drug therapy, resource utilization, and costs for a 6-month period in 2010. Outcomes for new MTM enrollees with congestive heart failure (CHF) or chronic obstructive pulmonary disease (COPD) were assessed. Improved medication adherence and the discontinuation of high-risk medications were seen consistently for those enrolled in MTM services, while the positive effects of reduced hospitalizations, emergency room visits, and costs were seen for some analyses but not others. For example, there were significant cost savings associated with all-cause hospitalizations but not with disease-specific (e.g., CHF-specific or COPD-specific) hospitalizations. Patients who received CMRs were more likely to benefit from MTM program participation across almost all outcomes relative to those in MTM programs who did not receive CMRs (http://innovation.cms.gov/Files/reports/MTM-Interim-Report-01-2013.pdf).

SUMMARY

Research describing and evaluating the provision of nondispensing clinically based pharmacy services has appeared in the literature since the 1970s. Both disease-specific and general pharmacy-related services have been described and are found under a variety of designations, such as cognitive services and pharmaceutical care services. A number of methods have been used to determine the economic value of pharmacy services. CV techniques have been used to elicit what patients would be willing to pay for these services, and dollar values of health care resources avoided because of pharmacist interventions have been estimated.

An American College of Clinical Pharmacy (AACP) task force has published three reviews of economic evaluation of services spanning different periods of time. Most of the articles reviewed assess services provided by a hospital or institution, but evaluations of community pharmacy services appear more frequently in the current literature.

The results of three prospective multipharmacy studies—the IMPROVE study, the Asheville Project, and the PSMP program—were summarized in this chapter. Certain issues related to pharmacy service research and its evaluation were discussed, including: the wide variation in services; the type of study (quasi or true CBA); the labor, overhead and opportunity cost measurements needed; the difficulty in determining the true cause and effect of services; and the drug budget silo mentality of insurers and providers.

The Medicare Modernization Act (MMA) created an outpatient prescription drug benefit that was implemented in January of 2006. This act requires contracted drug plans to provide MTM services for high-risk Medicare patients. Past research studies in outpatient settings that have indicated cost savings and improved patient outcomes as a result of the provision of pharmacy services (e.g., the multipharmacy studies referred to above) were conducted primarily at the local level and included face-to-face patient–pharmacist interactions. Preliminary surveys of drug plans, published in 2006, show that many insurance plans were fulfilling the MTM service requirements using mailings and in-house call centers instead of contracting with local pharmacists to provide direct patient care. The number of evidence-based evaluations of MTM services continues to expand. There is evidence that pharmacist-provided MTM services can have a positive impact on clinical outcomes for patients, and that payment for MTM services may be offset by savings on medical and hospital services. We also do not have a clear understanding of the relative effectiveness of differing models for MTM (e.g., face-to-face versus telephone; disease-focused versus holistic). More research is needed to further delineate patient risk stratification to identify specific cost savings on types of medical services; and to identify areas where high impact on cost savings can be realized.

COMPOSITE ARTICLE: PHARMACY SERVICES

Title: COST-BENEFIT ANALYSIS OF A PHARMACIST-RUN DIABETES CLINIC

BACKGROUND: Whitestock Healthcare (WH) system is a managed care network that provides health care to approximately 200,000 patients in central Texas. WH administrators were approached by the pharmacy department to discuss the development of a pharmacist-run clinic to manage the medication therapy of WH patients who had diabetes mellitus (DM). Many patients with DM have episodes of hypoglycemia or hyperglycemia that lead to emergency department (ED) visits or hospitalizations if their blood sugar is not adequately regulated. Administrators asked for an estimate of costs and savings to WH for the first 3 years of the clinic. Therefore, the objective of this study was to estimate the costs and economic benefits of a pharmacist-run diabetes clinic. The perspective of the study was the WH system.

METHODS: Past information on resource utilization of WH patients with DM and a review of existing literature were used for utilization and costs estimates. The WH accounting office was contacted to determine the labor, overhead, and supply costs associated with opening and operating a clinic. It was assumed that approximately 200 patients with DM would be enrolled in the clinic during its first year of operation and 400 patients would be enrolled in subsequent years. For the first year of operation, a pharmacist would spend about 15 hours per week in the clinic and 30 hours per week in subsequent years. Administrative support was budgeted to keep track of activities and appointments. It was proposed that a small private room in one of the main outpatient clinics be dedicated to this operation.

PHARMACY SERVICES PROVIDED: The pharmacist(s) chosen for this clinic would perform the following functions:

1. Identify DM patients in most need of drug therapy monitoring. The patients may include those with elevated hemoglobin-A1c laboratory values and those who had documentation of a recent hypoglycemic or hyperglycemic episode.
2. Contact each patient's physician to determine a treatment plan.
3. Contact the patient to schedule a medication consultation. This consultation would include review and documentation of the patient's medical and prescription history and would also include diabetes education. This consultation may result in higher compliance with medications (and thus increase the cost of medications) and higher utilization of laboratory monitoring.
4. Contact the physician for discussion and approval of any recommended medication changes.
5. Schedule follow-up consultations as needed.

RESULTS: Unit costs of health care resources based on WH averages are listed in Exhibit 12.1. Exhibits 12.2 and 12.3 list the 3-year estimated health care costs for "treatment as usual," without the pharmacy clinic, compared with cost estimates if the clinic was implemented. It is projected that patients who participate in the clinic will incur more medication and laboratory costs but will be less likely to have an ED visit or hospitalization, resulting in an overall estimated savings, discounted at 5%, of $305,780 compared with those who do not receive these services.

Exhibit 12.4 provides the estimated costs for 3 years of clinic operations, which when discounted at 5%, totals $254,097. The net benefit of the pharmacy clinic is $51,683 ($305,780 – $254,097), and the benefit-to-cost ratio is 1.20:1 ($305,780:$254,097), indicating that for every dollar spent on clinic operations, $1.20 is saved because of a decrease in costs associated with total health care services. If discounting is not performed, the net benefit would be $55,000 ($324,000 – $269,000), and the benefit-to-cost ratio would again be 1.20:1 ($324,000:$269,000).

DISCUSSION: The 3-year cost projections were well-received by WH administrators, and plans are being made to open a DM clinic soon. Costs specific to one health care system were used in these estimates and may not be generalizable to other sites.

EXHIBIT 12.1

Unit Cost Estimates for Diabetes

Diabetes-Related Health Care Resources	Unit Costs $	Estimated Change with Pharmacy Services
Oral antidiabetic agents (90% of patients)	100 per month per patient	10% increase
Insulin (10% of patients)	100 per month per patient	10% increase
Testing strips and supplies (10% of patients)	50 per month per patient	10% increase
Laboratory tests	50 per test (without service one test per year)	Twice per year test
Physician visits	150 per visit (two visits per year)	No change
ED visits	500 per visit (without service 30% of patients)	Reduction to 10% of patients
Hospitalizations	4,000 per stay (without service 15% of patients)	Reduction to 5% of patients

ED = emergency department.

EXHIBIT 12.2

Estimated Diabetes-Related Health Care Costs without Pharmacy Clinic

Diabetes-Related Health Care Services Without Pharmacy Service	Estimated Year 1 Costs (n = 200) ($)	Estimated Year 2 Costs (n = 400) ($)	Estimated Year 3 Costs (n = 400) ($)	Total Discounted Costs (Using a 5% Discount Rate) ($)
Oral antidiabetic agents (90% of patients)	216,000	432,000	432,000	1,019,265
Insulin (10% of patients)	24,000	48,000	48,000	113,252
Testing strips and supplies	12,000	24,000	24,000	56,626
Laboratory tests	10,000	20,000	20,000	47,188
Physician visits	60,000	120,000	120,000	283,129
ED visits (30% of patients)	30,000	60,000	60,000	141,565
Hospitalizations (15% of patients)	120,000	240,000	240,000	566,258
Total	472,000	944,000	944,000	2,227,284

ED = emergency department.

EXHIBIT 12.3

Estimated Diabetes-Related Health Care Costs with Pharmacy Clinic

Diabetes-Related Health Care Services with Pharmacy Service	Estimated Year 1 Costs (n = 200) ($)	Estimated Year 2 Costs (n = 400) ($)	Estimated Year 3 Costs (n = 400) ($)	Total Discounted Costs (Using a 5% Discount Rate) ($)
Oral antidiabetic agents (90% of patients)	237,600	475,200	475,200	1,121,192
Insulin (10% pts)	26,400	52,800	52,800	124,577
Testing strips and supplies	13,200	26,400	26,400	62,288
Laboratory tests	20,000	40,000	40,000	94,376
Physician visits	60,000	120,000	120,000	283,129
ED visits (10% of patients)	10,000	20,000	20,000	47,188
Hospitalizations (5% of patients)	40,000	80,000	80,000	188,753
Total	407,200	814,400	814,400	1,921,504
Cost savings (benefits)[a]	64,800	129,600	129,600	305,780

ED = emergency department.

[a]Difference in totals from Exhibit 12.2.

EXHIBIT 12.4

Estimated Costs and Benefits of Providing Diabetes Management Pharmacy Clinic Services

Cost Category	Estimated Year 1 Costs ($)	Estimated Year 2 Costs ($)	Estimated Year 3 Costs ($)	Total Discounted Costs (Using a 5% Discount Rate) ($)
Pharmacist time[a]	45,000	90,000	90,000	212,347
Administrative time[b]	5,000	10,000	10,000	23,594
Space and overhead	5,000	5,000	5,000	14,297
Materials/supplies[c]	2,000	1,000	1,000	3,859
Total costs of service	57,000	106,000	106,000	254,097
Cost savings (benefits)[d]	64,800	129,600	129,600	305,780

[a]Year 1: 15 hours per week; years 2 and 3: 30 hours per week at $50 per hour plus 15% fringe benefits.3.

[b]Year 1: 5 hours per week; years 2 and 3: 10 hours per week at $17 per hour plus 15% fringe benefits.4.

[c]Year 1 includes the purchase of a computer and printer.5.

[d]Difference in total costs of diabetes-related health care service versus without pharmacy services (see Exhibits 12.2 and 12.3).

WORKSHEET FOR CRITIQUE OF PHARMACY SERVICES COMPOSITE ARTICLE

1. Complete Title?

_____

_____

_____

_____

2. Clear Objective?

_____

_____

_____

_____

3. Appropriate Alternatives?

_____

_____

_____

_____

4. Alternatives Described?

_____

_____

_____

_____

5. Perspective Stated?

_____

_____

_____

_____

6. Type of Study?

_____

_____

_____

_____

7. Relevant Costs?

_____

_____

_____

_____

8. Relevant Outcomes?

_____

_____

_____

_____

9. Adjustment or Discounting?

_____

_____

_____

_____

10. Reasonable Assumptions?

_____

_____

_____

_____

11. Sensitivity Analyses?

_____

_____

_____

_____

12. Limitations Addressed?

_____

_____

_____

_____

13. Generalizations Appropriate?

_____

_____

_____

_____

14. Unbiased Conclusions?

_____

_____

_____

_____

CRITIQUE OF PHARMACY SERVICES COMPOSITE ARTICLE

1. **Complete Title:** The title did identify the type of study (i.e., CBA) and what was being assessed: a pharmacist-run diabetes clinic.

2. **Clear Objective:** The objective of this study was "to estimate the costs and economic benefits of a pharmacist-run diabetes clinic." This was clear.

3. **Appropriate Alternatives:** This was an example of a "with-or-without" study. The alternatives were to implement a diabetes clinic compared with providing usual diabetes care.

4. **Alternatives Described:** This is an important question for pharmacy services research because the set of activities may differ from one site to the next. This article provided some detail as to the services that would be provided in the clinic.

5. **Perspective Stated:** The perspective of the study was explicitly stated as that of the managed health care system (i.e., WH). Therefore, only direct costs to the system were estimated.

6. **Type of Study:** The study was correctly identified as a CBA because outcomes were valued in monetary units as cost savings. Some researchers would not consider the calculations of only direct medical costs and saving as a complete, or true, CBA because intangibles and indirect costs were not included and no dollar value was placed on improved health outcomes.

7. **Relevant Costs:** It may be more complex to answer this question about CBAs because both inputs and outcomes are measured in dollars. Input costs (left-hand side of the pharmacoeconomics (PE) equation; see Fig. 1.1 in Chapter 1) included the estimated costs of operating a diabetes clinic. These included labor, overhead, and supplies. Fringe benefits for both the administrative personnel and the pharmacist were included. Some researchers might have included the costs of the added laboratory studies or extra medication as an input cost because these were projected based on recommendations of the clinic pharmacist. If this had been done, the net benefit calculations would have been identical, but the benefit-to-cost ratios would have been different.

8. **Relevant Outcomes:** Based on the objective and perspective of the study, the difference in direct medical costs was estimated to determine the benefit of the clinic (right-hand side of the PE equation; see Fig. 1.1 in Chapter 1). No non-medical, indirect, or intangible costs were included.

9. **Adjustment or Discounting:** The cost and benefits were estimated for a 3-year period. Discounting at 5% was conducted. Because most costs (except for the computer in the first year) were recurring (versus start-up costs), discounting had little effect on the benefit-to-cost ratio.

10. **Reasonable Assumptions:** Because this was based on estimations and projections, all values were assumed to be accurate approximations. Because the estimated costs were detailed in the tables, other health care systems could calculate a ratio using their own estimates. Other assumptions included the number of patients who would participate in the clinic each year and the amount of time it would take the pharmacist to monitor and meet with each patient. Lastly, the assumption that ED visits and hospitalization would decrease substantially should have been documented based on past research on DM clinics.

11. **Sensitivity Analyses:** The only sensitivity analysis conducted was with regard to discounting (5% discounting versus no discounting [0%]). Other sensitivity analyses based on personnel time and reduction of ED visits and hospitalizations should have been conducted.

12. **Limitations Addressed:** The authors did address the limitation that these estimates were based on information from their own health care system and may not extrapolate to other systems. The lack of information (using past literature) on estimating the reduction of health care use should have been addressed.

13. **Generalizations Appropriate:** The authors did not try to extrapolate beyond their health care system.

14. **Unbiased Conclusions:** Conclusions were based on the estimates presented in detailed tables, but because no sensitivity analysis on these estimates or further documentation of effects of diabetes services were presented, the results should be interpreted with some caution.

QUESTIONS/EXERCISES

Based on the following abstract (condensed summary of a research article), please answer the following questions:

ABSTRACT

TITLE: Cost-Effectiveness Analysis of Medication Therapy Management Services Provided to Medicare Patients.

OBJECTIVE: The objective of this study was to determine the costs and effects of providing medication therapy management (MTM) services to Medicare patients for 1 year.

STUDY DESIGN: Redbud health plan is a health maintenance organization (HMO) located in Oklahoma. The HMO has a contract with Medicare as a Medicare Advantage Prescription Drug (MA-PD) plan and provides both medical services (Parts A and B) as well as outpatient prescription drug coverage (Part D) to its Medicare members. Any patients predicted to spend $4,000 or more on outpatient prescriptions per year were defined as high-risk patients and MTM services were provided for these patients. MTM services at clinic A consisted of patient-specific educational mailings and the provision of a toll-free number to call for counseling services from licensed pharmacists at a centralized call center. MTM services at clinic B consisted of patient-specific educational mailings and face-to-face consultations with licensed pharmacists at their clinic. If patients at clinic B were not able to come to the clinic for face-to-face counseling (e.g., they were not ambulatory), pharmacists from clinic B would provide counseling over the phone. The perspective was that of the HMO. The costs of providing MTM services were measured based on the time to produce patient-specific letters, mailing costs, phone charges, and the pharmacists' time spent counseling patients. Savings attributable to health care costs avoided and changes in medication costs as a result of the MTM services were also measured. All costs were based on 2008 cost estimates. Clinical outcomes were measured as the differences in SF-36 mental and physical health component summary scores given at the beginning and the end of the year.

RESULTS: A total of 206 Medicare patients were deemed "at risk" by the computer algorithm (102 at clinic A and 104 at clinic B).

Costs: The average costs of providing MTM services were $100 per patient at clinic A and $200 per patient at clinic B. Average costs for medications increased for both groups from the previous year (clinic A, increase of $200; clinic B, increase of $250). Average medical service costs increased by $500 for group A and $100 for group B. This resulted in an average total cost increase of $800 for clinic A and $550 for clinic B.

Outcomes: There were no significant baseline to end-of-year differences in the average mental health component summary score or physical health summary score for the patients in clinic A. There were no significant differences in the average mental health component summary score for patients in clinic B, but there was a 10% improvement in their physical health summary score.

CONCLUSIONS: In this analysis, the patients in clinic B who received individualized letters and counseling from local pharmacists (mostly face-to-face consultations) had a lower overall increase in costs and an improvement in their self-assessed physical functioning compared with patients in clinic A who received individualized letters and counseling by telephone from a centralized call center.

1. Was the title complete?

_____

_____

_____

_____

2. What were the alternatives? Were they appropriate?

_____

_____

_____

_____

3. Were pharmacy services adequately defined?

_____

_____

_____

_____

4. Was discounting needed? Was it conducted?

_____

_____

_____

_____

5. Was a sensitivity analysis conducted? If so, on what variables?

_____

_____

_____

_____

REFERENCES

1. Bootman JL, Townsend RJ, McGhan WF. Introduction to pharmacoeconomics. In Bootman JL, Townsend RJ, McGhan WF (eds). *Principles of Pharmacoeconomics* (3rd ed.). Cincinnati, OH: Harvey Whitney Books Co, 2005.
2. National Center for Health Services Research and Development. Report of the Task Force on the Pharmacist's Clinical Role. *Journal of the American Pharmaceutical Association* 11(9):482–485, 1971.
3. Bootman LJ, Wertheimer AI, Zaske D, Rowland C. Individualizing gentamicin dosage in burn patients with gram-negative septicemia: A cost-benefit approach. *Journal of the Pharmaceutical Sciences* 68(3):267–272, 1979.
4. Hepler CD, Strand LM. Opportunities and responsibilities in pharmaceutical care. *American Journal of Hospital Pharmacy* 47(3):533–543, 1990.
5. Centers for Medicare & Medicaid Services. Medication therapy management and quality improvement program. In *Medicare Prescription Drug Benefit Manual*. Available at http://www.cms.hhs.gov/PrescriptionDrugCovContra/Downloads/PDBManual_Chapter7.pdf; accessed January 2007.
6. Blumenschein K, Johannesson M. Use of contingent valuation to place a monetary value on pharmacy services: An overview and review of the literature. *Clinical Therapeutics* 21(8):1402–1417, 1999.
7. Suh DC. Consumers' willingness-to-pay for pharmacy services that reduce risk of medication-related problems. *Journal of the American Pharmacists Association* 40(6):818–827, 2000.
8. Rupp MT. Value of community pharmacists' interventions to correct prescribing errors. *Annals of Pharmacotherapy* 26(12):1580–1584, 1992.
9. Dobie RL, Rascati KL. Documenting the value of pharmacist interventions. *American Pharmacy* NS34(5):50–54, 1994.
10. Lee AJ, Boro MS, Knapp KK, et al. Clinical and economics outcomes of pharmacist recommendations in a Veterans Affairs Medical Center. *American Journal of Health-System Pharmacy* 59(2):2070–2077, 2002.
11. Willett MS, Bertch KE, Rich DS, et al. Prospectus on the economic value of clinical pharmacy services. *Pharmacotherapy* 9(1):45–56, 1989.
12. Schumock GT, Meek PD, Ploetz PA, Vermeulen LC. Economic evaluations of clinical pharmacy services: 1988–1995. *Pharmacotherapy* 16(6):1188–1208, 1996.
13. Schumock GT, Butler MG, Meek PD, et al. Evidence of the economic benefit of clinical pharmacy services: 1996–2000. *Pharmacotherapy* 23(1):113–132, 2003.
14. Posey LM. Proving that pharmaceutical care makes a difference in community pharmacy. *Journal of the American Pharmacist Association* 43(2):136–139, 2003.
15. Carter BL, Malone DC, Billups SJ, et al. Interpreting the findings of the IMPROVE study. *American Journal of Health-System Pharmacy* 58(14):1330–1337, 2001.
16. Cranor CW, Bunting BA, Christensen DB. The Asheville Project: Long-term clinical and economic outcomes of a community pharmacy diabetes care program. *Journal of the American Pharmacist Association* 43(2):173–184, 2003.
17. Bunting BA, Cranor CW. The Asheville Project: Long-term clinical, humanistic, and economic outcomes of a community-based medication therapy management program for asthma. *Journal of the American Pharmacists Association* 46(2):133–147, 2006.

18. Garrett DG, Bluml BM. Patient self-management program for diabetes: First-year clinical, humanistic, and economic outcomes. *Journal of the American Pharmacists Association* 45(2):130–137, 2005.

19. Rupp M. Analyzing the costs to deliver medication therapy management services. *Journal of the American Pharmacists Association* 51(3):e19, 2011.

20. Bluml BM. Definition of medication therapy management: Development of profession wide consensus. *Journal of the American Pharmacists Association* 45(5):566–572, 2005.

21. American Pharmacists Association and National Association of Chain Drug Stores Foundation. Medication therapy management in community pharmacy practice: Core elements of an MTM service (version 1.0). *Journal of the American Pharmacists Association* 45(5):573–579, 2005.

22. Academy of Managed Care Pharmacy. Sound Medication Therapy Management Programs, Version 2.0 with validation study. *Journal of Managed Care Pharmacy* 14(1 suppl B): S2–2S44, 2008.

23. Buffington DE. Pharmacist Current Procedural Terminology codes and medication therapy management. *American Journal of Health-System Pharmacy* 63(11):1008–1010, 2006.

24. Etemad LR, Hay JW. Cost-effectiveness analysis of pharmaceutical care in a Medicare drug benefit program. *Value in Health* 6(4):425–435, 2003.

25. Touchette DR, Burns AL, Bough MA, Blackburn JC. Survey of medication therapy management programs under Medicare Part D. *Journal of the American Pharmacists Association* 46(6):683–691, 2006.

26. Winston S, Lin YS. Impact on drug cost and use of Medicare part D of medication therapy management services delivered in 2007. *Journal of American Pharmacists Association* 49(6):813–820, 2009.

27. Hong S, Liu J, Wang J, Brown L, White-Means S. Conjoint analysis of patient preferences on Medicare medication therapy management. *Journal of the American Pharmacists Association* 51(3):378–387, 2011.

28. Oladapo A, Barner J, Rascati K. The need for more evidence-based studies to justify the economic value for the provision of medication therapy management and other clinical pharmacy services. *Clinical Therapeutics* 34(11):2196–2199, 2012.

SUGGESTED READINGS

Isetts B. Pharmaceutical care, MTM, & payment: The past, present, & future. *The Annals of Pharmacotherapy* 46(4), S47–S56, 2012.

Kuo GM, Buckley TE, Fitzsimmons DS, Steinbauer JR. Collaborative drug therapy management services and reimbursement in a family medicine clinic. *American Journal of Health-System Pharmacy* 61(4):343–354, 2004.

Padiyara RS, Rabi SM, Bruce SP, Jackson T. Physician perceptions of pharmacist provision of outpatient medication therapy management services. *Journal of the American Pharmacists Association* 46(6):660–667, 2006.

Reeder EG, Gagnon JP, Moore WM. Pharmacoeconomics and community practice. In Bootman JL, Townsend RJ, McGhan WF (eds). *Principles of Pharmacoeconomics* (3rd ed.). Cincinnati, OH: Harvey Whitney Books Co, 2005.

Schumock GT. Methods to assess the economic outcomes of clinical pharmacy services. *Pharmacotherapy* 20(10, pt 2):243S–252S, 2000.

Scott DM. Ambulatory care. In McCarthy RL, Schafermeyer KW (eds). *Introduction to Health Care Delivery: A Primer for Pharmacists* (3rd ed.). Sudbury, MA: Jones and Bartlett Publishers Inc, 2004.

Stebbins MR, Kaufman DJ, Lipton HL. The PRICE clinic for low-income elderly: A managed care model for implementing pharmacist-directed services. *Journal of Managed Care Pharmacy* 11(4):333–341, 2005.

Chapter 13

International Perspective

Objectives

Upon completing this chapter, the reader will be able to:

1. List the basic differences in health care expenditures between the United States and other nations.

2. Discuss the comparability of using pharmacoeconomic results from different countries.

3. Give a brief history on the development and use of pharmacoeconomic guidelines in Australia, Canada, and the United Kingdom.

4. Find updated references and websites on worldwide pharmacoeconomic guidelines.

♦ HEALTH CARE EXPENDITURES

As mentioned in Chapter 1, the United States spent about $2.7 trillion on health care in 2010, for an average of about $8,000 per person, or about 17% of the gross domestic product (GDP). About 12% (over $900 per person) of health care expenditures were for medications.[1] How does this compare with other countries? According to estimates by the Organization for Economic Cooperation and Development (OECD), the United States spends by far more per person on health care and, in turn, medication, than any other country (Table 13.1). In addition, the United States is one of the few industrialized countries where the federal government is not the primary payer for health care services.[1] Countries that fund most of their citizens' health care have an incentive to evaluate the value they are receiving for their tax dollars.

TABLE 13.1. COMPARISON OF HEALTH CARE SPENDING BY COUNTRY IN 2010

Country	Percent GDP Spent on Health Care (%)	Dollars per Capita Spent on Health Care ($)	Percent Paid by Public Resources (%)	Percent of Healthcare Dollars Spent on Prescription Drugs (%)	Dollars per Capita Spent on Prescription Drugs ($)
Australia	9.1	3,670	68.5	14.7	540.9
Austria	11.0	4,395	76.2	12.0	525.3
Belgium	10.5	3,969	75.6	15.8	626.2
Canada	11.4	4,445	71.1	16.7	740.7
Chile	8.0	1,202	48.2	11.1	134.7
Czech Republic	7.5	1,884	83.8	19.9	374.7
Denmark	11.1	4,464	85.1	7.4	330.9
Estonia	6.3	1,294	78.9	21.8	281.8
Finland	8.9	3,251	74.5	13.9	452.0
France	11.6	3,974	77.0	16.0	634.5
Germany	11.6	4,338	76.8	14.8	640.0
Greece	10.2	2,914	59.4	24.8	676.5
Hungary	7.8	1,601	64.8	33.6	538.4
Iceland	9.3	3,309	80.4	15.8	523.3
Ireland	9.2	3,718	69.5	18.5	686.4
Israel	7.5	2,071	60.5	NI	NI
Italy	9.3	2,964	79.6	17.2	510.8
Japan	9.5	3,035	80.5	20.8	630.2
Korea	7.1	2,035	58.2	21.6	439.8
Luxembourg	7.9	4,786	84.0	9.1	406.0
Mexico	6.2	916	47.3	27.1	249.9
Netherlands	12.0	5,056	85.7	9.5	481.2
New Zealand	10.1	3,022	83.2	9.4	285.4
Norway	9.4	5,388	85.5	7.3	394.9
Poland	7.0	1,389	71.7	22.7	314.8
Portugal	10.7	2,728	65.8	18.6	508.1
Slovak Republic	9.0	2,096	64.5	26.4	554.2
Slovenia	9.0	2,429	72.8	19.4	471.9
Spain	9.6	3,056	74.2	18.4	561.2
Sweden	9.6	3,758	81.0	12.6	474.4
Switzerland	11.4	5,270	65.2	9.7	510.4
Turkey	6.1	913	73.0	NI	NI
United Kingdom	9.6	3,433	83.2	11.8	369.4
United States	**17.6**	**8,233**	**48.2**	**11.9**	**983.1**
OECD AVERAGE	9.5	3,265	72.2	16.6	495

GDP = gross domestic product; NI = no information.

Organization for Economic Cooperation and Development. OECD Health Data 2012: Frequently Requested Data. http://www.oecd.org/health/health-systems/oecdhealthdata2012-frequentlyrequesteddata.html. Accessed February 2013.

✦ COMPARABILITY OF PHARMACOECONOMIC RESULTS BETWEEN COUNTRIES

This book is targeted toward students who plan to practice pharmacy in the United States, so the examples and composite articles in previous chapters were targeted with the US health care system in mind. Economic studies conducted in the United States may not transfer well to other countries. Although one can argue that a chemical entity (and thus a pharmaceutical product) is the same in any country, other factors come into play that limit the generalizability of pharmacoeconomic analyses of these products.[2] For example, immunization or screening programs are more cost-effective in countries with a higher incidence of the disease of interest. The availability (or lack thereof) of timely access to medical services can modify decision making. For example, if gastrointestinal endoscopies (used to detect stomach ulcers) are delayed or unavailable, the physician may prescribe a medication to treat ulcers without confirmation that the patient actually has an ulcer. Another factor is that a product may be licensed in some countries but not others or a generic version may be available in some countries but not others, so the alternatives chosen for comparison (current usual practice) may differ by country. Even though a small number of studies have shown that there is not a great difference in people's preferences or scores for different health states between Europeans and North Americans,[3,4] the dollar value placed on outcomes, such as a quality-adjusted life-year (QALY), by decision makers has been shown to differ by country.[5]

✦ HISTORY OF PHARMACOECONOMIC GUIDELINE DEVELOPMENT

Governments that finance the majority of health care in their countries are particularly motivated to extract value in return for their health care spending. This may be accomplished by adding another level of control, which might include price negotiation, price setting, or **formulary** management. When a country is the single payer for pharmaceuticals, it has more leverage to negotiate the price and formulary status of a medication. Some countries have developed and implemented pharmacoeconomic guidelines to aid pricing and reimbursement decisions. Others have created advisory bodies that recommend what medications should and should not be included on local and national formularies. These guidelines are a set of rules that outline the requirements and information needed from manufacturers that wish to have their product considered. The number of countries that have implemented guidelines, as well as the specific rules contained in these guidelines, change frequently. Some of these guidelines are mandatory, and others are voluntary. This chapter first briefly summarizes the guidelines from three countries and then provides Website addresses for the reader to find current information.

Australian Guidelines

In 1992, Australia was the first country to publish mandatory guidelines for the evaluation of pharmaceutical products (they became effective in 1993). The Pharmaceuticals Benefits Advisory Committee (PBAC) was created to help the federal government determine what medications should be listed on Australia's Pharmaceutical Benefits Scheme (PBS), indicating their use would be covered with public funds. The PBAC is an independent expert body appointed by the Australian

Government. Members include doctors, health professionals, health economists and consumer representatives. When recommending a medicine for listing, the PBAC takes into account the medical conditions for which the medicine was registered for use in Australia, its clinical effectiveness, safety and cost-effectiveness ("value for money") compared with other treatments. Manufacturers who want to seek to have their product listed on the PBS or change the current listing of their product (e.g., change the price or indication for use) are required to submit pharmacoeconomic data to the PBAC. The PBAC can either recommend that the medication be listed (or its listing changed), decide that it should not be listed (or changed), or defer its decision until more information is received.

Canadian Guidelines

The Canadian government does not mandate that provinces cover prescription medication for all of its citizens. Instead, each province or territory sets its own rules about who is eligible for coverage and which medications are covered. This is similar to the US Medicaid system, in which each state sets its own policies (within broader federal regulations) regarding who is eligible to receive Medicaid and what limits are set on medications. The first Canadian province to publish pharmacoeconomic guidelines was Ontario, in 1993. The first edition of national guidelines was published in 1994 (followed by a second edition in 1997) by the agency formerly known as the Canadian Coordinating Office for Health Technology Assessment (CCOHTA). In 2006, this agency, now known as the Canadian Agency for Drugs and Technology in Health (CADTH). Instead of submitting information to a variety of local drug plans, the pharmaceutical manufacturers now follow this one set of submission guidelines.[7] CADTH, in turn, analyzes these submissions and makes recommendations to the federal, provincial, and territorial publicly funded drug plans concerning their formularies. The results of the reviews are published on their Website. The drug plans incorporate other factors (e.g., local mandates, resources) along with CADTH recommendations when making formulary decisions, so although there is one nationally accepted set of submission guidelines, there is no uniform nationwide formulary.

United Kingdom (England and Wales) Guidelines

In the United Kingdom, health care services, including prescription medications, are regulated by the National Health System (NHS). In 1999, the National Institute for Clinical Excellence (NICE) was established, in part, to evaluate the clinical and economic benefits of new and existing health care technologies in England and Wales and to make recommendations to the NHS. Guidance on health care technologies (including medications) is developed by a variety of independent advisory bodies consisting of NHS staff, health care professionals, patients, advocacy groups, industry, and academicians. NICE advisory groups carry out their own data gathering and analyses of technologies, in contrast to the PBAC, which relies more on analyses conducted by the petitioning manufacturer. A publication describing how recommendations are reached, as well as a list of current guidance summaries is available online.[8] Although technically, following these recommendations is voluntary, local health care bodies are under budget constraints set by the NHS. An analysis of the impact of NICE guidelines on practice patterns found that they have had "an important, if uneven, impact on care in the NHS."[9]

Other Guidelines

A summary was published in 2001 that compared health economic guidelines from Europe, North America, and Australia.[10] It was determined that although there was good agreement between the various guidelines with regard to key factors such as type of analyses required (e.g., **cost-effectiveness** analysis or **cost-utility analysis**), treatment alternative (current practice), acceptance of modeling, and **discount rate**, there was also disagreement on other factors, such as the **perspective** and method used to value resources. Although the importance of the **societal perspective** was often mentioned, the focus of most guidelines was on **direct medical costs**.

As pointed out already, pharmacoeconomic guidelines around the world are modified frequently. The International Society for Pharmacoeconomics and Outcomes Research (ISPOR) provides information on pharmacoeconomic guidelines and lists current websites for a variety of countries.[11] When ISPOR was developing this framework, they used the following definition to determine what guideline summaries were included in the grid. "Pharmacoeconomic guidelines can be used as a reference for preparation of studies to be included in application for reimbursement, a guide for design and implementation of a study, or a template for evaluating economic study reports."[12] Thirty-three key points for more than 30 countries were summarized. For illustrative purposes, the key features from the Australian and UK submission guidelines are listed in Table 13.2.

TABLE 13.2. INFORMATION ON PHARMACOECONOMIC SUBMISSION GUIDELINES: ISPOR GRID—EXAMPLES FROM AUSTRALIA AND THE UNITED KINGDOM

Comparison of Submission Guidelines for Selected Countries on Selected Key Features

	Australia	England & Wales
Title and year of the document	Guidelines for Preparing Submissions to the Pharmaceutical Benefits Advisory Committee (December 2008)	Guide to the Methods of Technology Appraisals (June 2008)
Affiliation of authors	Pharmaceutical Benefits Advisory Committee (PBAC)	National Institute for Health and Clinical Excellence (NICE)
Purpose of the document	Provide manufacturers with guidance to prepare the clinical and economic data for submissions to the PBAC. PBAC and Economics Sub-Committee (ESC) making recommendations on the suitability of drug products for subsidy by the Australian Government.	To provide an overview of the principles and methods of health technology assessment and appraisal within the context of the NICE appraisal process. It describes key principles of appraisal methodology and is a guide for all organizations considering submitting evidence to the technology appraisal programme of the Institute.
Standard reporting format included	Yes	No, however developed a reference case for cost-effectiveness analysis.
Disclosure	Not stated	No
Target audience of funding/author's interests	Manufacturers preparation for submission	All organizations considering submitting evidence to the Technology Appraisal Program of the Institute

	Australia	*England & Wales*
Perspective	Societal and health care sector	For the reference case, the perspective on outcomes should be all direct health effects, whether for patients or, when relevant, other people (principally carers)
Indication	Approved one(s)	Clearly define the spectrum of diseases
Target population	Clearly specify. Justify trials population and target population for the PBS	Yes, includes age and sex distribution and comorbidities
Subgroup analysis	Yes	Yes
Choice of comparator	Analogue prescribed for the largest number of patients. Standard medical management. Similar formulation.	Relevant comparators for the technology being appraised are those routinely used in the NHS, and therapies regarded as best practice when this differs from routine practice.
Time horizon	Depends on the natural history of the disease and the study purpose.	The time horizon for estimating clinical and cost-effectiveness should be sufficiently long to reflect all important differences in costs or outcomes between the technologies being compared.
Assumptions required	Yes	Yes
Preferred analytical technique	Any one of CMA, CEA, CUA, CBA. Need justification.	For the reference case, cost-effectiveness (specifically cost-utility) analysis is the preferred form of economic evaluation.
Costs to be included	Direct medical costs, social services, indirect costs. Changes in productive capacity as an outcome of therapy are not encouraged in submission to the PBAC.	Potential direct and indirect resource costs for the NHS and PSS that would be expected.
Source of costs	Manual of Resource Items and Their Associated Costs, DRG lists	Current official listing published by the Department of Health and/or the Welsh Assembly Government
Modeling	Yes, requires details	Yes
Systematic review of evidences	Yes, Appendix J	Yes
Preference for effectiveness over efficacy	Yes. The listing of comparative RCTs must be complete	Yes
Preferred outcome measure	Effectiveness in natural and patient relevant units. Both general and disease-specific QoL instruments can be used, and are valid, reliable, and responsive ones.	Given its widespread use, the QALY is considered to be the most appropriate generic measure of health benefit that reflects both mortality and HRQL effects.
Preferred method to derive utility	Need to specify details	Patient derived EQ–5D values with UK societal tariffs applied; alternatively TTO valuation using a representative sample of the public

(continued)

TABLE 13.2. INFORMATION ON PHARMACOECONOMIC SUBMISSION GUIDELINES: ISPOR GRID—EXAMPLES FROM AUSTRALIA AND THE UNITED KINGDOM (Continued)

	Australia	England & Wales
Equity issues stated	Not specific	Yes, an additional QALY has the same weight regardless of the other characteristics of the individual receiving the health benefit
Discounting costs	Yes, 5%	Base: 3.5%; SA: 0~6%
Discounting outcomes	Yes, 0% or 5%	Base: 3.5%; SA: 0~6%
Sensitivity analysis-parameters and range	One-way SA must be conducted on all variables using extreme values. Conduct two-way SA on all variables shown to be sensitive in the one-way SA.	All inputs used in the analysis will be estimated with a degree of imprecision. Appropriate ways of presenting uncertainty in cost-effectiveness data parameter uncertainty include confidence ellipses and scatter-plots on the cost-effectiveness plane (when the comparison is restricted to two alternatives) and cost-effectiveness acceptability curves. The presentation of cost-effectiveness acceptability curves should include a representation and explanation of the cost-effectiveness acceptability frontier.
Sensitivity analysis-methods	One-way, and two-way SA	Probabilistic SA
Presenting results	Present the results firstly in disaggregated form, then in increasingly aggregated form. Present the appropriately aggregated and discounted results separately for outcomes and resources and separately for the proposed drug and its main comparator.	All data used to estimate clinical and cost-effectiveness should be presented clearly in tabular form and include details of data sources.
Incremental analysis	Yes	Yes
Total C/E	Yes	Yes
Portability of results (Generalizability)	Yes, in Appendix N	In NHS context
Financial impact analysis	Required, for the PBS and government health budgets, for two years horizon	Yes, the cost should be disaggregated by appropriate generic organization (NHS, PSS, hospital, primary care) and budgetary categories (drugs, staffing, consumables, capital).
Mandatory or recommended or voluntary		Recommended

Reprinted with permission from International Society for Pharmacoeconomics and Outcomes Research. Pharmacoeconomic Guidelines Around the World. Available at http://www.ispor.org/PEguidelines/index.asp; accessed February 2013.

CBA = cost-benefit analysis; C/E = Cost/Effectiveness; CEA = cost-effectiveness analysis; CUA = cost-utility analysis; DRG = diagnosis-related group; CMA = cost-minimization analysis; QoL = quality of life; PPS = prescription pricing service; RCT = randomized, controlled trial; SA = sensitivity analysis.

SUMMARY

In many countries around the world, their governments' prescription pricing services are the primary purchaser of health care for their citizens. As such, they are motivated to seek value for their expenditures by making use of their bargaining power with the manufacturers of health care technology (including pharmaceutical companies). Australia was the first country to publish national pharmacoeconomic guidelines. Pharmaceutical manufacturers must provide pharmacoeconomic justification to have their medications included on Australia's national drug formulary (and thus be covered). Canada and the United Kingdom (more precisely, England and Wales) have established evaluation teams that analyze clinical and economic information to make national recommendations that may be (or in some cases, may not be) incorporated into local health care reimbursement decisions. Because the development of new guidelines and revisions of current guidelines are taking place around the globe, the ISPOR offers an online grid that provides up-to-date information and links to guidelines from more than 20 countries.

Although the United States spends more per capita on health care and pharmaceuticals than any other nation, the federal government does not, in general, set reimbursement rates or provide a national formulary list for pharmaceutical products. The Department of Defense (DoD) and the Veterans Administration (VA), which are federal agencies, conduct their own internal pharmacoeconomic analyses to determine formulary selections and negotiate prices, but neither has published guidelines. In addition, the Academy of Managed Care Pharmacy (AMCP) organization has published a *Format for Formulary Submissions* that can be adapted by private insurers and managed care organizations in the United States.[13] This will be discussed in further detail in Chapter 14.

QUESTIONS/EXERCISES

Based on the following abstract (condensed summary of a research article), please answer the following questions:

ABSTRACT

TITLE: Cost-Effectiveness and Cost-Utility Analysis of WeightGone versus Placebo in the United Kingdom

BACKGROUND: It is estimated that the direct medical cost of treating obesity and its related health consequences in the United Kingdom is about £500 million per year. This figure does not include indirect costs (i.e., non-health sector costs) attributable to lost productivity. A new product, WeightGone (note: not a real product), has been recently introduced, and it works to decrease the appetite of obese patients.

PURPOSE: The purpose of this study was to assess the cost-effectiveness and cost-utility of using WeightGone compared with placebo in the United Kingdom.

METHODS: An economic analysis, following a methodology similar to that provided in the December 2006 NICE guidance on other weight-loss medications (orlistat and sibutramine; found at http://guidance.nice.org.uk/CG43/guidance/section6), was conducted. A total of 300 patients were randomized to receive WeightGone or placebo and were followed for 12 months. WeightGone treatment costs and outcomes (response to treatment for WeightGone and placebo treatment groups; health benefit expressed as quality-adjusted life years [QALYs] gained associated with weight loss) were measured. The baseline cost estimates of the medication and the baseline utility estimates were varied.

RESULTS: A total of 36 (24%) of the 150 patients taking WeightGone lost at least 10% of their beginning weight at 12 months compared with nine (6%) of the 150 patients taking the placebo. The increased cost of WeightGone over placebo is £60 per month (£720/year), so the incremental cost per patient who lost 10% of their body weight at 12 months was £4,000 (£720 × 150 patients increased cost / [36 – 9 successful patients]). For every kilogram lost, it was estimated that the patient gained 0.002 QALY. The baseline incremental cost per QALY was estimated to be £20,000. When the cost of the medication was varied, the results ranged from £10,000 to £30,000 per incremental QALY. When the utilities associated with weight loss were varied, the results ranged from £5,000 to £50,000 per incremental QALY.

CONCLUSIONS: Results from this study on WeightGone (range, £5,000 to £50,000 per additional QALY) were comparable to previous NICE findings for orlistat and sibutramine (range, £6,000 to £77,000 per QALY) and should therefore be recommended as an alternative treatment for obesity in the United Kingdom.

1. Was the title complete?

_____

_____

_____

_____

2. Were the alternatives (WeightGone versus placebo) appropriate?

_____

_____

_____

_____

3. What was the perspective?

_____

_____

_____

_____

4. Was a sensitivity analysis conducted? If so, on what variables?

_____

_____

_____

_____

5. Were limitations addressed?

_____

_____

_____

_____

REFERENCES

1. Organisation for Economic Cooperation and Development. OECD health data 2012. Available at http://www.oecd.org/health/health-systems/oecdhealthdata2012-frequently requesteddata.html; accessed February 27, 2013.
2. Drummond M, Pang F. Transferability of economic evaluation results. In Drummond M, McGuire A (eds). _Economic Evaluation in Health Care: Merging Theory with Practice_. Oxford: Oxford University Press, 2002.
3. Johnson JA, Luo N, Shaw JW, et al. Valuations of EQ-5D health states: Are the United States and United Kingdom different? _Medical Care_ 43(3):221–228, 2005.
4. Johnson JA, Ohinmaa A, Murti B, et al. Comparison of Finnish and U.S.-based Visual Analog Scale valuations of the EQ-5D measure. _Medical Decision Making_ 20(3):281–289, 2000.
5. Rascati KL. The $64,000 question: What is a quality-adjusted life-year worth? _Clinical Therapeutics_ 28(7):1042–1043, 2006.
6. Pharmaceutical Benefits Advisory Committee. Available at http://www.health.gov.au/internet/main/publishing.nsf/content/health-pbs-general-listing-committee3.htm; accessed February 2013.
7. Canadian Agency for Drugs and Technology in Health: Common Drug Review Procedure. Available at: http://www.cadth.ca/media/cdr/process/CDR_Procedure_e.pdf; accessed February 2013.
8. National Institute for Health and Clinical Excellence. Available at http://www.nice.org.uk; accessed February 2013.
9. Pearson SD, Rawlins MD. Quality, innovation, and value for money: NICE and the British National Health Service. _Journal of the American Medical Association_ 294(20):2618–2632, 2005.
10. Hjelmgren J, Berggren F, Andersson F. Health economic guidelines: Similarities, differences, and some implications. _Value in Health_ 4(3):225–250, 2001.
11. International Society for Pharmacoeconomics and Outcomes Research. Pharmacoeconomic guidelines around the world. Available at http://www.ispor.org/PEguidelines/index.asp; accessed February 2013.
12. Tarn TYH, Dix-Smith M. Pharmacoeconomic guidelines around the world. _ISPOR Connections_ 10(4):5–15, 2004.
13. Academy of Managed Care Pharmacy: AMCP Format for Formulary Submissions, Version 3.1, January 2013. Available at http://amcp.org/AMCPFormatforFormularySubmissions; accessed February 2013.

SUGGESTED READINGS

Anderson GF, Hussey PS, Frogner BK, Waters HR. Health spending in the Unites States and the rest of the industrialized world. *Health Affairs* 24(4):903–914, 2005.

Buxton M. Implications of the appraisal function of the National Institute for Clinical Excellence (NICE). *Value in Health* 4(3):212–216, 2001.

Dickson M, Bootman JL. Pharmacoeconomics: An international perspective. In Bootman JL, Townsend RJ, McGhan WF (eds). *Principles of Pharmacoeconomics* (3rd ed.). Cincinnati, OH: Harvey Whitney Books Co, 2005.

Glennie JL, Torrance GW, Baladi JF, et al. The revised Canadian guidelines for economic evaluation of pharmaceuticals. *Pharmacoeconomics* 15(5):459–468, 1999.

Henry DA, Hill SR, Harris A. Drug prices and value for money: The Australian Pharmaceutical Benefits Scheme. *Journal of the American Medical Association* 294(20):2630–2632, 2005.

Laupacis A. Incorporating economic evaluations into decision-making: The Ontario experience. *Medical Care* 43(7 suppl):II-15–II-19, 2005.

Miners AH, Garau M, Fidan D, Fischer AJ. Comparing estimates of cost effectiveness submitted to the National Institute for Clinical Excellence (NICE) by different organizations: A retrospective study. *British Medical Journal* 330(7482):65–68, 2005.

Rawlins M, Barnett D, Stevens A. Pharmacoeconomics: NICE's approach to decision-making. *British Journal of Clinical Pharmacology* 70(3):346–349, 2010.

Reinhardt UE, Hussey PS, Anderson GF. US health care spending in an international context. *Health Affairs* 23(3):10–25, 2004.

Wonder MJ, Neville AM, Parsons R. Are Australians able to access new medicines on the pharmaceutical benefits scheme in a more or less timely manner? An analysis of Pharmaceutical Benefits Advisory Committee recommendations, 1999–2003. *Value in Health* 9(4):205–212, 2006.

Chapter 14

Future Issues

Objectives

Upon completing this chapter, the reader will be able to:

1. Summarize the trends in the use of pharmacoeconomics in the United States.

2. List barriers to the use of pharmacoeconomics in the United States.

3. Be aware of the pharmacoeconomic educational opportunities.

4. Discuss future pharmacoeconomic issues.

◆ APPLICATION OF PHARMACOECONOMICS IN THE UNITED STATES

As mentioned in Chapter 13, although the United States spends more per capita on pharmaceuticals than any other nation, it lags behind many countries in the central standardization and application of pharmacoeconomics for decision making. The US health care system, which consists of a mix of public and private payers, is complex and fragmented. Policy decisions based on pharmacoeconomics can and do occur at the national !evel (e.g., federal agencies) or at a more local level (e.g., hospital systems and health plans). This chapter summarizes the current state of the use of pharmacoeconomics in the United States at both levels.

◆ FEDERAL AGENCIES

Food and Drug Administration

Although the Food and Drug Administration (FDA) does not require any economic analyses for a drug product to be approved for sale in the United States, it does oversee advertising claims for pharmaceuticals. Section 114 of the 1997 FDA Modernization Act (FDAMA) addresses economic and **health-related quality of life** (HRQoL) claims made by pharmaceutical manufacturers.[1] Although the FDAMA allows some latitude regarding economic and quality of life information provided by a manufacturer to a formulary committee (or similar entity) upon request by the committee (see Health Plan section below), when a drug company actively promotes its products—using, for example, brochures, press releases, or websites—these messages are monitored by the FDA for appropriateness." As mentioned in Chapter 8 on HRQoL, in 2009, the FDA provided guidance on the measurement of **patient-reported outcome** (PRO) instruments and their relationship to HRQoL measures. Interpretive guidance from the FDA on "economic claims" is still scant, although Stewart and Neumann[2] provide some insight into this regulation by summarizing the content of FDA warning letters sent to manufacturers for "misleading or unsubstantiated" economic claims.

The Department of Defense

Active duty military personnel and their families receive health coverage through the Department of Defense (DoD) Military Health System (MHS). The DoD created a centralized Pharmacoeconomic Center (PEC) in San Antonio, Texas. The PEC vision states that, "The Department of Defense (DoD) Pharmacoeconomic Center (PEC) is a customer oriented Center of Excellence implementing recognized state of the art pharmacoeconomic analysis for the purpose of improving readiness by increasing value, quality, and access to medical care and pharmacotherapy within the available resources of the Military Health System (MHS)."[3]

The Veterans Health Administration

The Veterans Health Administration (VHA) provides health care services to over 4 million military veterans. Before the development of the Veterans Administration National **Formulary** (VANF) in 1996, each VA medical center managed its own drug formulary. The VANF is available online.[4] Regional additions to this national formulary are allowed for each of the 17 Veterans Integrated Service Networks (VISNs).

Hospital Systems

Surveys of US hospital formulary processes have found that 85% to 96% of responding institutions use pharmacoeconomics in their medication formulary process.[5-7] A telephone survey of Pharmacy and Therapeutics (P&T) committee members in Florida hospitals reported that the majority of respondents (86%) said they used pharmacoeconomic data "very often" or "all of the time" and that its use was "somewhat important" or "very important" (87%). About 70% indicated that someone on their hospital staff had "pharmacoeconomic knowledge," and the most common sources of pharmacoeconomic data used by the P&T committee were a mix of in-house hospital data (76%) and published literature (57%).[7]

✦ PRIVATE HEALTH CARE PLANS

For many health plans, information gathering and analysis have been conducted in an informal and nonsystematic manner. In the late 1990s, one health plan, Regence BlueShield, developed guidelines requesting standardized summaries (i.e., dossiers) of clinical and economic information from pharmaceutical manufacturers.[8] The dossiers received from the pharmaceutical companies were used when considering formulary addition or changes. Based on these guidelines, the Academy of

Managed Care Pharmacy (AMCP) developed a similar document for use nation-wide. The first version of AMCP's *Format for Formulary Submissions* was published in 2000 and has since been updated. Version 3.1 was published in January 2013.[9] The *Format* assists health plans in making formal requests for dossiers from the manufacturers that include safety, efficacy, and economic information. The request asks for more information than is available through normal channels (e.g., publications), recommending that manufacturers include data from unpublished studies, off-label indications, and economic models. Many pharmacists and decision makers have been trained to adapt this format to their health setting, and the AMCP format (or a similar process based on the format) has been adopted by numerous private health plans as well as some government agencies. A group of researchers analyzed the dossier submissions to a large health plan in Washington State from 2002 to 2005.[10] The health plan requested that manufacturers use the AMCP dossier format when submitting their products for formulary review. Of the 115 dossiers received during this 3-year time frame, 53 (46%) included economic data. For these 53 dossiers, 106 economic evaluations were provided (some dossiers included analyses for different indications or used different economic methods). Many did not include standard economic information: for example—only 43% performed sensitivity analysis, and only 38% stated the study perspective. Dossiers of high costs medications (defined as ≥$1,000 per month) contained a higher quality of economic analyses, possibly indicating that manufacturers place a higher priority on developing the justification necessary to persuade the decision makers to cover these high-cost products.

✦ BARRIERS TO PHARMACOECONOMICS IN THE UNITED STATES

The adoption of pharmacoeconomics, specifically **cost-effectiveness analyses** (CEAs), by US decision makers has been slow compared with other countries. Barriers to the use of CEA have been discussed in the literature. Some of these barriers concern the information itself, which could be provided in a more unbiased and useful way. Mullins and Wang[11] indicate that pharmacoeconomic data would be more useful to decision makers and providers if the information was provided in a timelier manner (e.g., near the launch date of the product), based on head-to-head comparisons with competing products (versus placebo), peer reviewed, independently sponsored (versus industry sponsored), and applicable to relevant populations. Other criticisms include that often economic evaluations are not **transparent** (users do not know what data, including estimates and assumptions, went into the analyses) and do not include information on **budget impact** (the estimated effect on the overall cost of adding a product to the formulary).[12] Other reasons given for the slow acceptance of economic evaluations include the lack of expertise and the lack of national resources devoted to research.[13] (Educational issues are addressed in a later section of this chapter.) Although research is being sponsored and conducted by pharmaceutical companies, decision makers may mistrust the results of these studies.

Luce[14] maintains that the reluctance by US policy makers to embrace CEA is "more political than technical." CEA is seen by many as "rationing," which is politically unacceptable to Americans. Neumann[15] points to "America's deep-seated distaste of limits and of the corporate or government officials who impose them." Many Americans do not want to acknowledge that resources are limited nor do they want to make tradeoffs.

This reluctance by the US government to support explicit economic analysis of health care interventions was highlighted in recent legislation. In 2010, the Affordable Care Act (ACA) was a major shift in legislating health care reform for US citizens.[16] One of the goals of the ACA was to promote the use of **comparative effective research**. As mentioned previously, "**efficacy**" (can the drug work) research is essential to get a drug approved by the FDA for sale in the US. "**Effectiveness**" (does the drug work in usual practice) research is important for health care practitioners and payers. **Comparative effectiveness research** takes this one step further—to ask "How well does the new drug work compared with other established options?" ACA established The Patient-Centered Outcomes Research Institute (PCORI) to coordinate federal funding of comparative effectiveness research. PCORI's research is intended to give patients a better understanding of the prevention, treatment, and care options available.[17] Prospectively comparing similar products in "head-to-head" trials can be very resource intensive. Other research methods that can be used for comparative effectiveness research (e.g., meta-analysis, retrospective analyses) are being advanced. While comparing clinical outcomes between competing alternatives is a great stride forward in ensuring that new products improve health, economic analyses of the value of these products is not supported. The new PCORI initiative specifically prohibits the use of QALYs to set a dollar threshold for coverage or reimbursement decisions. Many believe this ban on cost analyses is due to political pressure, for example, concern about "death panels" or "rationing" based on age or disability level.[18,19]

Another offshoot of the ACA was the development of pilot programs called Accountable Care Organizations (ACOs). ACOs are a grouping of doctors, hospitals, and other health care providers who agree to provide coordinated care, and assume financial responsibility for their patients. A Wall Street Journal editorial questions whether ingrained physician and patient behaviors can change enough for the ACOs to be effective at reducing costs.[20] The effect of ACOs on accessibility, costs, and quality of health care will be important to monitor.

✦ OTHER FUTURE ISSUES

Pharmacogenomics

Pharmacogenomics is a new science that predicts an individual patient's response to medication therapy based on his or her genetic makeup. Pharmacogenomics has the potential to improve the cost-effectiveness of a product in two ways. Genetic testing may help predict which subset of patients will be more likely to respond to therapy or which subset of patients may be less likely to suffer adverse events from the therapy. If a medication is given only to patients likely to benefit from treatment, overall costs would be reduced (i.e., not spent on nonresponders), and the percent effectiveness for those who receive the medication would increase, thus affecting both the numerator (costs) and denominator (effectiveness) of the **incremental cost-effectiveness ratio** (ICER) in a beneficial manner. Similarly, if the medication were not given to patients who would be likely to have toxic side effects, overall costs to treat side effects would be reduced. On the other hand, the costs of developing and testing medications based on genetic markers and the cost of administering genetic tests to patients may increase the overall costs associated with these products. Beaulieu et al. performed a systematic review of pharmacoeconomic studies of pharmacogenomic tests. Key parameters that impacted the cost-effectiveness ratios included marker prevalence, population ethnicity, pharmacogenomic treatment effect, and cost of genomic data collection and analysis.[21] Another review by Vegter et al. found that most economic analyses reported that genetic screening was cost-effective or even dominated existing nonscreening strategies. However, there was a lack of standardization regarding aspects such as the association between genotype and phenotype, the perspective of the analysis, the variables used in sensitivity analyses, and discount rates.[22]

Education in Pharmacoeconomics

Because pharmacoeconomics is a global and multidisciplinary topic, educational opportunities in this area are diffuse and (similar to guidelines) not standardized.[23] In addition to pharmacy, pharmacoeconomic topics are included in a variety of disciplines, including medicine, nursing, public health, epidemiology, psychometrics, health economics, and biostatistics. These topics are taught using different approaches; as part of a degree, fellowship, or certificate program; as a short-course, workshop, or continuing education offering by professional societies; and via the internet.[24] Surveys that have been conducted to determine the extent of pharmacoeconomic education in US schools and colleges of pharmacy[25-27] have found that the vast majority (98% by the year 2011) of US colleges of pharmacy offer at least some class hours devoted to pharmacoeconomics, although the number of classroom hours (2 to 60 hours) and course objectives varied considerably. This education is found to a lesser extent in other countries. Nwokeji and Rascati[28] conducted an e-mail survey in 2004 directed toward colleges of pharmacy outside of the United States. Respondents from 90 colleges of pharmacy representing 43 countries provided usable responses, and about 50% ($n = 47$ from 28 countries) indicated they provided some level of pharmacoeconomics education.

The extent of phamacoeconomic education beyond the PharmD degree has also been studied. A survey was sent to 30 eligible US programs that conferred a PhD in pharmacoeconomics, pharmaceutical outcomes research, or a related field, and 16 (53%) programs completed the survey. The majority (75%) were located in a school of pharmacy.[29] The extent of pharmacoeconomics and outcomes research (PEOR) fellowships was also examined. Over 50 fellowships were publicized on the Web, by organizations such as the American College of Clinical Pharmacy (ACCP), the International Society of Pharmacoeconomics and Outcomes Research (ISPOR), and the AMCP. These fellowships are offered by sponsors in a variety of environments (e.g., academia, industry, consulting services, United States managed care, and government). Guidelines for these types of fellowships have recently been revised.[30]

SUMMARY

In the United States, although there is no central independent regulatory or accrediting agency charged with assessing economic evaluations of health care technology, an ongoing increase in the use of these evaluations has been seen by a variety of national and local decision makers. Although inherent limitations in the methods of economic evaluations have been cited as a barrier, the slow uptake of centralized evaluations by the United States has been driven more by cultural and political factors.

A continued increase in the use of pharmacoeconomics is projected based on the ever-increasing costs of pharmaceuticals in the United States, new pharmacogenomic and biologic products, and health care reform initiatives. Resources are limited, and today few would argue that economic evaluations have no place in health care decisions. The challenge is to increase the **transparency** and open discussion regarding the use of these evaluations (which currently play more of a behind-the-scenes or implicit role) while understanding political pressures to avoid the stigma of "rationing" of health care services.

QUESTIONS/EXERCISES

1. Using an internet-based medical search engine, such as MEDLINE:
   a. Search for the number of articles using the term "cost-minimization" in their abstracts.
   b. Search for the number of articles using the term "cost-effectiveness" in their abstracts.
   c. Search for the number of articles using the term "cost-utility" in their abstracts.
   d. Search for the number of articles using the term "cost-benefit" in their abstracts.

   Based on these numbers, what is the most common type of analysis? What is the second most common?

2. Using an internet-based medical search engine, such as MEDLINE:
   a. Search for the number of articles with "pharmacoeconomic*" in their abstracts.
   b. How many have both "pharmacoeconomic*" and "Medicare" in their abstracts?
   c. How many have both "pharmacoeconomic*" and "pharmacogenomics*" in their abstracts?
   d. How many have both "pharmacoeconomic*" and "education*" in their abstracts?

REFERENCES

1. Food and Drug Administration Modernization Act (FDAMA) of 1997. Available at http://www.fda.gov/RegulatoryInformation/Legislation/FederalFoodDrugandCosmeticActFDCAct/SignificantAmendmentstotheFDCAct/FDAMA/default.htm; accessed February 2013.
2. Stewart KA, Neumann PJ. FDA actions against misleading or unsubstantiated economic and quality of life promotional claims: An analysis of warning letters and notices of violation. *Value in Health* 5(5):389–396, 2002.
3. Department of Defense Pharmacoeconomic Center. Available at http://www.pec.ha.osd.mil; accessed February 2013.
4. Veterans Administration National Formulary. Available at http://www.pbm.va.gov/National-Formulary.aspx; accessed February 2013.
5. Pedersen CA, Schneider PJ, Scheckelhoff DJ. ASHP national survey of pharmacy practice in hospital settings: Prescribing and transcribing, 2004. *American Journal of Health-System Pharmacy* 62(4):378–390, 2005.
6. Anagnostis E, Wordell C, Guharoy R, Beckett R, Price V. A national survey on hospital formulary management processes. *Journal of Pharmacy Practice* 24(4):409–416, 2011.
7. Odedina FT, Sullivan J, Nash R, Clemmons CD. Use of pharmacoeconomic data in making hospital formulary decisions. *American Journal of Health-System Pharmacy* 59(15):1441–1444, 2002.

8. Fullerton DS, Atherly D. Formulary development at Regence BlueShield: A formula for success. *Value in Health* 5(4):297–300, 2002.

9. AMCP Format for Formulary Submissions, Version 3.1. Available at http://amcp.org/AMCPFormatforFormularySubmissions; accessed February 2013.

10. Colmenero F, Sullivan S, Palmer J, et al. Quality of clinical and economic evidence in dossier formulary submissions. *The American Journal of Managed Care* 13(7):401–407, 2007.

11. Mullins CD, Wang J. Pharmacy benefit management: Enhancing the applicability of pharmacoeconomics for optimal decision making. *Pharmacoeconomics* 20(1):9–21, 2002.

12. Drummond M, Brown R, Fendrick AM, et al. Use of pharmacoeconomics information: Report of the ISPOR task force on use of pharmacoeconomic/health economic information in health-care decision making. *Value in Health* 6(4):407–416, 2003.

13. Fry RN, Avey SG, Sullivan SD. The Academy of Managed Care Pharmacy Format for Formulary Submissions: An evolving standard—A Foundation for Managed Care. Pharmacy Task Force Report. *Value in Health* 6(5):505–521, 2003.

14. Luce BR. What will it take to make cost-effectiveness analysis acceptable in the United States? *Medical Care* 43(7 suppl):II-44–II-48, 2005.

15. Neumann PJ. Why don't Americans use cost-effectiveness analysis? *American Journal of Managed Care* 10(5):308–312, 2004.

16. The Affordable Care Act: A brief summary. Available at: http://www.ncsl.org/portals/1/documents/health/hraca.pdf; accessed February 2013.

17. Patient-Centered Outcomes Research Institute PCORI. Available at http://www.pcori.org/about-us/; accessed February 2013.

18. Neumann P, Weinstein M. Legislating against use of cost-effectiveness information. *The New England Journal of Medicine* 363(16):1495–1497, 2010.

19. Chambers J, Neumann P. US healthcare reform: Implications for health economics and outcomes research. *Expert Review of Pharmacoeconomics & Outcomes Research* 10 (3):215–216, 2010.

20. Christensen C, Flier J, Vijayaraghavan V. The Coming Failure of 'Accountable Care.' *Wall Street Journal.* February 18, 2013.

21. Beaulieu M, de Denus S, Lachaine J. Systematic review of pharmacoeconomic studies of pharmacogenomic tests. *Pharmacogenomics* 11(11):1573–1590, 2010.

22. Vegter S, Boersma C, Rozenbaum M, Wilffert B, Navis G, Postma M. Pharmacoeconomic evaluations of pharmacogenetic and genomic screening programmes: A systematic review on content and adherence to guidelines. *Pharmacoeconomics* 26(7), 569–587, 2008.

23. Rascati KL, Drummond MF, Annemans L, Davey PG. Education in pharmacoeconomics: An international multidisciplinary view. *Pharmacoeconomics* 22(3):139–147, 2004.

24. International Society for Pharmacoeconomics and Outcomes Research/Education Index Page. Available at http://www.ispor.org/education/EducationIndex.asp; accessed February 2013.

25. Rascati KL, Conner TM, Draugalis JR. Pharmacoeconomic education in US schools of pharmacy. *American Journal of Pharmaceutical Education* 62(2):167–169, 1998.

26. Reddy M, Rascati K, Wahawisan J, Rascati M. Pharmacoeconomic education in US colleges and schools of pharmacy: An update. *American Journal of Pharmaceutical Education* 72(3):51, 2008.

27. Makhinova T, Rascati KL. An update (2011) on pharmacoeconomic education in US schools and colleges of pharmacy (submitted to AJPE). Abstract available at *American Journal of Pharmaceutical Education* 76(5):95–96, 2012.

28. Nwokeji ED, Rascati KL. Pharmacoeconomic education in colleges of pharmacy outside of the United States. *American Journal of Pharmaceutical Education* 69(3):348–355, 2005.

29. Slejko J, Libby A, Nair K, Valuck R, Campbell J. Pharmacoeconomics and outcomes research degree-granting PhD programs in the United States. *Research in Social & Administrative Pharmacy: RSAP* 9(1):108–113, 2013.

30. Kane-Gill S, Reddy P, Gupta S, Bakst A. Guidelines for pharmacoeconomic and outcomes research fellowship training programs: Joint guidelines from the American college of clinical pharmacy and the international society of pharmacoeconomics and outcomes research. *Pharmacotherapy* 28(12):1552, 2008.

SUGGESTED READINGS

Bala MZ, Zarkin GA. Pharmacogenomics and the evolution of health care: Is it time for cost-effectiveness analysis at the individual level? *Pharmacoeconomics* 22(8):495–498, 2004.

Berger ML, Teutsch S. Cost-effectiveness analysis: From science to application. *Medical Care* 43(7 suppl):II-49–II-53, 2005.

Clough J, Crawford A, Nash DB. The future of economic evaluation within the United States. In Pizzi LT, Lofland JH (eds). *Economic Evaluation in US Health Care: Principles and Applications.* Sudbury, MA: Jones and Bartlett Publishers, 2006.

Drummond M, Sculpher M. Common methodological flaws in economic evaluations. *Medical Care* 43(7 suppl):II-5–II-14, 2005.

Helfand M. Incorporating information about cost-effectiveness into evidence-based decision-making: The evidence-based practice center (EPC) model. *Medical Care* 43(7 suppl):II-33–II-43, 2005.

La Caze A. Does pharmacogenomics provide an ethical challenge to the utilization of cost-effectiveness analysis by public health systems? *Pharmacoeconomics* 23(5):445–447, 2005.

Luft HS. What works and what doesn't work well in the US healthcare system. *Pharmacoeconomics* 24(suppl 2):15–28, 2006.

Lyles A. Formulary decision-maker perspectives: Responding to changing environments. In Pizzi LT, Lofland JH (eds). *Economic Evaluation in US Health Care: Principles and Applications.* Sudbury, MA: Jones and Bartlett Publishers, 2006.

Mather D. Do decision makers really need health economic data? *Value in Health* 6(4):404–406, 2003.

McGhan WF, Bootman JL. Pharmacoeconomics, health policy, and limited resources. In Bootman JL, Townsend RJ, McGhan WF (eds). *Principles of Pharmacoeconomics* (3rd ed.). Cincinnati, OH: Harvey Whitney Books Co, 2005.

Neumann PJ. *Using Cost-Effectiveness Analysis to Improve Health Care: Opportunities and Barriers.* Oxford: Oxford University Press, 2005.

Pizzi L, Singh V. Pharmacoeconomics is coming of age. *Clinical Pharmacology and Therapeutics* 84(2):188–190, 2008.

Shih Y-CT, Pusztai L. Do pharmacogenomic tests provide value to policy makers? *Pharmacoeconomics* 24(12):1173–1177, 2006.

Siegel JE. Cost-effectiveness analysis in US healthcare decision-making: Where is it going? *Medical Care* 43(7 suppl):II-1–II-4, 2005.

Stefanacci RG, Lofland JH. The U.S. regulator's perspective in determining and improving the value of healthcare interventions. In Pizzi LT, Lofland JH (eds). *Economic Evaluation in US Health Care: Principles and Applications.* Sudbury, MA: Jones and Bartlett Publishers, 2006.

Walley T, Breckenridge A. Pharmacoeconomics comes of age? *Clinical Pharmacology and Therapeutics* 84(2):279–280, 2008.

Glossary

Absorbing state: Used in developing a Markov model. Patients in this type of health state cannot reasonably move to a different health state in a future cycle.

Adjustment of costs: A method used to value costs that are collected over 1 year to one point in time. See *Standardization of costs*.

Allowable charge: The amount that a payer "allows" to be charged for a specific product or service; the monetary amount the payer agrees to reimburse (pay).

Assumptions: Estimates or "best guesses" of variables used to conduct analyses.

Average manufacturer's price (AMP): The list price estimating the pharmacy acquisition costs based on actual costs charged by manufacturers.

Average wholesale price (AWP): The list price established by the manufacturer (usually higher than the price actually paid by pharmacies).

Benefit-to-cost ratios: The benefit in monetary terms divided by the costs in monetary terms.

Budget impact: The estimated effect on the overall cost to an organization or health plan if changes in interventions were made.

Channeling bias: A type of selection bias in which patients with certain characteristics are more likely to get channeled to (prescribed) one medication over another.

Charge: The monetary amount billed to a payer for a product or service.

Claims data: Data that are collected from health care providers by the insurance plan to reimburse them.

Cohort simulation: A group (cohort) of patients starts out in the same health state and transitions according to preset specific probabilities. These simulations do not take into account the variability of estimates. May be used in Markov models.

Contingent valuation (CV): A method used to determine the value placed on a good or service using hypothetical (contingent) scenarios. See *Willingness to pay*.

Cost analysis: The measurement and comparison of the costs of various options without the measurement of outcomes.

Cost-benefit analysis (CBA): A comparison in which both inputs and outcomes are measured in monetary units.

Cost-consequence analysis (CCA): A comparison in which inputs are measured in monetary values and outcomes are listed in a variety of ways.

Cost-effectiveness analysis (CEA): A comparison in which inputs are measured in monetary units and outcomes are measured in natural units of effectiveness.

Cost-effectiveness grid: A 3 × 3 table used to compare costs (higher cost, same cost, lower cost) with outcomes (better outcome, same outcome, worse outcome).

Cost-effectiveness plane: A two-dimensional graphical depiction of cost-effectiveness comparisons, using quadrants.

Cost-effectiveness ratio (CER): Total costs of an intervention divided by units of effectiveness of the intervention.

Cost-minimization analysis (CMA): A comparison in which inputs are measured in monetary values and outcomes are assumed to be identical.

Cost-of-illness analysis (COI): A method used to estimate the total economic burden (including prevention, treatment, losses because morbidity and mortality, and so on) of a particular disease on society.

Costs: The resources (or inputs) that are used in the production of a good or service.

Cost-to-charge ratio: A ratio used to estimate the actual costs to a provider or institution; the costs per department or facility are divided by the amount charged to payers.

Cost-utility analysis (CUA): A comparison in which inputs are measured in monetary units and outcomes are measured as patient preference–weighted extensions of life.

Cycle: The time period used in a Markov model that is determined to be clinically relevant to the specific disease or condition.

Decision analysis: The application of an analytical method for systematically comparing different decision options.

Deterministic analysis: Costs and outcomes are determined using point estimates (does not include data on variability of estimates).

Diagnosis-related group (DRG): The method used to classify clinically cohesive diagnoses and procedures that use similar resources.

Direct benefits: Savings attributable to avoiding indirect costs.

Direct costs: Costs of input used directly to provide the treatment. These can be medically related (e.g., hospitalization) or nonmedical (e.g., transportation to clinic visit).

Direct elicitation preference-based measures: Utility measures attained in response to health states presented to the respondents using methods such as time trade off or standard gamble.

Direct medical benefits: Savings attributable to avoiding direct medical costs.

Direct medical costs: Costs of medically related inputs used directly to provide a treatment.

Direct nonmedical costs: Costs to patients and their families that are directly associated with treatment but are not medical in nature.

Discounted: Monetary amounts that have been calculated to take into account their present value.

Discounting: The process of converting monetary amounts, either paid or received, over time periods of more than 1 year, to their present value.

Discount rate: Approximates the cost of capital by taking into account the interest rates of borrowed money.

Disease-specific measures: Instruments or questionnaires that measure important effects of specific health conditions or diseases and their treatment.

Disease-specific per diem: Uses an overall estimate of costs for a day in the hospital for a specific disease or condition.

Domain: Aspect, dimension, or concept. Common domains measured by health-related quality-of-life instruments include physical functioning, psychological functioning, and social or role functioning.

Dominant: Used to indicate that the treatment of interest is both more effective and less expensive than a comparator treatment.

Dominated: Used to indicate that the treatment of interest is both less effective and more expensive than a comparator product.

Dossier: Information packet provided by a drug manufacturer to a formulary committee or health plan upon request that includes clinical and economic data from published and unpublished studies.

Effectiveness: Outcomes measured in the "real world" or routine clinical practice.

Efficacy: Outcomes measured under controlled conditions (usually randomized, controlled trials).

External validity: Valid in a broader range of the population; "external" to the specific study population.

Formulary: A list of medications compiled by an institution or health care plan that contains which drugs are approved for use and which are reimbursed.

Formulary committee: The committee that determines what is included in a formulary or drug list.

Generalizablility: The degree to which findings from a specific study population can be extrapolated to an entire (general) population.

Generic or general measures: Instruments or questionnaires that measure health in general terms.

Half-cycle correction: May be used in developing a Markov model. Because all patients do not transition from one cycle to another at the same time during the cycle (e.g., at the end of the cycle), this calculation adjusts for an overestimation of costs and outcomes.

Health care sector costs: Medical resources consumed by health care entities; these do not include direct medical costs paid for by the patient or other sectors.

Health status: A description of the physiologic and psychological effects of a disease or condition on an individual.

Health-related quality of life (HRQoL): The functional effect of an illness and its consequent therapy upon a patient, as perceived by the patient.

Health-related quality of life (HRQoL) measures: These are generally used to represent a patient's estimation of his or her own health at a point in time.

Human capital (HC): Estimates of wages and productivity losses to value changes in illness, disability, or death.

Hurdle rate: The minimum expected monetary return rate expected before an investment would be considered.

Incremental cost-effectiveness ratio (ICER): The ratio of the difference in costs divided by the difference in outcomes.

Incremental costs: The difference in estimated costs between two or more interventions.

Incremental net benefit (INB): A monetary estimate of the value for health benefits (outcomes, or lambda) is substituted into an incremental cost-effectiveness analysis. See *Net monetary benefit*.

Indirect benefits: Increases in productivity or earnings because of a program or intervention.

Indirect costs: Costs that result from the loss of productivity because of illness or death.

Indirect elicitation preference-based measures: Utility measures attained using algorithms based on population preferences used to weight summary scores of health states.

Insensitive: The results do not vary depending on the range of a variable, thereby strengthening confidence in the study results.

Intangible benefits: Benefits caused by a decrease in intangible costs (e.g., decrease in pain, anxiety, or discomfort).

Intangible costs: Costs that are difficult to put a monetary value on, such as the costs of pain, suffering, anxiety, or fatigue that occur because of an illness or the treatment of an illness.

Internal rate of return (IRR): The rate of return that equates the present value of benefits to the present value of costs.

Internal validity: Validity in the specific study population studied in randomization and controlled conditions.

Lambda: An estimate of the value for health benefits (outcomes) that is used in incremental net benefit or net monetary benefit calculations to estimate a payer's maximum acceptable willingness to pay for an outcome.

Marginal cost: The change in total costs that arises when the quantity produced changes by one unit.

Markov analysis: An analysis that uses Markov modeling.

Markovian assumption: A cited disadvantage to Markov models. These models assume that the probability of a patient moving from one health state to another is not based on experiences from former cycles.

Markov model or modeling: A type of decision analysis used when patients transition (move) from one health state to another.

Markov or Markovian chain: A Markov model that uses the assumption that the probability of transitioning from one health state to another is constant over time from one cycle to the next.

Markov or Markovian process: A Markov model that incorporates changes in the probability of transitioning from one health state to another for different cycles.

Markov states: Used in developing a Markov model. A list of mutually exclusive health states that delineate different scenarios a patient might reasonably experience.

Medication therapy management (MTM): Services that include a broad range of professional activities and may occur in conjunction with or independently from the dispensing of a medication.

Micro-costing: Collecting information on resource use for each component of an intervention.

Minimally Important Difference (MID): The smallest difference in a measure that represents a clinical change in the patient's health.

Monte Carlo simulation: May be used in Markov models. This type of analysis takes into account patient-level and parameter variability.

Net benefit: Calculation of monetary benefits minus costs.

Net monetary benefit (NMB): A monetary estimate of the value for health benefits (outcomes, or –lambda) is substituted into an incremental cost-effectiveness analysis. See *Incremental net benefit*.

Nonutility measures: Measures that are generally used to represent a patient's estimation of his or her own health at a point in time. Also referred to as health-related quality of life measures.

Non-preference-based measures: Measures that are generally used to represent a patient's estimation of his or her own health at a point in time. Also referred to as health-related quality of life measures.

Observational study: A research method that documents the costs or outcomes of actual medical practice (does not use randomization or controlled experimental design).

Opportunity costs: The value of the best-forgone option; the value of the "next best option."

Other sector costs: Costs related to a disease but not medical in nature, such as housing, homemaking services, and educational services.

Patient and family costs: Costs to the patient and his or her family without regard to whether they are medical or nonmedical in nature.

Patient-reported outcome (PRO): The measurement of any aspect of a patient's health status that comes directly from the patient.

Per diem: An overall estimate of costs for a day in the hospital without regard to the reason for the hospitalization. This is the least precise method of estimating hospital costs.

Perspective: An economic term that describes whose costs are relevant (being measured) based on the purpose of the study.

Pharmaceutical care: The responsible provision of drug therapy for the purpose of achieving definite outcomes that improve a patient's quality of life.

Pharmacogenomics: A new science that predicts an individual patient's response to medication therapy based on his or her genetic makeup.

Preference-based measures: Also referred to as utility measures. Respondents are asked to imagine possible health states and record their scores (usually from 1.0 to 0) to reflect their preferences for the various scenarios.

Present value (PV): The value of money at a current point in time. Future costs or revenues are discounted (reduced) to account for the time value of money.

Productivity costs: Costs related to missing work or being less productive because of health conditions. See *Indirect costs*.

Prospective study: Study that involves the collection of data forward in time.

Protocol-driven costs: Costs that occur because of the research protocol of a randomized control trial that would not occur in everyday practice.

Publication bias: Bias based on the premise that only research papers with positive results are submitted for publication.

Quality-adjusted life year (QALY): An outcome measured as life years gained adjusted (weighted) by patient preferences for various health states.

Quality of life (QoL): Overall well-being. This may be related to health factors (see *Health-related quality of life*) or nonhealth factors such as environmental, economic, and political components.

Randomization: Process in which subjects are assigned to a category (or treatment group) in a random manner solely based on chance.

Randomized, controlled trial (RCT): Study of safety and efficacy of treatments in which patients are selected based on prespecified criteria and placed randomly into different treatment arms.

Rating scale (RS): Method used to measure health preferences. Respondents are asked to indicate where various diseases or condition would fall on a line with scaled markings from 100 (or 1.0) indicating perfect health to 0 indicating death.

Reimbursed costs: Amount actually paid for a product or service.

Reliable or reliability: Degree of constancy or stability.

Responsiveness: The ability to detect a change in outcomes.

Retrospective data or database: Data used in a study that have been collected previously, usually for other purposes, such as reimbursement.

Retrospective study: Study that involves the analysis of data already existing in a database.

Robust: Capable of coping well with variations. See *Insensitive*.

Selection bias: Bias that occurs when patients with certain characteristics are more likely to be selected for inclusion or more likely to receive one treatment over another.

Sensitive: The results vary depending on the range of a variable, thereby weakening confidence in the study results.

Sensitivity analysis: Allows one to determine how the results of an analysis would change when "best guesses, "or assumptions, are varied over a relevant range of values.

Silo mentality: When a decision maker considers only one budget or silo rather than overall resource use.

Societal costs: Costs to all sectors such as costs to the insurance company, costs to the patient, other sector costs, and indirect costs because of the loss of productivity.

Societal perspective: Measuring all costs to all sectors. See *Societal costs*.

Standard gamble (SG): Method used to measure health preferences. Respondents are asked to choose (hypothetically) between taking a risk on a treatment versus living with the disease or condition.

Standardization of costs: A method used to value costs that are collected over 1 year to one point in time. See *Adjustment of costs*.

Stochastic analysis: Statistical variations in estimates that are used when comparing costs and outcomes.

Symptom-free days (SFDs): An outcome measure used to indicate how many days an individual has no symptoms related to the disease of interest.

Threshold analysis: Analysis that calculates the level within the range of estimates at which a decision switches from one option to another.

Time tradeoff (TTO): Method used to measure health preferences. Respondents are asked to choose (hypothetically) between living with a disease or condition for a specified amount of time versus living in perfect health for a shorter period of time.

Tornado diagram: Diagram used to compare the impact of various one-way sensitivity analyses. The range that has the biggest impact on the answer is placed at the top of the graph and the rest appear below in descending rank (hence the funnel or tornado look).

Transition: A change from one health state to another health state.

Transition probabilities: Used in developing a Markov model. These probabilities are used to estimate the percent of patients that are likely to move from one health state to another during each cycle.

Transparent: Information presented to the reader or user that makes it easy to determine where the information came from and how the analysis was performed.

Tunnel states: An advanced computation used to overcome the Markovian assumption. It allows for integration of information on previous health experiences from former cycles.

Utility or utilities: A measure of the relative preference for various options or satisfaction gained.

Utility measures: Also referred to as preference-based measures or quality-adjusted life-year measures. Respondents are asked to imagine possible health states and record their scores (usually from 1.0 to 0) to reflect their preferences for these various scenarios.

Valid or validity: The extent to which instruments actually measure concepts they are designed to measure.

Willingness to pay (WTP): The estimate of how much people are willing to pay to reduce the chance of an adverse health outcome. See *Contingent valuation*.

Work measurement: A method for estimating how much time it takes to complete a task or job.

Index